Next Step In Management
2nd Edition
USMLE Step 3

Amninder S. Dhesi, MD

ISBN : 978-0-578-14301-9

Note to Reader

Although the information, ideas, management, in this book is carefully reviewed for correctness, neither authors or editors nor the publisher can accept the legal responsibility for any errors or omissions that maybe made. Neither the publisher nor editor makes any warranty, expressed or implied, with respect to the material contained herein.

ISBN-13: 978-0-578-14301-9

DEDICATION

To my family: my mother, father, brother and sister for continuous support and encouragement. To my loving wife for her love, support and steady inspiration

TABLE OF CONTENTS

TABLE OF CONTENTS

CCS CASES APPROACH

Step 1: Read the case carefully, and check if the patient is stable, unstable or has any life-threating condition such as MI, thoracic aorta dissection or asthma exacerbation. Further management is as follow:

    1a. If the patient is **stable** and has **no life-threatening** condition, then proceed to do a **full physical exam**.

    1b. If the patient is **unstable** or **has a life-threatening** condition, then stabilize the patient first by ordering the **followings**:

- IV access
- IV fluids
- Oxygen saturation
- Oxygen
- Vital sign monitor
- IV morphine, if patient is in pain
- IV promethazine, if patient is vomiting
- Additionally, order emergency measures based on the organ of chief complaint. For example, if a patient is presenting with angina type chest pain, then order EKG, aspirin, oxygen, nitroglycerin

Step 2: Physical exam
- If the patient is **stable**, then order a **complete physical exam**. However, avoid rectal, genital and breast exam, unless it is needed
- If the patient is **unstable or has a life-threatening** condition, then order **focused physical exam** (heart, lungs and the organ of chief complaint). Rest of the physical exam can be performed, while waiting for the lab results.

Step 3: Labs
    3a. For all of the cases order the following labs:
- CBC
- UA
- BMP
- Beta-hCG for all reproductive age women
- Chest X-ray, but it is imperative to rule out pregnancy in a reproductive age women with urine beta-hCG before ordering chest X-ray

3b. Additional labs are based on the **organ of chief complaint** and additionally labs for **differential diagnosis**

3c. If labs were ordered in step 1, then move the clock forward to get the results

Step 4: Medications
- If the diagnosis is at this point, then **prescribe the medicine** However, make sure that the patient is not allergic that medicine
- If patient needs to be hospitalized, then **switch oral medicines to IV**
- Check if any **medicine needs to be stopped**. For example, stop metformin if a patient needs an angiography.

Step 5: Location

5a. If a patient is **stable,** then make a **follow-up appointment** after all the labs results are available, and send them home.

5b. If the patient is **unstable or requires additional hospital monitoring,** then transfer the patient to the following location:
- If the patient is still unstable, then keep the patient in **ER**
- If the patient had life-threatening conditions such MI, or Diabetic ketoacidosis, then transfer the patient to **ICU**
- If the does not have any life- threatening, but needs further hospital monitoring, for conditions such as osteomyelitis or meningitis, then transfer the patient to the hospital **ward**

Step 6: If the patient needs hospital monitoring (ER, ICU, or ward), then make sure to order the followings:
- NPO or a type of diet patient needs to be on such as low sodium diet
- Bed rest with bathroom privilege or strict bedrest
- Pneumatic compression to prevent DVT
- Vital check every 8 hours or 4 hours

Step 7: Labs
- If the patient **came back** for a follow-up appointment, then see if more labs are needed to **confirm the diagnosis**. For example, if initial CT or X-ray shows a mass, then you may need to order biopsy of that mass

- If the lab results of **culture and sensitivity** are available, then see if the medicine needs to be switched based on culture sensitivity
- If the patient was already in the hospital, then check if the patient **needs additional labs to determine the severity of the condition.** For example, a patient with MI may need **angiography or a patient carotid stenosis may need carotid angiography**

Step 8: Consultation
- Anytime you **order invasive procedure or biopsy**, order consultation of specialist such as cardiologist for angiography or pulmonologist for lung biopsy

Step 9: Check if the patient needs, reassurance, additional medicines, interval follow-ups, discharged or surgery,
- If the patient needs **reassurance**, then reassure the patient and make a follow-up appointment. For example, patient with IBS may need reassurance
- If the patient needs medicine based on culture or sensitivity, then **switch the medicine based on culture** and make a follow-up appointment
- If one medicine is not able to control symptoms, then **add or switch the medicine**. For example if patient's HTN is not controlled with on medicine, then add the second medicine
- If the patient needs hospital **follow-ups**, then follow-up every 8 hours until patient gets better
- If the patient is feeling better and the labs are normal, then discharge the patient and make a follow-up appointment. Make sure to cancel, hospital diet, monitoring, switch IV medicine to oral medicine
- If the patient needs **surgery**, then order pre-surgery preparations such as PT, PTT, INR, IV antibiotics, IV painkillers, and then move the clock forward to get the surgery results

Most of the **CCS cases end after step 9**

Step 10: On two-minute screen order the followings:
- **Basic counseling** such as wear seat belt, while driving, no smoking, no drinking, no drugs, safe sex

- **Age and gender-specific counseling** such as colonoscopy, PAP smear, mammogram
- **Advance directive** for all elderly
- **Immunization**, a needed
- **Case specific counseling** such as, patient with HNT should be told to stay on low salt diet, no smoking, low fat diet, exercise, strict glucose control, weight
- **Suicide contract**, if patient is depressed

Guide to CCS cases

Real time is the time given to solve the case.
Case time is the time to diagnose and treat the condition. You can only move this forward.

In a nutshell: It is like a time travel game, which you can play for 15 minutes **(real time)** and in that 15 minutes period you were allowed to move your life ahead to the next hour, days, months or even years ahead **(case time)** to see what you will look like at that time. Just like the time travel game, in CCS, you perform patient's physical exam and move the clock forward to get physical exam results, and then order labs, and subsequently manage the patient based on physical exam and labs.

Orders are usually placed under **stat option or routine option**
- Orders are placed under stat option if the results are needed fast. It is usually used in emergency cases
- Orders are places under routine option in stable cases.

CARDIOLOGY

CHEST PAIN

CHEST PAIN DIFFERENTIAL DIAGNOSIS

1.   **Pericarditis:** Chest pain in pericarditis is characterized by sharp chest pain, which is worst when patient is supine and relives with leaning forward.
Diagnosis: EKG shows **ST elevation in all leads**
Treatment: **NSAIDs**, but if it is ineffective, then give **prednisone**

2.   **Costochondritis:** Chest pain in costochondritis is characterized by localized, and stabbing chest pain, which can be **reproduced by physical motion.**
Diagnosis: clinical diagnosis, physical exam shows chest wall tenderness. EKG is usually normal
Treatment: **NSAIDs**

3.   **GERD:** Chest pain in GERD is felt after eating certain foods and it gets better with antacids. Proton **pump inhibitors are diagnostic and therapeutic**

4.   **Esophageal spasm:** Chest pain in esophageal spasm is felt after drinking cold water or beverage
Diagnosis: best initial test is barium swallow, and most accurate test is esophageal manometry
Treatment: Calcium channel blocker or nitrates

5.   **Aortic dissection:** Chest pain is aortic dissection is characterized by sharp, tearing chest pain, **radiating to the back.** It is mostly seen after trauma, motor vehicle accident at the speed > 45mph or collagen vascular disease, such as Marfan syndrome, Ehlers–Danlos syndrome.
Diagnosis:
   • Physical exam shows **different blood pressure in each arm**
   • Chest X-ray shows widened mediastinum
   • Most accurate test is CT angiography

Treatment: beta-blockers such as **labetalol or esmolol** are the first line of treatment to lower the blood pressures, followed by vasodilators such as **sodium nitroprusside**, and then **surgery**

6.   **Pneumothorax:** It is mostly seen in young patients. Patient usually presents with **sudden onset of chest pain and shortness of breath**. Diagnosis:
- **Clinical diagnosis:** physical exam shows JVD, and auscultation of lungs shows absent breath sounds on the affected side of the lungs

Treatment:
- Immediate chest decompression with a needle insertion in the 2nd **intercostal space mid-clavicular line**

7.   **Cocaine abuse:** Cocaine abuse may cause angina. Look for other clues such as history of drug abuse, nosebleed, or pupillary dilation. Treatment: **Calcium channel blockers**

8.   **Panic attacks:** Chest pain in panic attacks is felt suddenly after feeling overwhelming sense of fear. **Treatment: Clonazepam**

CHARACTERISTICS OF CHEST PAIN IN A MI
Three main characteristics of chest pain in a MI are:
- Substernal chest pain that may radiate to left arm, shoulder, or jaw
- Chest tightness or pressure sensation
- Chest pain that is not reproducible by body motion

Note: Diabetics, postmenopausal women, elderly and heart transplant patients likely to have silent MI or atypical symptoms such as nausea, dyspnea, weakness or confusion

RISK FACTORS FOR CORONARY ARTERY DISEASE (CAD)
- Cigarette smoking
- Diabetes mellitus
- BP > 140/90 or on BP medications
- HDL < 40
- Male > 45 years, or female > 55 years of age
- First-degree male relative < 55 years of age with CAD, or first-degree female relative < 65 years of age with CAD

Note: Diabetes mellitus is the **greatest risk factor** for CAD, and cigarette-smoking cessation is the **most preventable** CAD risk factor.

Cardiac enzymes

Enzyme	Detectable after infarction
Myoglobin	• Is detectable within 1-4 hours
CK-MB	• Is detectable within 4-6 hours, peaks in 12-24 hours and normalizes within 2-3 days • Is also used to detect MI **re-infraction**
Troponin	• Is detectable within 3-4 hours, peaks in 12-16 hours and remains elevated for up to 2 weeks

TYPES AND MANAGEMENT OF ANGINA

1. STABLE ANGINA
Stable angina occurs due to poor blood flow through the coronary arteries, which are either blocked or narrowed

Mechanism: Blocked or narrowed coronary arteries may supply enough blood to the heart when the oxygen demand is less such as while sitting, walking or working at normal pace. However, during physical exertion or stress blocked arteries are unable to meet heart's oxygen demand, and that leads to stable angina.

Si/Sx: chest pain or discomfort with **predictable amount of exertion and relieved by rest or nitroglycerin**

Diagnosis: EKG shows ST depression and inversion or flattening of T-wave.
Note: EKG may be normal when patient's heart is not stressed anymore. In that case, patient's heart is stressed with a stress test, and EKG is monitored for any changes. (Stress test is discussed in details below)

Stress test *(High-yield for step 3)*
In a stress test patient's heart rate is raised to his maximum heart rate (maximum heart rate= 220 – patient's age) via treadmill stress test or chemical stress test, and heart activity is monitored. Which stress test is appropriate for a particular patient is determined based on the followings:

- If patient can walk and has no pre-existing baseline EKG changes, then do **treadmill stress**
- If patient cannot walk or has pre-existing baseline EKG changes, then do **one of following chemical stress test**:

Types of stress test and indications

Type of stress test	Indications
Dipyridamole, or adenosine thallium	• If patient is deconditioned, cannot walk due to lower extremity defect, amputations, peripheral vascular diseases (PVD), weakness
Dobutamine stress echo	• If patient has COPD, asthma, 2nd or 3rd degree heart block
Nuclear stress test (exercise thallium)	• If patient has preexisting **baseline EKG changes,** such as: Left bundle block, left ventricular hypertrophy, taking digoxin, pacemakers implanted

Stress test interpretation:
- Treadmill stress test is considered positive, if a patient shows ≥ 2mm ST-segment depression and/or a drop in systolic BP > 10mmHG
- Dobutamine stress echo test shows **abnormal wall motion** in ischemic area
- Exercise thallium and adenosine thallium tests show **decreased isotope uptake** in ischemic area

Angiography is performed after an EKG or stress test is positive for unstable angina. It is done to check the extent of coronary artery occlusion, and number of coronary arteries occluded, which helps determining whether or not a patient needs coronary artery bypass grafts (CABG)

Treatment for stable angina is as follow:

Acute treatment: If **a patient is presenting** with anginal chest pain, then give **morphine, oxygen, sublingual nitroglycerin, aspirin and beta-blockers,** even before doing EKG or other tests. As this management lowers the mortality by preventing further blood from clotting, opening the arteries and lowering the oxygen demand. Further management may include PCI or CABG (discussed below):

- **Percutaneous coronary intervention (PCI),** commonly known as coronary angioplasty, is a standard care
- **Coronary artery bypass graft (CABG)** is indicated when any of the following is present:
  1. Angiography shows any of the followings:
     - Significant stenosis of the left main coronary artery
     - > 70% stenosis of proximal LAD and left circumflex
     - 3-vessels occluded in a patient with CAD or 2-vessels occluded in a patient with DM
  2. Ejection fraction <25%
  3. Medicine failure

> Internal mammary **artery** grafts are preferred over saphenous vein because they lasts 10 years, whereas saphenous **vein** grafts lasts 5 years

Long-term treatment is focused towards reducing the future MI risks such as diet modification, lower diabetes, lower cholesterol levels, lower the risk of clot formation
- Aspirin (if a patient is allergic to aspirin, then give clopidogrel)
- Statins
- Long-acting nitroglycerin
- Beta-blockers (metoprolol or carvedilol)
- Life style modification such as stop smoking, exercise
- Diet modification

2.   ACUTE CORONARY SYNDROME (ACS)

Acute coronary syndrome refers to a group of heart conditions that are caused by obstruction (atherosclerosis or clot) of the coronary artery. ACS should be distinguished from stable angina, which occurs predictable amount of exertion and relieves by rest or nitroglycerin

ACS is classified into two main groups according to the ST-segment on EKG
1. **ST-segment elevation MI (STMI)**
2. Non-ST-segment elevation coronary syndrome, which is further sub-divided into two, based on cardiac enzymes
2a. **Non-ST-segment elevation MI (NSTMI), in which cardiac enzymes are elevated**
2b. **Unstable angina** in which **cardiac enzymes are absent**

In a nutshell: ACS refers to three types of MI: ST-segment elevation MI (STMI), Non-ST-segment elevation MI (NSTMI), and unstable angina, which are **diagnosed based on EKG and cardiac enzymes**

STMI is defined as symptoms consistent of ACS, and any of the followings:
*   ST elevation in ≥ 2mm in two contiguous chest leads, or ≥ 1 mm in two contiguous limbs leads
*   Q wave
*   New left bundle branch block (LBBB)

Cause: NSTMI and unstable angina are caused by obstruction of coronary arteries by **atherosclerosis**, and **STMI** is caused by obstruction of coronary arteries by a **clot.**

Si/Sx: Chest pain, heaviness, tightness, pressure, pain radiating to left arm, shoulder or jaw, which is **not relieved by rest or nitroglycerin**

STMI area of infarction & blood supply

ST elevation, T wave inversion on EKG	Heart infarction area	Blood supply
II, III, aVF	Inferior	Right coronary artery
I, V4, V5, V6, aVL	Lateral	Left anterior descending
V1, V2	Posterior	Posterior descending
V1, V3	Anteroseptal	Left anterior descending
V2, V4	Anterior	Left anterior descending

(High-yield for step 3)

Management: all patients are given morphine, oxygen, aspirin and beta-blockers even before an EKG. Rest of the management is as follow:

Note: **do not wait for the cardiac enzymes** results to start treatment because they may take hours to be detectable

- **Acute treatment** for **NSTMI and unstable angina** is heparin and / or PCI and adjuvant treatment

- **Acute treatment** for **STMI** is PCI or thrombolytics and adjuvant therapy
  - PCI is proven to be superior to thrombolytics. The standard care is to perform PCI within 90 minutes, " door-to-ballon time". However, if PCI is delayed for some reasons, then give thrombolytics. Furthermore, make sure that the patient does not have any contraindications for thrombolytics.
  - **Adjuvant treatment for ACS includes aspirin, ACE-inhibitors and GIIa/IIIb inhibitors. Clopidogrel and heparin are added only if PCI is planned**

Contra-indications for thrombolytics (tPAs)

Absolute contraindications	Relative contraindications
• Intracranial hemorrhage • Ischemic stroke within last 6 months • Aortic dissection • Active bleeding • Surgery within last 2 weeks	• BP> 180/110 mmHg at the time of presentation • Prolong CPR (>10 minutes) within 2-4 weeks • Active peptic ulcer disease • Major surgery within 3 weeks • INR> 2.0 • Pregnancy

Important: tPAs are beneficial only in STMI because STMI is caused by a clot in a coronary artery, and tPAs **restore the perfusion by lysing the clot.**

Summary of acute treatment of different types of angina

Medication	Stable angina	NSTMI and Unstable angina	STMI
Aspirin	Yes	Yes	Yes
Nitroglycerin	Yes	Yes	Yes
Beta-blocker	Yes	Yes	Yes
Morphine	Yes	Yes	Yes
ACEIs*	Yes	Yes	Yes
Clopidogrel	No	Yes, if PCI is planned	Yes if PCI is planned
Low-molecular weight heparin	No	Yes, if PCI is not planned	Yes, if PCI is planned
IV heparin	No	Yes, if PCI is planned	Yes, but only after tPA
GP IIb/IIIa	No	Yes (Tirofiban or eptifibatide)	Yes, abciximab if PCI is planned
Thrombolytics (tPAs)*	No	No	Yes (only if PCI is delayed or cannot be performed)

*ACEIs prevent cardiac remodeling. They also lower the mortality in patients with ejection fraction (EF) < 45%. ACEIs are given to a patient with stable angina if patient has CHF, systolic dysfunction or EF< 45%.

* tPAs can be given up to 12 hours of onset of symptoms of STMI or new LBBB

Long-term treatment of ACS:

- Aspirin (if a patient is allergic to aspirin, then give clopidogrel)
- Clopidogrel for 9-12 months
- Statins
- Short-acting nitrates
- Beta-blockers (metoprolol or carvedilol)
- Life style and diet modification

KEY MANAGEMENT STEPS OF ANGINA

Chest pain in **stable angina** occurs with a predictable amount of exertion and **relieves by rest or nitroglycerin.** In contrast chest pain in **ACS** occurs suddenly, often with rest or minimal exertion, and **does not relieve with nitroglycerin**

1. If a patient presents with a chest paint that has characteristics of angina, then manage the patient as follow:
   1a. Give Morphine, Oxygen, nitroglycerin and aspirin. A classic mnemonic to remember that, is **MONA**
   1b. Get EKG
   1c. If EKG is inconclusive, then do a stress test. If EKG shows stable angina or any of the stress test is positive, then do angiography
   1d. If EKG shows STMI, then treatment options include PCI or thrombolytic, and adjunct therapy. PCI is a preferred treatment, but if it is delayed for > 90 minutes or the hospital has **no PCI lab, and** then give tPAs.
   1e. If EKG shows NSTMI coronary syndrome (NSTMI or unstable angina), then treatment options include PCI and/ or heparin and adjunct therapy.

Remember:
- Do not wait for cardiac enzyme to start the treatment because they may take hours to be detectable
- Always check for tPAs contraindications before giving them to a patient
- Even if PCI is delayed for some reasons, it is still the definitive treatment for STMI. Give patient tPAs and arrange for PCI
- If patient is allergic to aspirin, then give clopidogrel

(High-yield for step 3)
Drugs that lower the mortality in ACS are:
- Metoprolol
- Clopidogrel
- Aspirin
- Thrombolytic
- Statins
- ACE-Inhibitors (ACEIs)
- Angiotensin receptor blockers (ARBs)

(High-yield for step 3)

LIPIDS GOAL IN A POST-MI PATIENT

1. LDLs goals are as follow:
   - LDLs goal in a patient with **CAD or CAD equivalents alone** is < 100 mg/dl
   - LDLs goal is a patient with **CAD plus diabetes** is <70 mg/dl
2. Triglycerides goal is <150 mg/dl
3. HDLs goal is > 40 mg/dl

CORONARY ARTERY DISEASE (CAD) EQUIVALENTS:

- Diabetes
- Peripheral artery disease
- Aortic artery disease
- Carotid disease

LDLs goals and management

Risk factors	Lifestyle modification	Initiate drug treatment
0-1 risk factor for CAD	≥ 160 mg/dl	>190 mg/dl
≥ 2 risk factor for CAD	≥ 130 mg/dl	≥160 mg/dl
CAD or CAD equivalents	≥ 100 mg/dl	≥130 mg/dl

Note: If the patient has **CAD and diabetes, then** initiate drug treatment and do lifestyle modifications to keep LDLs **<70 mg/dl.**

RISK FACTORS FOR CORONARY ARTERY DISEASE (CAD)

- Cigarettes smoking
- Diabetes mellitus
- BP > 140/90 or on BP medications
- HDL < 40
- Male > 45 years, or female > 55 years of age
- First-degree male relative < 55 years of age with CAD, or first-degree female relative < 65 years of age with CAD

Lipid lowering medications

Medication	Effects	Side effects
Statins	Lowers LDL & triglyceride	Increases liver enzymes (AST, ALT), myositis
Fibric acid derivatives	Lowers triglyceride & increases HDL	Myositis, GI upset
Ezetimibe	Lowers LDL	Diarrhea, abdominal pain
Bile acid resins	Lowers LDL	Flatus & abdominal cramping, myalgia
Niacin	Lowers LDL & increases HDL	Skin flushing, pruritus

POST-MI COMPLICATIONS

Post MI complication	Diagnosis	Treatment
Cardiogenic shock	Echocardiography, right heart catheter	ACEIs, dobutamine, urgent surgery
Myocardial wall rupture	Physical exams shows distance heart sounds, JVD, hypotension	Pericardiocentesis, urgent surgical repair
Cardiac valve rupture	2D echocardiography	ACEIs, nitroprusside, urgent surgery
Cardiac septal rupture	Holosystolic murmur best heard at **the left lower sternal border,** echocardiography, Right heart catheter shows **increased oxygen saturation in right ventricle and pulmonary artery**	ACEIs, nitroprusside, urgent surgery
Right-sided heart failure	Physical exam shows **clear lung,** Echocardiography	**IV fluids** and catheterization,
Left-sided heart failure	Physical exam shows **dullness on percussion** at lung bases, Echocardiography	**Intra-aortic balloon pump** and catheterization or ACEIs, dobutamine, and catheterization
Myocardial rupture	Persistent ST elevation on EKG, echocardiography	Warfarin to lower the clot formation, and in rare case, surgery

- Other post-myocardial complications include **ventricular arrhythmias (most common cause of death in a post-MI patient)**, first-, second, and third-degree heart block. Late complication of MI is Dressler's syndrome

CARDIAC ARRHYTHMIAS AND CONDUCTION ABNORMALITIES

A normal heart rate is 60-100 beats per minute (bpm)
- Bradycardia: heart rate < 60 bpm
- Tachycardia: heart rate > 100 bpm

Note: some people have arrhythmia that occurs only during a particular activity. Moreover, EKG does not detect heart rhythm abnormalities that do not occur during the test. In that case, patient may need a **Holter monitor** (stable, outpatient) **or telemetry monitor** (unstable or hospitalized patients). These are medical deceives that continuously monitor the heart rate and rhythm for 24 -72 hours. Please note that these are not used to detect stable angina.

1. SINUS BRADYCARDIA
Sinus bradycardia is referred to a heart rate that originates from the sinus node and has a **heart rate < 60 bpm**
Cause: Medicines (beta-blockers, calcium channel blockers, digitalis and antiarrhythmics), sinus node dysfunction, increased vagal tone, hypothyroidism
Si/Sx: some patients may be asymptomatic, but symptoms may include lightheadedness, shortness of breath, dizziness, hypotension
Diagnosis:
- EKG shows **heart rate < 60 bpm**, with **normal P wave, PR interval and QRS complexes**

Treatment: treatment depends on symptoms
- **No treatment** is required for a **asymptomatic patient**
- **Atropine or pacemakers** for **symptomatic** patient

Note Beta-blockers, and calcium channel blockers medicines should be avoided in sinus bradycardia because both of these may slow the heart conduction and worsen the symptoms

2. FIRST-DEGREE HEART BLOCK

In a first-degree heart block, electric impulse moves slower than normal through the AV node.

Cause: it can occur in a normal individual, but risk factors include increased vagal tone, drugs (beta-blockers, calcium channel blockers digoxin, amiodarone), acute myocardial infarction, myocarditis

Si/Sx: Asymptomatic

Diagnosis:

- EKG shows normal sinus rhythm with prolong **PR interval (>. 02ms)**

Treatment: treatment depends on symptoms

- **No treatment** is required for **asymptomatic patient**
- **Atropine or pacemakers** for **symptomatic** patient

Note: Beta-blockers, calcium channel blockers medicines should be avoided in first-degree heart block because both of these slow the heart conduction and can worsen the symptoms

3. SECOND-DEGREE HEART BLOCK

Second-degree heart block is sub-classified into two types:

- Second-degree type I heart block
- Second-degree type II heart block

3a. SECOND-DEGREE TYPE I HEART BLOCK

In a second-degree type I heart block (also known as Mobitz Type I or Wenckebach's block), the electric signals moves slower and slower with each heartbeat until the heart skips a heartbeat.

Cause: increased vagal tone, medicine (beta-blockers, calcium channel blockers, digoxin)

Si/Sx: some patients may be asymptomatic, but symptoms may include lightheadedness, dizziness, syncope

Diagnosis:

- EKG shows **progressive prolonged PR intervals until a nonconducted P wave**

Treatment:

- Stop the offending drug
- Atropine or pacemaker is only for symptomatic patients

3b. SECOND-DEGREE TYPE II HEART BLOCK

In a second-degree type II heart block (also known as Mobitz Type II), some electrical signals move normally between atria and ventricles, while other signals are blocked.

Cause: Anterior septal MI, fibrosis of conducting system, inflammatory conditions (rheumatic fever, Lyme disease), autoimmune (SLE, systemic sclerosis), infiltrative myocardial disease (amyloidosis, sarcoidosis)

Si/Sx: light-headedness, dizziness syncope

Diagnosis:
- EKG shows **normal PR intervals with unexpected non-conducted P wave**

Treatment:
- **Transvenous** pacemakers for **stable patients**
- **Transcutaneous** pacemakers for **unstable patients**
- **Intra-cardiac** pacemaker is the best **long-term management**

Complication: second-degree type II heart block can progress to 3rd degree heart block

4. THIRD-DEGREE HEART BLOCK

In a third-degree heart block (also known as complete heart block) all electric signals are blocked from atria to ventricles. As a result, both **atria** and **ventricles** are contracting at **their own rate**.

Cause: acute MI, inferior MI, second-degree type II heart block, Lyme disease

Si/Sx: Syncope, dizziness, hypotension, acute heart failure

Diagnosis:
- EKG shows **uncoordinated P waves and QRS complexes**

Treatment:
- **Transvenous** pacemakers for **stable patients**
- **Transcutaneous** pacemakers for **unstable patients**
- **Intra-cardiac** pacemaker is the best **long-term management**

5. VENTRICULAR FIBRILLATION (VF)

Ventricular fibrillation is uncoordinated contractions of ventricle muscles of the heart

Cause: CAD, MI, heart surgery, heart muscle disease

Si/Sx: Syncope, hypotension, pulselessness, sudden death

Diagnosis: EKG shows **disorganized heart rhythm**

Treatment: VF is a life threatening condition; it can lead to death within few minutes if the patient is not treated quickly. **Unsynchronized defibrillation (200-300-360 J)** is the primary standard care

6. VENTRICULAR TACHYCARDIA (VT)

Ventricular tachycardia is defined as rapid high heartbeat (>100 bpm) that starts in the ventricles, and has least 3 consecutive premature ventricular contractions (PVCs)

Cause: CAD, MI, myocarditis, cardiomyopathy, valvular heart disease, anti-arrhythmic medicines

Si/Sx: Most of the patients are asymptomatic, but symptoms may include palpitations, angina, syncope, shortness of breath, light-headedness

Diagnosis:

- EKG shows **wide QRS complex with ventricular rate > 100 bpm,** 3 or more consecutive PVCs

Treatment: Treatment depends on symptoms

- If a patient is **unstable,** then do **synchronized defibrillation**
- If a patient is **stable,** then **check BP and pulse:**
  - If patient has **normal BP** and **pulse,** then treat the patient with **amiodarone or lidocaine**
  - If patient is **hypotensive** or has **no pulse,** then do **synchronized defibrillation**

7. ATRIAL FIBRILLATION (A-fib)

Atrial fibrillation is uncoordinated contractions of atrial muscles of the heart

Cause: pulmonary disease, ischemia, rheumatic heart disease, anemia, atrial myxoma, thyrotoxicosis, ethanol, sepsis

Si/Sx: most of patients are asymptomatic, but symptoms may include hypotension, tachycardia, chest pain, palpitations, **irregularly irregular pulses**

Diagnosis:
- EKG shows **absent P wave, variable and irregular QRS complex**

Management: is as follow:
1. **Control the heart rate**
- If a patient is **hemodynamic unstable** (lightheadedness, confusion, CHF, hypertension, or chest pain), then do **synchronize electrical cardioversion.**
- If a patient is **stable,** then **slow the heart rate** with **calcium channel blockers** (diltiazem, verapamil), **beta- blocker** (metoprolol, esmolol), or digoxin

Note: calcium channel blockers are the first-line treatment, beta-blockers are second, and digoxin is the third choice to control HR in A-fib

2. **Restore the heart rhythm**
After controlling the HR in A-fib, it is important to **restore the heart rhythms.** It can achieve by **medicine** such as IV procainamide (1st choice), sotalol or amiodarone, or **cardioversion** (200-300-360 J):
- If A-fib is lasted **< 48 hours,** then **medicine treatment** is preferred
- If A-fib lasted **> 48 hours,** then either give patient an **anticoagulant** (warfarin or aspirin) for a month, and then give **medicine or do cardioversion,** or perform **transthoracic echocardiography to exclude a clot,** and then give **medicine or do cardioversion**

Complication: Patients with atrial fibrillation are at increased risk of embolic stroke. To lower the risk, he/she should be given anticoagulants **(warfarin or aspirin) to maintain INR 2-3 indefinitely.** Anticoagulants is given **based on total risk,** also known as **CHADS2** score (discussed below)

Risk factor	Relative risk
CHF	1
HTN	1
Age > 65	1
Diabetes	1
Previous stroke	2

- **For score** 0 or lone A-fib, give **aspirin**
- **For scores 1-2,** give **aspirin or warfarin**
- **For score 3 or higher,** give **warfarin**

For example:
- A patient with CHF and HTN has a CHADS2 score: 1+1= 2
- A patient with CHF, HTN and previous stroke has a CHADS2 score: 1+1+2 =4

8. ATRIAL FLUTTER
Atrial flutter is uncoordinated contractions of atrial muscles of the heart. Atrial rate is usually 250-300 bpm in atrial flutter
Cause: COPD, CHF, ASD, surgically repaired congenital heart disease
Si/Sx: most of patients are asymptomatic, but symptoms may include hypotension, tachycardia, chest pain or palpitations
Diagnosis: EKG shows regular rhythm with **"saw tooth appearance"** of P wave
Treatment: same as A-fib

9. SUPRAVENTRICULAR TACHYCARDIA (SVT)
Supraventricular tachycardia is a fast heart rhythm that originates at or above the atrioventricular node
Si/Sx: palpitation, **tachycardia,** syncope
Diagnosis: EKG shows **narrow QRS complex with ventricular rate 160- 180 bpm**
Treatment: depends on patient's symptoms:
- **Synchronized** cardioversion is performed in an **unstable patient**
- **A stable patient** can be treated with **carotid massage, Valsalva maneuver, or ice water face immersion**. If this is ineffective, then use **IV adenosine**
- **Radiofrequency catheter** ablation is the best long-term management

10. MULTIFOCAL ATRIAL TACHYCARDIA
Multifocal atrial tachycardia is a rapid heart rate that occurs when multiple electric signals are sent from atria to ventricles
Cause: COPD, hypoxemia, reentrant pathway
Si/Sx: most of the patients are asymptomatic, but symptoms may include hypotension, tachycardia, chest pain, palpitations
Diagnosis:
- EKG shows **multiple P waves** with heart **rate > 100 bpm**

Treatment: start with **oxygen**, then give calcium channel blockers (verapamil, diltiazem) or beta-blockers, correct electrolytes imbalance and treat the underlying cause

11. WANDERING PACEMAKER
Wandering pacemaker (also known as atrial arrhythmia) occurs when heart pacemaker site shifts from SA node to atria, and or AV node
Diagnosis:
- EKG shows **multiple P waves** with heart **rate of < 100 bpm**

Treatment: None

12. WOLFF–PARKINSON–WHITE SYNDROME (WPW)
Wolff–Parkinson–White syndrome is a heart condition caused by an abnormal extra electrical pathway in the heart that allows the electrical signal to bypass the AV node.
Cause: " short-circuit" conducting system that bypasses the AV node and allow reentrant
Diagnosis:
- EKG shows **delta wave** (slurred upstroke of QRS complex)
- Most accurate test is electrophysiology

Treatment:
- Initial treatment is procainamide
- **Radiofrequency catheter** ablation is the best long-term management

---

KEY MANAGEMENT POINTS OF ARRHYTHMIAS

1. EKG is the best initial to for arrhythmia, but if it is inconclusive, then portable device heart monitor such as **Holter or telemeter monitor may be needed.**

2. Patients with bradycardia, first-, and second-degree type I heart block usually require no treatment, but if they are symptomatic, then treat them with atropine, if that is ineffective, then put pacemakers

3. Patients with second-degree type II and third-degree heart block are treated as follow:

- Transvenous pacemakers for **stable patients**
- Transcutaneous pacemakers for **unstable patients**
- Intra-cardiac pacemaker is best **long-term management**

4. Ventricular fibrillation is treated with **unsynchronized defibrillation (200-300-360 J)**

5. Patient with ventricular tachycardia is treated as follow:
   - If the patient is unstable, has low BP or pulseless, then do **synchronized defibrillation**
   - **If the patient is stable, then treat the patient with amiodarone or lidocaine**

6. Patient with a-fib or atrial flutter is managed as follow:
   - If the patient is hemodynamic **unstable** then do **synchronized cardioversion.** However, if the patient is **stable,** then slow the heart rate with **calcium channel blocker, beta-blocker or digoxin.**
   - Once the heart rate is controlled, then **control the heart rhythm.** If arrhythmia lasted < 48 hours, then give IV procainamide (1st choice), sotalol or amiodarone. However, if it lasted for more> 48 hours, then patient can be managed with either medication or cardioversion, which is given after one month treatment with anticoagulant or immediately after excluding the presence of a clot in the heart with transthoracic echocardiography

7. Patient with SVT is treated as follow:
   - If patient is unstable, then give **synchronized cardioversion**
   - If the patient is stable, then the best initial treatment is carotid massage, Valsalva maneuver or ice water face immersion. If that is ineffective, then give IV adenosine.

In a nutshell: if the patient is hemodynamic unstable then do synchronized defibrillation, except for ventricular fibrillation, which is treated with unsynchronized defibrillation. If a patient is stable, then treat with medicines.

HEART VALVE LESIONS

Valvular lesions and effects of maneuvers

Valvular lesions	Squatting/ leg Raise	Standing/ Valsalva
AS, AR, **MS**, MR, VSD	Murmur increases	Murmur decreases
MVP, HOCM	Murmur decreases	Murmur increases

Valvular lesions and effects of maneuvers

Valvular Lesion	Hand grip	Amyl Nitrate
AR, MR, VSD	Murmur increase	Murmur decrease
AS, MVP, HOCM	Murmur decreases	Murmur increases
MS	Minimal effect	Minimal effect

AS= Aortic stenosis, AR= Aortic regurgitation, MS=Mitral stenosis, MR= Mitral regurgitation, VSD= Ventricular septal defect, HOCM=Hypertrophic subaortic stenosis

SYSTOLIC MURMUR GRADES:
- I/VI is barely audible
- II/VI is faint, but audible
- III/VI is loud, but without a palpable thrill
- IV/VI is loud with palpable thrill
- V/VI is loud that it can be heard with the stethoscope lightly placed on the chest
- VI/VI is so loud that it can be heard even without a stethoscope

Innocent murmurs are systolic murmur, I/VI or II/VI grade murmur.

SUMMARY OF HEART MURMUR LOCATIONS
- Aortic stenosis: 2nd right intercostal space radiating to the carotid arteries
- Aortic regurgitation, tricuspid murmur: left lower sternal border
- Mitral regurgitation: 5th intercostal space, below the left nipple
- Pulmonic valve: 2nd left intercostal space

1. AORTIC STENOSIS (AS)
Aortic stenosis is characterized by abnormally narrowed opening of aortic valve. This leads to lower blood flow from heart to the body

Cause: most common cause in a young patient is **congenital bicuspid valve**, and in an old patient (>60 years of age) is **calcification of normal aortic valves**

Si/Sx: angina-type chest pain, syncope, exertional dyspnea, palpitation

Diagnosis:

- Physical exam shows peripheral pulses that are weak and late compared to heat sounds (pulsus parvus et tardus)
- Auscultation of heart usually shows midsystolic **crescendo-decrescendo systolic** murmur heard at **second right intercostal space radiating to the carotid arteries and apex**, paradoxically split S2
- ECG shows **left ventricular hypertrophy**
- **Best initial test** diagnostic test is **transthoracic echocardiography**
- **Most accurate test** is **left heart catheterization**

Treatment:

- **Diuretics**
- **Valves are replaced** in all symptomatic patients or when valve area is < .8cm^2. Two main types of valve replacements options include:
  - **Mechanical** valves, which **do not have to be replaced again,** but they **require anticoagulant** indefinitely to maintain INR 2.0-3.0
  - **Bioprosthetic** valves, which have to be **replaced every 10 years,** but **do not require** anticoagulant
- If a patient cannot tolerate valve replacement, then do **balloon valvuloplasty**

Note: Beta-blockers or afterload reducers should be avoided

Prognosis of AS with concomitant other conditions:

- Patient with AS and coronary artery disease has average survival time of 3-5 years
- Patient with AS and syncope has average survival time of 2- 3 years
- Patient with AS and CHF has average survival time of 1.5 - 2 years

2. AORTIC REGURGITATIONA (AR)

Aortic regurgitation is caused by improper closure of aortic valves. This leads to backward flow of blood from aorta to ventricle during ventricular diastole

Cause: Most common cause is hypertension; other causes may include endocarditis, Marfan syndrome, syphilis, ankylosing spondylitis, aortic dissection

Si/Sx: Patients often are asymptomatic, but symptoms may include shortness of breath, bounding pulses, fatigue, fatigue, shortening of breath

Diagnosis:

- Physical exam may show:
  o Corrigan pulse: **rapid rise** and **fall of pulses**
  o Duroziez sign: **diastolic murmur** heard over **femoral artery**
  o De Musset sign: **head-bobbing** with each pulse
  o Hill sign: **systolic blood pressure > 30 mmHg** higher in **lower extremities compared to upper extremities**
  o Quincke pulse: **pulsation in fingernails**
- Chest auscultation shows **diastolic murmur** over left lower sternal border
- EKG shows **left ventricular hypertrophy**
- **Best initial test diagnostic** test is **transthoracic echocardiography**
- **Most accurate test** is **left heart catheterization**

Treatment:

- Decrease the afterload with ACE-inhibitors, ARBs, or vasodilators such as Nifedipine, hydralazine
- Aortic valve are replaced if any of the following is present:
  o Symptomatic patient
  o If echocardiograph shows **ejection fraction (EF) <50% or left ventricular end systolic diameter > 5.0 cm**

3. MITRAL REGURGITATION (MR)

Mitral regurgitation is caused by improper closure of mitral valve. This lead to backward flow of blood from ventricle to atrium during ventricular systole

Cause: Mitral valve prolapse, ischemic heart disease, collagen vascular disease, papillary muscle dysfunction

Symptoms: dyspnea on exertion, orthopnea, paroxysmal nocturnal dyspnea, pulmonary edema

Diagnosis:

- Chest auscultation shows **holosystolic murmur heard** at 5th intercostal space **below left nipple radiating to axilla**
- **EKG** shows left atrial enlargement
- Most **accurate test is transesophageal echocardiography**

Treatment:

- Asymptomatic patients are treated with ACE-inhibitors, ARBs, or vasodilators such as Nifedipine, hydralazine
- Mitral valve are replaced if any of the following is present:
  - Symptomatic patient
  - If echocardiograph shows **ejection fraction (EF) <60% or left ventricular end systolic diameter > 4.0 cm**

4. MITRAL STENOSIS

Mitral stenosis is characterized by abnormally narrowed opening of mitral valve. This leads to lower blood flow from ventricle to atrium

Cause: rheumatic fever disease is the most common cause

Si/Sx: most of the patients' stay asymptomatic until A-fib develops or woman becomes pregnant. Symptoms may include:

- **Dysphagia,** which is caused by left atrium pressure on esophagus
- **Hoarseness,** which is caused by left atrium pressure on recurrent laryngeal nerve

Diagnosis:

- Chest auscultation shows **opening snap** followed by **mid diastolic rumble,** loud S1
- Chest X-ray shows **elevation of left main bronchus & straightening of left heart border**
- **EKG** shows left atrial enlargement
- Most **accurate test is transesophageal echocardiography**

Treatment:

- Beta-blockers and digitalis are given to control the heart rate
- **Best initial treatment** is diuretics and salt reduction to lower the fluid overload
- Most effective treatment is **balloon valvuloplasty; it is well tolerated even in pregnancy**
- Surgical valve are replaced in refractory cases

- Anticoagulants (warfarin) is given for embolus prophylaxis, maintain INR 2-3

Complication of mitral stenosis is stroke

5. MITRAL VALVE PROLAPSE (MVP)

Mitral valve prolapse is caused by improper closure of mitral valve. This leads to backward flow of blood from ventricle to atrium during ventricular systole

Risk factor: MVP is seen in 7 % of the population, mainly in young women

Cause: connective tissue disorder especially Marfan syndrome, and in rare genetic disorders

Si/Sx: most of the patients are asymptomatic, but symptoms may include lightheadedness, palpitations, syncope, chest pain

Diagnosis:

- Chest auscultation shows **late systolic murmur with midsystolic click**
- **Echocardiography can be used to confirm diagnosis**

Treatment:

- Usually no treatment is required
- Beta-blockers or valve replacement is for symptomatic patient

---

KEY MANAGEMENT POINT OF HEART VALAVE LESIONS

- In aortic regurgitation and mitral regurgitation valves are replaced when patient is symptomatic or when echocardiography shows the followings: see table below

	Aortic regurgitation	Mitral regurgitation
Ejection fraction	**<50%**	**<60%**
Left ventricular end systolic diameter	**> 5.0 cm**	**> 4.0 cm**

- Most effective treatment of mitral stenosis is **balloon valvuloplasty, which is well tolerated even in pregnant women**

- **Aortic valves can be replaced with mechanical or bioprosthetic valves. Mechanical** valves **do not have to be replaced again**, but they **require anticoagulant** indefinitely to maintain INR 2.0-3.0 **Bioprosthetic valves** have to be **replaced every 10 years**, but they **do not require** anticoagulant

---

CONGESTIVE HEART FAILURE (CHF)

Congestive heart failure is a heart condition in which heart is unable to pump enough blood to the rest of the body.

Types: CHF can be right-side heart failure, left-side heart failure, both sided heart failure, systolic dysfunction, or diastolic dysfunction

Causes: CAD, MI, HTN, faulty heart valves, arrhythmias, hypo/hyperthyroidism, cardiomyopathy, myocarditis, congenital heart defects, pulmonary HTN

Si/Sx: discussed in the table below

Right and left-sided heart failure symptoms

Right-sided heart failure symptoms	Left-sided heart failure symptoms
• JVD • Hepatomegaly • Hepatojugular reflex • Bipedal edema • Cyanosis • Weight loss	• Bilateral rales • S3 Gallops • Pleural effusion • Pulmonary edema • Orthopnea • Exertional dyspnea • Paroxysmal nocturnal dyspnea

New York Heart Association (NYHA) Functional Classification Of CHF

NYHA class	Symptoms
I	CHF, but no symptoms and no limitation with normal physical activity
II	Mild symptoms and slight limitation with normal physical activity
III	Marked limitation in activity due to symptoms, even with mild activity. Comfortable only at rest
IV	Severe limitations, symptoms, experienced even while resting. Patient are mostly bedbound

Diagnosis:

- Chest x-ray shows cardiomegaly, effusion, cephalization of pulmonary vessels, pulmonary vascular congestion
- EKG: Arrhythmias, sinus tachycardia
- **Echocardiograph** is the only test which helps differentiate systolic from diastolic dysfunction; ejection fraction is **< 45 % in systolic dysfunction, and > 45 % in disystolic dysfunction**
- **Brain natriuretic peptide (BNP)**
- **Most accurate test is MUGA scan** (nuclear ventriculography)

Management: as follow

- **If patient has pulmonary edema, then** have patient sit in upright position and give oxygen, and then furosemide, followed by nitrate and morphine (morphine mobilizes the fluid, reduced pain and anxiety
- **If ejection fraction is < 35 %, then use implantable cardioverter-defibrillator**
- **If ejection fraction is < 25 %, then perform angiography**
- If EKG shows **QRS interval > 130 msec,** then implant **biventricular pacemaker**
- **Chronic treatment** for a stable CHF patient depends on the type of dysfunction, discussed below:

Chronic CHF treatment

Systolic dysfunction	Disystolic dysfunction
- ACE-inhibitor or ARBS (lowers the mortality) - Beta-blockers such as metoprolol or carvedilol (Lowers the mortality) - Spironolactone (lowers the **mortality in class III and IV CHF)** - Digoxin (**reduces the hospitalization)** - Furosemide	- Beat-blockers (metoprolol or carvedilol) - Diuretics

Note: If a patient cannot tolerate ACE inhibitor, then use hydralazine and isosorbide dinitrate

PULMONARY EDEMA

Pulmonary edema is characterized by abnormal fluid buildup in the air sacs of the lungs

Cause: CHF is the most common cause; other less common causes include kidney failure, lung damage, high altitude exposure

Si/Sx: SOB, pink frothy sputum, nocturnal dyspnea, orthopnea

Diagnosis:

- Clinical diagnosis
- Physical exam show rales or crackles on lung exam, JVD
- Chest X-ray show Kerley B lines, effusion, dilated pulmonary vessels

Management:

Initial step is to have patient sit in **upright position** and give **oxygen**, and then **furosemide**, followed by **nitrate and morphine** (morphine mobilizes the fluid, reduced pain and anxiety)

CARDIOMYOPATHY

1. DILATED CARDIOMYOPATHY

Dilated cardiomyopathy is a condition in which heart muscles become weakened and enlarged, mainly the left ventricle. As a result, heart cannot pump enough blood to the body.

Cause: ischemia is the most common cause; other causes include Infection (Chagas' disease, HIV, Coxsackie virus), medicines (Adriamycin doxorubicin), alcohol, beriberi,

Si/Sx: same as CHF

Diagnosis:

- Echocardiography shows decreased ejection fraction (systolic dysfunction)
- **Most accurate test is MUGA scan** (nuclear ventriculography)

Treatment: stop the offending agent or treat the underlying condition. And, treat the patient as per **systolic dysfunction CHF**

2. HYPERTROPHIC OBSTRUCTIVE CARDIOMYOPATHY (HOCM)

Autosomal dominant trait that causes the thickening of the interventricular septum. Thickened septum bulges into the ventricle and blocks the blood outflow from ventricle. It is the **most common cause of death in young athletes.**

Si/Sx: Chest pain, palpitation, dyspnea

Diagnosis:

- Physical exam shows systolic murmur, which **increases with Valsalva & amyl nitrite, and decreases with handgrip, leg raise & squatting**
- EKG shows left ventricular hypertrophy
- Most **accurate test is transesophageal echocardiography**, it shows decreased diastolic function

Treatment:

- Best initial treatment is **beta-blockers or verapamil**
- If drug therapy is ineffective, then give pure alcohol injection in septal arteries
- Myomectomy is a last resort
- Patients should be advised against intense training or exercise
- AICD (Automatic Implantable Cardioverter Defibrillator) should be placed if any of the following is present:
  - Family history of sudden death at young age
  - Unexplained syncope

3. RESTRICTIVE CARDIOMYOPATHY

Restrictive cardiomyopathy is a condition in which heart size is normal or slightly enlarged, but heart muscles are stiff and cannot relax during diastole. As a result, heart does not fill and pump enough blood to the body

Cause: amyloidosis, hemochromatosis, radiation, sarcoidosis, scleroderma, glycogen storage disease

Si/Sx: Combination of right and left-sided heart failure

Diagnosis:

- Physical exam shows increased jugular venous pressure (JVP) with inspiration (**Kussmaul's sign)**
- Chest X-ray shows cardiomegaly
- EKG shows low-voltage QRS complex
- Most accurate test is **endomyocardial biopsy**

Treatment: salt restriction, diuretic for fluid overload and treat the underlying cause

Note: Kussmaul's sign is present in restrictive cardiomyopathy and constrictive pericarditis.

PERICARDIAL DISEASE

1. CONSTRICTIVE PERICARDITIS

Constrictive pericarditis is a chronic inflammation of the pericardium that leads to calcification, fibrosis and stiffening of the heart muscles

Causes: tuberculosis, radiation therapy of chest, heart surgery, mesothelioma

Si/Sx: similar to right-sided heart failure (JVD, lower extremity edema, hepatomegaly)

Diagnosis:

- Physical exam shows increased jugular venous pressure (JVP) with inspiration **(Kussmaul's sign)**, and **pericardial knock**, an extra diastolic apical sound due to thickened pericardium
- Chest X-ray shows **pericardium calcification**
- CT or MRI of chest show thickened pericardium

Treatment: low sodium diet and diuretic and pericardiectomy

2. PERICARDITIS

Pericarditis is an inflammation of the pericardium

Causes: viral infection is the most common cause; other causes include fungal, bacterial, rheumatoid arthritis, MI, trauma, drugs

Si/Sx: retrosternal pain, which is **worst when patient is supine** and **relieves** with **leaning forward and sitting up.** Pain is not affected by activity or food.

Diagnosis:

- Physical exam shows **pericardial friction rub**
- EKG shows **ST elevation in all leads and PR depression** (PR depression very specific, but is not always present)

Treatment:

- NSAIDs is given for **viral pericarditis**, but if NSAIDs is ineffective, then give prednisone
- For **post-myocardial** pericarditis **high-dose aspirin**
- Pericarditis caused by other causes is treated by treating the underlying cause

3. PERICARDIAL TAMPONADE

Pericardial tamponade is pressure on the heart due to blood or fluid buildup in pericardial sac (space between the heart muscles and pericardium)

Cause: infections (viral, bacterial), metastatic cancer, trauma, dissecting thoracic aorta aneurysm, heart surgery, SLE

Si/Sx: chest pain, palpitations, rapid breathing, difficulty breathing, light-headedness

Diagnosis:

- Physical exam shows **Pulsus paradoxus** (blood pressure decreases > 10 mmHg during inspiration), **Beck's triad** (distance heart sounds, JVD, and hypotension)
- EKG shows **low voltage QRS and electrical alternans** (beat-to-beat height difference of QRS complex axis)
- Most accurate test is echocardiography, which shows **diastolic collapse of** right atrial and right ventricular

Treatment:

- Give **IV fluids** to maintain blood pressure, and then **immediate pericardiocentesis**; needle drainage of the fluid from the pericardial sac
- Pericardial window (the most effective treatment) or pericardiectomy may be done in a recurrent case

Note: Pulsus paradoxus is not diagnostic for pericardial tamponade because it is also seen in CHF and asthma

CARDIOLOGY INFECTIOUS DISEASES

ENDOCARDITIS

Endocarditis is an inflammation of the inner lining of the heart (endocardium). It usually involves the heart valves, but it may also involve other structures inside of the heart such as interventricular septum, chordae tendineae

Causes: most common cause is infection from bacteria, virus or fungus. Which most likely entered the bloodstream during central venous line access, injection drug use (IV drug abuse) or dental surgery. Other causes include SLE, cancer

Types:

1. **Acute bacterial** endocarditis affects the **healthy heart valves. It is** common in IV **drug abusers. Patient usually** develops symptoms **within days to weeks** after the exposure of infection. **S. Aureus and Strep. Pneumonia** is the most common causes.

2. **Subacute bacterial** endocarditis affects **previously damaged** heart valve. It is caused by **Streptococcus viridian.**

3. **Culture negative endocarditis** is caused organisms that are hard to culture known as the HACEK group: H. Parainfluenzae, Actinobacillus, Cardiobacterium, Eikenella, Kingella kingae

4. Systemic lupus erythematosus (SLE) also causes endocarditis known as Libman-sacks endocarditis, which is probably due to autoantibody mediated damage of heart valves

5. Marantic endocarditis (also known as non-bacterial thrombotic endocarditis) is causes by metastatic cancer

Si/Sx: fever and new murmur are the most common symptoms, but other symptoms may include:

- **Splinter hemorrhage** (red brown streak in nail beds)
- **Osler nodes** (painful nodules on fingers and toes)
- **Roth spots** (retinal hemorrhage with clear central area)
- **Janeway lesions** (dark spots on palms and soles)

Diagnosis: it is diagnosed based on Duke criteria: 2 major or 1 major + 3 minors or 5 minor, which is as follow: see table below

Major Criteria	Minor Criteria
• 2 positive blood cultures growing same organism • Positive echocardiography* or onset of new murmur	• Presence of predisposing valve abnormality • Fever >38 C or 100.4 F • Embolic disease • Immunologic phenomena, such as Osler nodes, Roth spots • 1 positive blood culture

* Transesophageal echocardiography is preferred over transthoracic echocardiography because it is more sensitive than transthoracic echocardiography

Note: If the blood culture comes back positive for Streptococcus bovis, then make sure to do **colonoscopy**, because it is associated with colorectal carcinoma

Treatment:
- Empiric treatment with IV vancomycin and gentamicin, until the culture and sensitivity results are available. Organism specific treatment is discussed in a table below
- Surgical valve replacement if any of the following is present:
  - Abscess is on the valves
  - Prosthetic valves are involved
  - AV block
  - Recurrent emboli

Organism specific therapy of endocarditis

Organism	Native valves	Prosthetic valves
S.Aureus	Nafcillin + gentamicin	Nafcillin + gentamicin +**rifampin**
Step. Viridian	Penicillin or ceftriaxone + gentamicin	Penicillin or ceftriaxone + gentamicin
Enterococcus	Penicillin or ampicillin + gentamicin	Penicillin or ampicillin + gentamicin

Note: If a patient is allergic to penicillin or Methicillin-resistant Staphylococcus aureus (MRSA) is found on culture and sensitivity, then substitute penicillin, nafcillin and ampicillin with **vancomycin**

ENDOCARDITIS PROPHYLAXIS

Endocarditis prophylaxis is given to patients who are at risk to have endocarditis

Risk factors:

- If a patient is going to have dental procedures, respiratory tract procedures, or surgery of infected skin.
- Heart conditions such as prosthetic valves, previous endocarditis unrepaired cyanotic heart disease, or heart transplant recipient who develops valve disease

Prophylaxis medication:

- Amoxicillin prior to the procedure
- Penicillin allergic patient are given clindamycin, macrolide or cephalosporin

KEY MANAGEMENT POINT OF ENDOCARDITIS

- If the blood culture is positive, then next step in management is to do echocardiography. Transesophageal echocardiography is more sensitive than transthoracic echocardiography.
- If blood culture is positive for S. bovis, then next step in management is to get **colonoscopy**
- Remember, blood culture may not be positive in all cases of endocarditis, because it may also be caused by culture negative organisms known as HACEK group

CARDIOVASCULAR SURGERY

THORACIC AORTA DISSECTION
Thoracic aorta dissection is a transverse tear in the intima of the aorta in the chest area

Risk factors: Most common risk factor is hypertension

Types: Two types of thoracic aorta dissections are:
- Type A, which affects the ascending aorta
- Type B, which affects the descending aorta

Si/Sx: chest pain radiating thorough the back between **scapula's**

Diagnosis:
- Physical exam shows **different high blood pressure** in **each arm**
- Best initial test is **chest X-ray, which** shows **widening of mediastinum**
- Most accurate test is **chest CT angiography**

Treatment: treatment depends on the type of dissecting aorta, which is a follow:
- Descending aortic dissection: control the blood pressures with **beta blockers** (IV labetalol or esmolol) or nitroprusside, unless life-threatening condition arise
- Ascending aortic dissection is a surgical emergency, it is managed as follow: beta-blockers such as **labetalol or esmolol** are the first-line treatment to control the blood pressures, followed by vasodilators such as **sodium nitroprusside**, and **surgery**

ABDOMINAL AORTA ANEURYSM (AAA)
Abdominal aorta aneurysm is characterized by aneurysm of aorta in abdomen area

Risk factors: smoking (the most common cause), male gender, obesity, high blood pressure, high cholesterol

Si/Sx: most of the patients are asymptomatic, but symptoms may include pain in the abdomen or back, clammy skin, dizziness, shock

Diagnosis:
- Physical exam usually shows pulsatile abdominal mass or abdominal bruits.
- Diagnosis is confirmed with ultrasound

- CT is performed to determine the size to AAA

Management is as follow:

- AAA < 4 cm: annual imaging
- AAA> 5 cm: surgically repair
- AAA 4-5 cm: follow-up every 6 months
- Ruptured AAA requires immediate surgical intervention

Screening for AAA: USPSTF recommends one-time ultrasound screening for men between 65- 75 years of age who have smoked at least 100 cigarettes in their lifetime

PERIPHERAL VASCULAR DISEASE

Peripheral vascular disease is characterized by narrowing of arteries by atherosclerotic plaque of arteries outside of the heart and brain

Risk factors: hypertension, diabetes, smoking, elevated blood cholesterol, obesity

Si/Sx: Depends on the location and extent of the blocked artery, but common symptoms includes Intermittent claudication, smooth shiny skin,

Diagnosis:

- Complete physical exam, palpitations of pluses & auscultation for bruits
- **Ankle-brachial index (ABI)**: normal ABI is >1.0.
- **Doppler ultrasounds of legs** is done to find the pressure gradient
- **Angiography,** is performed after doppler shows the pressure gradient, it is done to find the location of occlusion

Treatment:

- Smoking cessation
- Exercise, as tolerated
- Aspirin
- ACE to decrease the blood pressure
- Cilostazol
- Statins to keep LDL <100
- **If symptoms are severe or medical therapy is ineffective, then PVD is managed as follow:**
  - Short segment PVDs are managed by angioplasty
  - Large segment PVDs are managed with bypass graft repair

SUBCLAVIAN STEAL SYNDROME

Subclavian steal syndrome is characterized by occlusion of subclavian artery proximal to the origin of the vertebral artery. In this syndrome blood is reversed from the vertebrobasilar artery to supply arm during arm exercise

Si/Sx: **Arm claudication, confusion**, nausea, syncope, and supraclavicular bruits

Diagnosis: Angiography

Treatment: Bypass graft

Note: Arm claudication without confusion is symptoms of **thoracic outlet syndrome**

LOWER EXTREMITY EMBOLIZATION

Lower extremity embolization is characterized by embolic arterial occlusion of the extremities

Cause: thrombosis from the heart, usually due to A-fib. , is the most common cause

Si/Sx: Sudden onset of **painful, cold, pale, pulseless, paresthesia and paralysis of lower extremity**

Diagnosis: Doppler ultrasound

Treatment;

- Early intervention with thrombolytics
- Late intervention includes embolectomy and fasciectomy

ARTERIAL ULCERS

Arterial ulcers occurs because of inadequate perfusion of skin and subcutaneous tissue, they are usually found on **lower leg and lateral ankle**

Cause: secondary to atherosclerotic plaque of the arteries

Risk factors: Smoking, diabetes with poor glycemic control, inadequate footwear

Si/Sx: Painful ulcers on lower leg and lateral ankle, absent pulses, claudication

Diagnosis: same as PVD

Treatment: same as PVD

VENOUS ULCERS

Venous ulcer are usually found **above the medial ankle and below knees**

Risk factors: DVT, varicose veins, incompetent valves, obesity,

Si/Sx: Painless ulcers usually located above medical ankle and below knees, contain bleeding granulation tissues

Diagnosis: Doppler of legs

Treatment: elevation of the affected leg to reduce the swelling, Unna's boot, and compression stocking

CARDIOLOGY CCS

Case introduction
A 59-years old African-American man comes to the ER because of chest pain that started 70 minutes ago.

Initial vitals signs
Temperature: 37.2 degrees
Pulse 85 beats/min, regular rhythm
Respiration rate: 21/ minutes

Blood pressure, systolic 140 mm Hg
Blood pressure, disystolic, 85 mm Hg

Height: 67.8 inches
Weight 134 labs

History of present illness (HPI)
A 59-years old African-American man comes to the ER because of chest pain that started 70 minutes ago. The pain started when he was moving his house furniture. He describes the pain as crushing sensation that radiates to his left shoulder and jaw. He rates his pain 7 on the scale of 10. He has had three similar episodes 3 three months ago but resolved with ant-acids, but this time pain did not go away with them. He has past medical history of HTN and diabetes, for which he is taking captopril and metformin.

Past medical history
Hospitalization: None
Other medical condition: DM and HTN
Current medication: captopril, metformin
Allergies: None
Vaccination: up to date

Family history
Father died of lung cancer at age 65. Mother is alive and well.

Social history

Marital history: Married; 1 child

Occupation: Bank teller

Recreational: watching movies, travel

Personal habits: Does not smoke, drink alcoholic beverage and use drugs

Review of system:

General: see HPI

Skin: see HPI

HEENT: see HPI

Musculoskeletal: see HPI

Cardiology: see HPI

Abdominal: see HPI

Genitourinary: see HPI

Approach for case 1: Please see pages 1-5   for general CCS cases approach

Step 1: Order the followings
- IV access
- IV normal saline
- Pulse oxy
- Oxygen
- Aspirin (ASA)
- Nitroglycerine
- Morphine
- EKG & EKG monitor
- BP & BP monitor

Step 2: order targeted physical exam, heart and lungs, and then move the clock forward to get the results, which shows:
- Patient is in pain and uncomfortable
- Heart and lung exam are normal

Step 3: order the following labs
- CBC
- UA
- BMP
- Portable chest x-ray
- CK-MB, Troponin × 8
- Fecal occult blood test (FOBT), it is usually done before starting heparin
- PT/PT/INR
- NPO

And then move the clock forward to get results, which shows:
- FOBT negative
- PT/PTT/INR is WNL
- EKG shows ST depression (3mm) and T inverted in leads 1, V4, V5, V6, aVL

Step 4: Treatment
- **Adjunct therapy** (discussed on page 10), and order **angiography** (don't forget to stop metformin, if applicable)

Step 5: Transfer the patient to ICU
- **Move the clock** forward to get angiography results, which shows Left main artery is 80% stenosis

Step 6: NPO

Step 7: order **Catheterization/ balloon angioplasty**

Step 8: **cardiology consultation** (type consult for angioplasty)

Step 9: **Move the clock** forward to get the cardiology consult, and then move clock angioplasty results

Case should end here

Two minutes screen counseling
- Order basic counseling (no smoking, drugs, alcohol, safe sex)
- Cardiac diet
- Order lipid panel

Diagnosis: stable angina

CASE # 2

Case introduction

A 66-years old woman with past medical history of uncontrolled hypertension comes to the ER after sudden onset of severe, anterior chest pain

Initial vitals signs

Temperature: 37.2 degrees
Pulse 85 beats/min, regular rhythm
Respiration rate: 21/ minutes

Blood pressure, systolic 140 mm Hg
Blood pressure, disystolic, 85 mm Hg

Height: 67.8 inches
Weight 134 labs

History of present illness (HPI)

A 66-years old woman with past medical history of uncontrolled hypertension comes to the ER after sudden onset of severe, anterior chest pain. She says her pain started 20 minutes ago and it is going through her back. She rates her pain 8 on the scale of 10. She has had chest pain few months before but that resolved with ant-acids, but this time pain did not go away with them. On examination she is alert and oriented. Her blood pressure shows that there is 20 mm difference in the systolic difference in both arms.

Past medical history

Hospitalization: None
Other medical condition: DM and HTN
Current medication: captopril, metformin
Allergies: None
Vaccination: up to date

Family history

Father died of lung cancer at age 65. Mother is alive and well.

Social history
Marital history: Married; 1 child
Occupation: Bank teller
Recreational: watching movies, travel
Personal habits: Does not smoke, drink alcoholic beverage and use drugs

Review of system:
General: see HPI
Skin: see HPI
HEENT: see HPI
Musculoskeletal: see HPI
Cardiology: see HPI
Abdominal: see HPI
Genitourinary: see HPI

Please see pages 1-5 for general CCS cases approach

Step 1: Thoracic aorta dissection is a life threatening, order the following, under " sat" option
- IV access
- IV normal saline
- Pulse oxy
- Oxygen
- EKG & EKG monitor
- BP & BP monitor
- Portable Chest X-ray
- Beta-blockers, IV labetalol or esmolol

Step 2: order targeted physical exam, heart and lungs, and then move the clock forward to get the results, which shows:
- Physical exam of upper extremities: Different high blood pressure in each arm
- Rest of the physical exam WNL

Move clock forward to get EKG and chest X-ray results, which shows:
- Chest x-ray shows widened mediastinum

Step 3: order the following labs:
- NPO
- CBC
- UA
- BMP
- CT angiograph or TEE

Move the clock forward to get the labs results, which shows:
- CT angiography suggests thoracic aorta dissection

Step 4: IV nitroprusside

Step 5: Transfer the to ICU

Step 6: order NPO

Step 7: order pre-surgery labs
- PT/INR
- PTT
- Blood type and cross match
- IV antibiotics

Step 8: order vascular surgery consultation

Step 9: order thoracic aorta repair surgery

Move the clock forward to get the lab results, consult, and then procedure results, which shows
- PT/PTT/INR is WNL
- Blood type: O negative
- Surgery is scheduled

Case should end there

Step 10: on 2-minutes screen order the followings:
- Order basic counseling (NO smoking, drugs, alcohol, safe sex)
- Diet modification
- Age specific screening

Diagnosis: **Thoracic aorta dissection**

CASE # 3

Case introduction
A 55-years old white man come to ER because of chest pain that started 70 minutes ago. He says the pain started when he was moving his house furniture

Initial vitals signs
Temperature: 37.2 degrees
Pulse 85 beats/min, regular rhythm
Respiration rate: 21/ minutes

Blood pressure, systolic 140 mm Hg
Blood pressure, disystolic, 85 mm Hg

Height: 67.8 inches
Weight 134 labs

History of present illness (HPI)
A 55-years old white man come to ER because of chest pain that started 70 minutes ago. He says the pain started when he was moving his house furniture. He described his pain as sharp pain, does not radiate to arm and or jaw. He rates his pain 8 on the scale of 10. He has past medical history of unstable angina two years ago. His father died of MI at the age of 80. On examination he is alert and oriented. He has recent medical history of " flu-like" symptoms one month ago.

Past medical history
Hospitalization: None
Other medical condition: DM and HTN
Current medication: captopril, metformin
Allergies: None
Vaccination: up to date

Family history
Father died of lung cancer at age 65. Mother is alive and well.

Social history
Marital history: Married; 1 child
Occupation: Bank teller
Recreational: watching movies, travel
Personal habits: Does not smoke, drink alcoholic beverage and use drugs

Review of system:
General: see HPI
Skin: see HPI
HEENT: see HPI
Musculoskeletal: see HPI
Cardiology: see HPI
Abdominal: see HPI
Genitourinary: see HPI

Please see pages 1-5 for general CCS cases approach

Step 1: Chest pain in pericarditis may mimic MI, and it is not possible to differentiate them without an EKG, so it is important to start patient on following management:
- IV access
- IV normal saline
- Pulse oxy
- Oxygen
- EKG & EKG monitor
- Aspirin

Step 2: order focused physical exam, heart and lung, and then move the clock forward to get results, which shows:
- Chest exam: pain worst when supine and relives with leaning forward and sitting up. Pericardial friction rub is also present

Step 3: Labs
  3a. Move the clock forward to get labs results of labs ordered in step 1, which shows
  - EKG shows **ST elevation in all leads, PR depression**
  3b. Order the following labs:
  - CBC
  - UA
  - BMP
  - Portable chest x-ray
  - CK-MB, every 8 hours
  - Troponin, every 8 hours
  - Echocardiogram

Step 4: Order IV aspirin or other NSAIDs
- Discontinue oxygen if pulse oxy saturation is normal

Step 5: Transfer to wards

Step 6: order

- Bed rest with bathroom privileges
- Normal diet

Step 7: none

Step 8: Cardiologist consultation

Step 9: Follow up patient every day
- If patient gets better in two days discharge the patient, otherwise add prednisone and follow up every day.

Case usually ends here

Step 10: One two-minutes screen
- Order basic counseling (NO smoking, drugs, alcohol, safe sex, wear set belts)
- Age specific counseling and screening
- Gender specific counseling and screening

Diagnosis: Pericarditis

HYPERTENSION

HYPERTENSION SCREENING
Current USPSTF recommends that every patient > 18 years of age should be screened for HTN at each visit

HYPERTENSION (HTN)
Hypertension is defined as systolic BP> 140 mmHg and diastolic BP >90 mm Hg

Cause:

- **Primary hypertension** or essential hypertension, accounts for 90-95 % of the cases of hypertension. There is no known cause for primary hypertension, but risk factors may include obesity, high sodium diet, alcohol, smoking, advanced age, family history of HTN or heart disease and race (African-Americans)
- **Secondary hypertension** accounts for remaining 5-10 % of the cases of hypertension (discussed below)

Causes of secondary HTN and specific findings

Cardiology	• Coarctation of aorta: BP is higher in upper extremity compare to lower extremity
Renal	• Renal artery stenosis: **abdominal bruits** • PCKD
Endocrine	• Pheochromocytoma: **episodic HTN** • Conn syndrome and Cushing syndrome: HTN with **hypokalemia** • Hyperthyroidism: **isolated systolic HTN** • Acromegaly
Drugs	• NSAIDs, OCPs, glucocorticosteroids

Si/Sx: most of the patient may have no symptoms and HTN is usually diagnosed incidentally during routine screening. But, even silent HTN can slowly lead to heart diseases, kidney diseases, or visual problems

Diagnosis: HTN is diagnosed based on the following:
- 3 separate measurement, taken at 4-weeks intervals
- Resting quietly for 5 minutes, before measuring BP
- Seated with arm at heart level
- Blood pressure cuff should encircle 80% of the arm

As discussed that silent HTN can cause other problems. Therefore, a patient diagnosed with HTN should also have following tests:
- Urinalysis (UA)
- Eye exam
- Cardiac exam & EKG
- Serum potassium & BUN/Cr
- Blood glucose and plasma lipids
-

Treatment: treatment **depends on the cause** of HTN (discussed below)

1. Treatment of **primary hypertension** is as follow:

HTN stage	BP range	Treatment
Normal BP	<120/80	None
Pre-HTN	120/80 –139/89	**Lifestyle modification** for 3-6 months, if this fails, then start HTN medication*
HTN stage 1	140/90 –159/99	**Lifestyle modification** for 3-6 months, if this fails, then start HTN medication*
HTN Stage 2	>160/100	**Life style modification and combination of 2 HTN medications****

* Best initial treatment is thiazide diuretics. If thiazide is ineffective, then add ACEIs, ARBs, beta-blockers or calcium channel blockers.

** 2-medicines combination usually includes thiazide + ACEIs, ARBs, beta-blockers or calcium channel blockers.

Lifestyle modifications and its benefits on BP is as follow:
- **Weight reduction** lowers systolic BP by **5-20 mmHg**
- **Healthy diet** lowers systolic BP **up to 14** mmHg
- **Exercise** lowers systolic BP by **4- 9** mmHg
- **Reduced sodium** lowers systolic BP **by 2-8** mm Hg
- **Limit alcohol** lowers systolic BP by **2-4** mmHg

Note: If a patient has comorbid disease(s), then start the medical treatment at the first visit, rather than waiting 3-6 months to check effect of lifestyle modifications

Compelling indications and contraindications for HTN medicines

Medicine	Indications	Contraindications	Side effects
Thiazide diuretics	• **No comorbid disease** • **Osteoporosis**	• Gout • Diabetes	• Hyperglycemia • Hyperlipidemia • Hyperuricemia
β-blockers	• MI • CHF • Migraine • Hyperthyroid -ism	• COPD • Diabetes • Hyperkalemia	• Asthma • Hypertriglyceridemia • Bradycardia
Calcium channel blockers	• Systolic HTN • Angina • Depression • Migraine	• Heart block	• **Peripheral edema** • **Constipation**
ACEIs	• **Diabetes** • CHF • HTN caused by **scleroderma**	• Pregnancy • Renal artery stenosis • Renal failure	• **Cough** • **Angioedema**
α− blockers (Prazosin, terazosin	• BPH	• Orthostatic hypotension	• **Postural hypotension** • **Headaches**

2. **Treatment for secondary HTN:** treat the underlying cause

HYPERTENSIVE URGENCY

Hypertensive urgency is defined as BP> 220/110 mm Hg **without the evidence of end-organ damage**

Treatment: oral blood pressure medicine such beta-blockers (labetalol), clonidine or ACEI, with the goal of slowly lowering the BP over several days

HYPERTENSIVE EMERGENCY

Hypertensive emergency is defined as BP> 220/110 mm HG with the **evidence of end-organ damage** such as acute renal failure, CHF, ischemia, encephalopathy

Treatment: hypertensive emergency is a medical emergency. Start the patient on **IV nitroprusside, nitroglycerin, labetalol, or nocardin,** but do not lower the BP more than 25 % within first 1-2 hour, otherwise patient may develop cerebral hypoperfusion or coronary insufficiency

---

KEY MANGEMENT STEPS OF HTN

- Patient with pre-HTN or stage 1 HTN is usually managed with lifestyle modification for 3-6 months. However, if the patient has any comorbid condition, then medication is started at the first visit.
- Best initial treatment is thiazide diuretic. However, if the patient has any compelling indication to start a particular medication, then start medication based on that. As discussed on the previous page
- Patient with HTN urgency is usually treated with oral blood pressure medication
- Patient with HTN emergency is usually treated with IV medication, but do not lower the BP more than 25% within first 1-2 hours otherwise patient will stroke out.
- Weight reduction is the most effective lifestyle modification to lower the HTN

HEMATOLOGY

ANEMIA

Anemia is a condition in which the body does not have enough red blood cells (RCBs) to carry oxygen to body tissues. It may also be defined as **hemoglobin < 14 mg/dl or hematocrit < 41 % in men, and hemoglobin < 12 mg/dl or hematocrit <36 % in women**

Cause: There are many causes of anemia, which can be divided into three main groups:

1) Decreased red blood cell production in conditions such as Iron – deficiency anemia, Sickle cell anemia, Vitamin deficiency and bone marrow problem
2) Blood loss from conditions such as ulcer, hemorrhoids, menstruation and NSAIDs.
3) Destruction of red blood cells in conditions such as infection, autoimmune hemolytic diseases and prosthetic heart valves.

Si/Sx: Signs and symptoms depend on the severity of anemia. Patents with **mild anemia may not have any symptoms**. As **anemia progress** patient may feel weak, tired even with usual activity, and problem with concentration. In **severe anemia** patient may experience shortness of breath, brittle nail, pale skin, chest pain and even MI in some cases.

Diagnosis:

- **Complete blood count** (CBC) with peripheral smear is the **best initial test** for all forms of anemia
- Reticulocytes count
- Iron study
- LDH and indirect bilirubin
- Haptoglobin
- Urinalysis

Treatment:

- Treat the underlying cause
- **Blood transfusion is required in a young patient when hematocrit level < 20 %, an elderly when hematocrit is < 30%, or a patient with heart disease who has hematocrit level < 30%.**

Mean Corpuscular Volume (MCV) and Anemia Differential Diagnosis

MCV < 80 (Microcytic anemia)	MCV 80 -100 (Normocytic anemia)	MCV > 100 (Macrocytic anemia)
• Iron deficiency anemia • Anemia of chronic disease • Thalassemia • Sideroblastic anemia • Lead poisoning	• Acute blood loss • Sickle cell anemia • Hereditary spherocytosis • Autoimmune hemolysis • Drug Induced hemolysis • Glucose-6-phosphate dehydrogenase • Paroxysmal nocturnal hemoglobinuria • Aplastic anemia • Renal failure	• Vitamin B 12 deficiency • Folate deficiency • Alcoholism • Liver disease • Hypothyroidism • Medicine (Metformin, methotrexate, phenytoin, zidovudine, and Bactrim) • Myelodysplastic syndrome

Reticulocyte count: it measures the percentage of immature red blood cells in the blood.

Differential diagnosis of reticulocyte count

Low reticulocytes count	High reticulocytes count
• All types of macrocytic anemia • All types iron deficiency except thalassemia • Bone marrow failure • Radiation therapy	• Acute bleeding • Hemolytic anemia • Thalassemia

SPECIFIC CAUSES OF ANEMIA

MICROCYTIC ANEMIA (MCV <80)

1. IRON DEFICIENCY ANEMIA

Iron deficiency anemia is an anemia that is caused by inadequate iron in the body. Iron helps make red blood cells. Insufficient iron in the body will result in reduced RBCs production or reduced RBCs size

Cause: Many things can cause iron deficiency anemia. Most common cause according to age groups is:
- In infants, feeding cows milk before six months of age
- In adults, celiac sprue disease
- In women, pregnancy, breastfeeding and blood loss during menstruation
- In elderly, colon cancer until proven otherwise

Si/Sx: symptoms of anemia depends on the severity of anemia. However, a classic clue often given on the boards in **pica**

Diagnosis:
- CBC with peripheral smear is the **best initial test**
- Best **initial diagnostic test** is **iron studies**, which shows:
  - **Low ferritin,** iron & iron saturation
  - **Increased** red cell distribution (RDW) and total iron binding capacity (TIBC)
- Bone marrow biopsy is the **most accurate test**, which shows decreased stainable iron

Treatment:
- Treat the underlying cause. Oral ferrous sulfate is often needed to replenish the iron body stores
- Blood transfusion in patients with severe anemia

Other *high-yield* anemia related points :
- If an elderly (> 60 years of age) presents with symptoms of anemia, then make sure to rule out colon cancer with **FOBT, followed by colonoscopy**
- If a patient has iron deficiency anemia and dysphagia, then the diagnosis is **Plummer-Vinson syndrome**

---

2. ANEMIA OF CHRONIC DISEASE

Anemia of chronic disease is caused by certain chronic medical conditions
Risk factors: end-stage renal disease, cancers, liver cirrhosis, and autoimmune disease such as Crohn's disease, ulcerative colitis, rheumatoid arthritis or systemic lupus erythematosus.
Si/Sx: symptoms of anemia depends on the severity of anemia

Diagnosis:
- CBC with peripheral smear is the **best initial test**
- Best **initial diagnostic test** is **iron studies**, which shows:
  - **Increased ferritin**
  - **Decreased** iron, iron saturation and total iron binding capacity (TIBC)

Treatment: Treat the **underlying cause**. However, anemia of chronic disease associated with end-stage renal disease is treated with **erythropoietin**.

3. SIDEROBALSTIC ANEMIA

Sideroblastic anemia is a condition in which **bone marrow** produces **ringed sideroblasts** (erythroblast with ferritin granules) rather than normal red blood cells. It results from **ineffective erythropoiesis** that is caused by a **defect in porphyrin pathway**

Cause: Two main causes of sideroblastic anemia are:
1. Inherited due to ALA synthase deficiency
2. Acquired cause such as alcohol abuse, lead poisoning or Isoniazid

Si/Sx: symptoms of anemia dependence on the severity of anemia

Diagnosis:
- CBC with peripheral smear is the **best initial test**
- Best **initial diagnostic test** is **iron studies**, which shows:
  - **Increased** Iron and ferritin
  - **Normal or low TIBC**
- Most accurate test is bone marrow biopsy with **Prussian blue stain**, which shows ringed sideroblasts

Treatment: depends on the cause
- ALA synthase deficiency is treated with pyridoxine (vitamin B 6).
- Acquired sideroblastic anemia is treated by treating the underlying cause

4. THALASSEMIA

Thalassemia is an inherited blood disorder in which abnormal hemoglobin is produced

Types: Hemoglobin is made up of alpha and beta chains. 4 genes are involved in the synthesis of alpha-hemoglobin chain and 2 genes are involved in the synthesis of beta-hemoglobin chain. Mutation in any gene(s) can lead to different symptoms.

Risk factors:

- Alpha-thalassemia is more common in Asian, African and Mediterranean
- Beat-thalassemia is more common in Mediterranean and African descent

Diagnosis:

- CBC with peripheral smear is the **best initial test,** which usually shows very low MCV (<70) and target cells on peripheral smear
- Best **initial diagnostic test** is **iron studies,** which shows
  - Normal ferritin, TIBC, iron, iron saturation, and RDW
- **Most accurate test is gel electrophoresis**
  - HgF and HbA, which are **increased in beta thalassemia,** but **normal in alpha thalassemia**
- Definitive test is **DNA**

Si/Sx: See tables below and on the next page
Treatment: See table below

Alpha –thalassemias, symptoms and treatment

Number of alpha genes mutated	Diagnosis	Symptoms	Treatment
1	Silent carrier	Usually asymptomatic	No treatment
2	α-Thalassemia minor	Mild anemia symptoms	No treatment, but may need iron pills
3	HbH disease	Mild to moderate anemia, splenomegaly	Periodic blood transfusion
4	Hydrops fetalis	Fetus usually dies before the delivery	No treatment

Beta-thalassemia symptoms and treatment

Number of beta genes mutated	Diagnosis	Symptoms	Treatment
1	Thalassemia-minor	Mild symptoms	No treatment
2	Thalassemia-major	**Newborn is asymptomatic for first 6 months of life.** They develop symptoms after that time due to **switch of γ- Hb to adult β –Hb**	Aggressive transfusion and splenectomy to enhance RBC survival. Deferoxamine to prevent iron overload

In a nutshell: only alpha-thalassemia HbH disease and beta-thalassemia major require blood transfusion, rest of the thalassemias require no treatment.

Other *high-yield* thalassemia related points are:

- Multiple blood transfusion recipients are susceptible to infection from yersinia enterocolitica, listeria monocytogenes
- Multiple blood transfusion recipients are at risk of acquiring secondary hemochromatosis from iron overload. However, women are at less risk than men due to monthly menstrual blood loss

MACROCYTIC ANEMIA (MCV > 100)
Vitamin B- 12 deficiency and folate deficiency are the leading cause of macrocytic anemia

1. VITAMIN B 12 DEFICIENCY

Vitamin B 12 plays an important role in red blood cell production. Deficiency of vitamin B 12 leads to megaloblastic anemia. Megaloblastic anemia is characterized by **large red blood cells (RBCs)**

Cause: malabsorption, autoimmune disease, pernicious anemia, atrophic gastritis

Si/Sx: Fatigue, **peripheral neuropathy (most common presentation)**, loss of position and vibration sense, smooth tongue, diarrhea, psychosis and dementia **(least common presentation)**

Diagnosis:

- Best initial test is **CBC with peripheral smear**, which shows MCV > 100, **macroovalocytes with hypersegmented neutrophils**
- Most **accurate test** is **Vitamin B 12 level**. However, not all cases show a low level of Vitamin B- 12 level, its level can be normal in acute phase reactant and elevated in stress, infection or cancer. In that case, **methylmalonic acid levels** may help.
- **Anti-parietal cell antibodies** and **anti-intrinsic factor** are used to **confirm the diagnosis of pernicious anemia**
- **Schilling test is last option, it is performed when all the other test are inconclusive**

Treatment: Vitamin B 12 replacement

Other *High-yield* vitamin B12 related points are:

- Most common complication of vitamin B 12 treatment is **hypokalemia**. Vitamin B12 increases the production of DNA that increases the production of new cells that take up potassium and lowers the extracellular potassium
- Vitamin B12 deficiency can cause type B gastritis
- Terminal ileum disease such as Crohn's disease reduces the absorption of vitamin B12 and leads to vitamin B12 deficiency. This form of vitamin B 12 deficiency can only be treated with **IM vitamin B12**

---

2. FOLATE DEFICIENCY ANEMIA

Folate plays an important role in red blood cell production. Folate deficiency can also lead to megaloblastic anemia

Cause: Causes of folate deficiency anemia include inadequate folic acid intake (diet, during pregnancy, sickle cell anemia), reduced absorption, medicines such as phenytoin, methotrexate

Si/Sx: fatigues, lightheaded, forgetfulness, trouble concentrating

Diagnosis:

- Best initial test is CBC with peripheral smear, which shows MCV > 100, macroovalocytes with hypersegmented neutrophils
- Folic acid levels

Treatment: Folic acid replacement

Note: Neurologic abnormalities are seen in vitamin B 12 deficiency, whereas, no neurologic abnormalities seen in folate deficiency anemia.

NORMOCYTIC ANEMIA (MCV 80- 100)

HEMOLYTIC ANEMIA

Hemolytic anemias are caused by increased destruction of RBCs, which may be intracellular or extracellular

Cause: sickle cell anemia, hereditary spherocytosis, cold-agglutinin hemolysis, Warm-autoimmune hemolysis, G6PD deficiency

Si/Sx: based on severity of anemia

Diagnosis: All hemolytic anemias shows:

- Normal MVC (80 -100)
- Increased reticulocytes, LDH, and indirect bilirubin
- Decreased haptoglobin

1. SICKLE CELL ANEMIA

Sickle cell is an autosomal recessive trait, caused by point mutation, which results in **glutamic acid being substituted for valine at position 6 of the beta chain or change in base pair thiamine for adenosine**

Si/Sx:

- Dehydration, hypoxia, infection, or acidosis, cause sickling of deoxygenated RBCs. These sickle **shaped cells obstructs the blood vessels and restricts the blood flow to organs**, which leads to ischemia, pain, necrosis and other conditions such as stroke, retinal infarctions, priapism and pulmonary infarction
- Autosplenectomy
- Aplastic crisis
- Intravascular hemolysis
- Avascular necrosis of the femoral head
- Osteomyelitis

Diagnosis:

- Best **initial test** is CBC with peripheral smear. Peripheral smear shows sickling of RBCs and Howell-jolly bodies
- Reticulocytes are usually increased by 10- 20 % from baseline
- Most **accurate test** is hemoglobin electrophoresis

Management:

- **Acute painful crisis** is managed with oxygen, IV hydration and analgesia. IV ceftriaxone or levofloxacin is added to the treatment if the patient has a fever
- Exchange transfusion, if the patient has acute chest syndrome, eye infarction, lung infarction or stroke.
- Folic acid replacement to prevent aplastic crisis
- **Hydroxyurea** is given to prevent **recurrent vaso-occlusive painful crisis**
- Patients with autosplenectomy should receive H. Influenza and pneumococcal vaccine to prevent infections from encapsulated organisms

---

KEY MANAGEMENT STEPS OF ACUTE SICKLE CELL CRISIS

1. Best initial step treatment is oxygen, IV hydration and analgesia. IV ceftriaxone or levofloxacin is added to the treatment if the patient has a fever
2. Check the **reticulocytes count**, they are usually increased by 10-20% in sickle cell anemia
2.a If reticulocytes count is **low, then do RBC transfusion**

2.b If reticulocytes count is **high** and causing acute chest syndrome, eye infarction, lung infarction or stroke, then do **exchange transfusion**

2.c If reticulocytes count is **zero** (aplastic crisis), then this could be either due to **folic acid deficiency or infection from parvovirus B19**.

- o Parvovirus is diagnosed with **PCR-DNA**, and treated with **transfusion plus IVIG**
- o Folic acid deficiency is diagnosed with folate levels and treated **transfusion and folic acid**

Other *High-yield* Sickle cell anemia related points are:

1. Best initial test is CBC with peripheral smear
2. Quick screening test is sickeldex or sickle prep
3. Specific test is hemoglobin electrophoresis
4. Most common cause of mortality is acute chest syndrome
5. All patients should be on folic acid replacement to prevent the risk of aplastic anemia
6. Patient should have yearly ophthalmology exam and transcranial Doppler
7. Patient with sickle cell anemia are at increased risk of osteomyelitis from Salmonella, but S.Aureus is still the most common cause of osteomyelitis in sickle cell anemia patients
8. Patients are at increased risk of aseptic necrosis of femoral head
9. Pregnant woman with sickle cell anemia is at increased risk to have spontaneous abortion, low birth weight baby
10. Patients with auto-splenectomy are at increased risk of infection from encapsulated bacteria such as S. Pneumococcus, H. influenza, N.meningitidis

---

2. HEREDITARY SPHEROCYTOSIS

Hereditary spherocytosis is characterized by the formation of RBCs that are sphere-shaped rather than bi-concave disk shaped. Sphere-shaped RBCs become trapped in the spleen, and spleen destroys them (hemolysis)
Cause: Autosomal dominant defect in spectrin gene

Si/Sx: Recurrent episodes of hemolysis, jaundice, pigmented gallstones, splenomegaly

Diagnosis:

- **Best initial test is CBC with peripheral smear:**
  - CBC shows low MCV and increased mean corpuscular hemoglobin concentration (MCHC)
  - Peripheral blood smear shows spherocytes with **no central pallor** of normal RBCs
- **Negative coombs' test**
- Most accurate test is **osmotic fragility test**. When patient's RBCs are placed in a hypotonic solution, RBCs absorb the solution until the RBCs cell membrane bursts (cell lysis)

Treatment: There is no cure for hereditary spherocytosis,

- Mild spherocytosis is treated with **folic replacement**, which support the RBCs production
- Severe spherocytosis is treated by surgical removal of spleen **(Splenectomy),** which stops the further hemolysis

3. COLD-AGGLUTININ HEMOLYSIS

Cold-agglutinin hemolysis is a rare form of autoimmune hemolytic anemia caused by cold-reacting autoantibodies, usually **IgM.** Cold-reacting autoantibodies bind to the cell membrane of RBCs and cause premature lysis of RBCs.

Cause: For most of the cases there is no known cause (idiopathic). Some known causes are **Mycoplasma pneumonia, mononucleosis, Epstein-Barr virus, cytomegalovirus or Waldenströn macroglobulinemia.**

Si/Sx: anemia occurs after body is exposed to cold temperature or following upper respiratory tract infection (URI). **Pain and purple discoloration** of body parts **exposed to cold temperature** such as the nose, ears, and fingers, which **resolves in warm temperature.**

Diagnosis:

- Direct coombs' test shows positive Anti-C3d, negative anti-IgG
- Most accurate test is **cold agglutinins titer (IgM)**

Treatment:

- **Supportive treatment**, avoid cold weather, and treat the underlying cause
- Rituximab (anti-CD 20 monoclonal antibody)

- In a case of **severe hemolysis** adjunct treatment with **plasmapheresis** can be done to **remove IgM antibodies**
- **Immunosuppressive** agents such as cyclophosphamide, azathioprine, interferon and fludarabine may be given to **stop IgM antibody synthesis**

Note: Prednisone and splenectomy are not useful for cold-agglutinin disease. However, these can be used if IgG co-antibodies are present.

4. WARM AUTOIMMUNE HEMOLYSIS

Warm autoimmune hemolysis occurs when body immune system directs antibodies against its own RBCs. It is usually **IgG mediated**

Cause: most of the cases are idiopathic. Some known causes include lymphoproliferative disorders (CLL, lymphoma), autoimmune disorders (Lupus, scleroderma, rheumatoid arthritis), and drugs (alpha-methyldopa, penicillin, rifampin)

Si/Sx: dark urine, fatigue, jaundice, shortness of breath

Diagnosis:

- **Best initial test is CBC with peripheral smear**
  - o Peripheral blood smear shows spherocytosis
- Most accurate test is positive direct coombs' test

Treatment:

- **Prednisone** is the **best initial treatment**
- **Intravenous immunoglobulin** (IVIG) is used if acute hemolysis is not responding to prednisone. IVIG reduces hemolysis by **reducing the interaction between spleen macrophage and antibody coated RBCs**
- If the patient has recurrent episodes of hemolysis, then do splenectomy
- Rituximab, azathioprine, cyclophosphamide, or cyclosporine are used in refractory cases

5. GLUCOSE-6-PHOSPHATE DEHYDROGENASE (G6PD) DEFICIENCY

G6PD deficiency is X-linked recessive hereditary disease

Precipitating factors: Fava beans and drugs such as sulfa drugs, primaquine, dapsone, nitrofurantoin, quinidine, quinine, and NSAIDs

Si/Sx: dark urine, fatigue, pallor, jaundice, and shortness of breath **after exposure of precipitating factor**

Diagnosis:
- **Best initial test is peripheral blood smear**, which show **Heinz body** (hemoglobin precipitates) and **bite cells** (damaged RBCs are removed by macrophages in the spleen)
- **Most accurate test** is G6PD level, which are measured 2-3 months after an acute episode of hemolysis

Treatment: There is no cure for G6PD deficiency. **Mild hemolysis is** treated with **supportive care (IV fluids) and removing the precipitating** factor. **Severe hemolysis is treated with blood transfusion**

6.   PAROXYSMAL NOCTURNAL HEMOGLOBINURIA (PNH)

Paroxysmal nocturnal hemoglobinuria (PNH) is an acquired RBCs membrane **defect in phosphatidylinositol glycan A (PIG-A)** that allows RBCs to bind to complements and cause intravascular hemolysis.

Complement lysis mostly happens in an acidic environment. Every one is mildly acidotic while sleeping because a relative hypoventilation; as a result, most of the patient present with nocturnal or early morning hemoglobinuria.

Si/Sx: nocturnal or early morning hemoglobinuria, shortness of breath, headaches

Diagnosis: Most **accurate test** is CD 55 and CD 59 levels or flow cytometry for CD 55 and CD 59

Treatment:
- Prednisone is the best initial treatment.
- Eculizumab is used for long-term treatment. It protects RBCs from immune destruction by inhibiting the complement pathway (inactivating C5 complement pathway)

Other *high-yield* **PNH related points are**:
- **Large venous thrombosis is the most common cause of death**
- PNH is an acquired RBCs stem cell defect; therefore, patient is at increased of acquiring ALL, aplastic anemia, blood clots, or myelodysplasia.

---

7.   MICROANGIOPATHIC HEMOLYTIC ANEMIA

Microangiopathic hemolytic anemia is a subgroup of hemolytic anemia in which **RBCs are destroyed by coagulation factors** in the small capillaries. It is seen in conditions such as hemolytic uremic syndrome (HUS), disseminated intravascular coagulation (DIC), thrombotic thrombocytopenia purpura (TTP) and malignant hypertension.

Differential diagnosis of microangiopathic hemolytic anemia

Condition	HUS	TTP	DIC
Cause	E. coli 157: H7, shigella, salmonella	HIV infection, SLE and drugs such as OCP, ticlopidine, or clopidogrel	Sepsis, trauma, septic abortion, trauma
Si/Sx	Anemia, thrombocytopenia, acute renal failure,	Anemia, thrombocytopenia, acute renal failure, **fever and neurological abnormalities**	**Bleeding from any site of the body**, acute renal failure, jaundice and **confusion**
Diagnosis	Normal PT/PTT	Normal PT/PTT and **increased bleeding time**	Increased PT/PTT and increased bleeding time. **Increased D-Dimer and fibrin split product. Decreased fibrinogen**
Treatment	**IV fluids for mild symptoms,** and **Plasmapheresis** for **severe** symptoms. Dialysis, if needed	Same as HUS	Treat the underlying cause. Fresh frozen plasma and platelet transfusion, as needed

Important: Antibiotics are not given to a patient with HUS because they can worsen the HUS

MYELOPROLIFERATIVE DISORDERS

1. POLYCTHEMIA VERA

Polycythemia Vera is a disorder of the bone marrow in which production of RBCs, WBCs and platelets are increased, but RBCs are produced more than WBC s and platelets

Types and Causes:

- **Primary polycythemia vera** is caused by mutation in **JAK protein**
- **Secondary polycythemia** is caused by **hypoxia** (COPD, smoking, high altitude)

Si/Sx: headache, dizziness, vision problem, shortness of breath, **itchiness after warm showers**, fatigue, and splenomegaly

Diagnosis:

- Best initial test is CBC, which shows:
  - Low MCV
  - Increased RBC
  - Increased hemoglobin: >18.5 g/dl in men and >16.5 g/dl in women
  - Increased hematocrit: > 52 % in men and >48% women
- Best **initial diagnostic test** is Erythropoietin (EPO) levels, which is:
  - **Low** in **primary** polycythemia
  - **High** in **secondary** polycythemia
  - **Normal** in **myeloid metaplasia**

Treatment:

- Best initial treatment is **Phlebotomy,** it lower the blood volume, and reduces the risk of thrombotic events. The goal is to **keep hematocrit < 45% in men, and < 42 % in women**
- Aspirin is also added to the treatment to reduce the risk of thrombotic events
- Allopurinol if the patient develops gout
- Hydroxyurea is also given if patient has any of the followings:
  - Can not tolerate phlebotomy
  - Patient is > 70 years of age
  - Platelet count is > 1.5 million
  - Cardiovascular disease

Complication: patient should have **hematocrit checked regularly**, because high hematocrit level increases the risk of thrombotic event, which in turns increases the risk of TIA, stroke, PE and MI

2.   ESSENTIAL THROMBOCYTHEMIA

Essential thrombocythemia is characterized by overproduction of platelets in the absence of any other cause, such as cancer, infection, or iron deficiency.

Si/Sx: headache, vision disturbance, tingling of the hands and feet, weakness, chest pain, nosebleeds, bruising

Diagnose:

- Platelet count > 450,000
- JAK mutation is present in 50 % of the cases

Treatment:

- If **platelets count is > 1.5 million**, then perform **plateletpheresis**
- If the patient is **symptomatic, > 65 years of age or has history of thrombosis**, then give **hydroxyurea and aspirin**
- If the patient is **asymptomatic, < 65 years of age and no history of thrombosis**, then no **treatment is required**

3.   MYELOFIBROSIS

Myelofibrosis is a disorder of the bone marrow, in which bone marrow is replaced by **fibrosis tissue**. This results in decreased production of RBCs, WBCs and platelets. Hematopoiesis shifts to the liver and spleen, and causes hepatosplenomegaly.

Si/Sx: fatigue, shortness of breath, pallor, bruising, easy bleeding, **hepatosplenomegaly**

Diagnosis:

- **Best initial test** is CBC with peripheral blood smear, which shows **pancytopenia** (low RBCs, WBCs, and platelets) and teardrop cell
- **Most accurate test** is **bone marrow biopsy**, which shows fibrosis of the bone marrow

Treatment:

- Bone marrow transplant (**BMT**) is the best treatment for patients **< 60 years of age and healthy enough to have BMT.**
- **Thalidomide** or **lenalidomide** is the best treatment for patients **> 60 years of age or are not healthy enough to have BMT.**

APLASTIC ANEMIA

Aplastic anemia is a condition in which bone marrow **does not produce** enough **RBCs, WBCs, and platelets**

Cause: idiopathic, chemotherapy, radiation, parvovirus B 19, lupus, and drugs (Sulfa drugs, chloramphenicol, phenytoin)

Si/Sx: fatigue, shortness of breath, pallor, bruising, easy bleeding due to low platelets, infections due to low WBCs

Diagnosis:

- Best initial test is CBC, which shows pancytopenia (low RBCs, WBCs, and platelets count)
- Most accurate test is bone marrow biopsy, which shows fewer-than-normal blood cells and an **increased amount of fat**

Treatment:

- Supportive treatment (IV fluids, antibiotics, blood transfusion and platelets), and treat the underlying cause.
- Bone marrow transplant (**BMT**) is recommended; if the patient is **< 45 years of age, has matched done and is in good health** to have BMT. However, if the patient **does not meet** this criterion, then give **anti-thymocyte globulin, cyclosporine and prednisone.**

LEUKEMIA

Leukemia is a cancer of white blood cells (WBCs), in which white blood cells are overproduced. WBCs grow faster and bigger and do not work as normal WBCs.

Over time, leukemia cell overcrowds the bone marrow that interferes with normal blood cell production, which can lead to other problems, such as anemia, infection and bleeding.

Types: four main types of leukemia are:

- Acute lymphoblastic leukemia (ALL)
- Acute myelogenous leukemia (AML)
- Chronic lymphoblastic leukemia (CLL)
- Chronic myelogenous leukemia (CML)

1. ACUTE LYMPHOBLASTIC LEUKEMIA (ALL)

ALL is the most common leukemia in children **between 2-5 years of age.**

Si/Sx: fever, fatigue, weight loss, **bruising, petechia, bone pain, infection, lymphadenopathy and hepatosplenomegaly**

Diagnosis:

- **Best initial test is CBC with peripheral smear,** which shows leukemic blast
- Bone marrow biopsy shows leukemic blast (WBC >20%)
  - Leukemic blast (WBC >20 %) on **peripheral smear and bone marrow biopsy confirms the diagnosis**
- Immunochemistry may reveal **PAS +, TdT +, CALLA +**
- Some patients may have cytogenic translocation t (9; 22) or t (4; 11)

Treatment:

- Best initial treatment for **ALL is induction chemotherapy with daunorubicin, asparaginase, vincristine and steroids.** Chemotherapy in ALL consists of three phases: induction, consolidation and maintenance therapy, which are as follow:
  - Induction therapy, its purpose is to kill tumor cells rapidly
  - **Consolidation therapy,** its purpose is to further kill any cancer cells that may be left in the body. It important to give **intrathecal chemotherapy (methotrexate)** during this phase to prevent CNS relapse of ALL
  - Maintenance therapy - to kill any residual tumor cells.
- Bone marrow transplant (**BMT**) is performed, if the patient **relapses after chemotherapy** or **has a bad prognosis.**

Bad prognosis is defined by the presence of any of the followings:
- Patient is less than 1 year of age at the time of diagnosis
- Patient is more than 10 years of age at the time of diagnosis
- Cytogenic translocation such as t (9; 22)
- WBCs more than 100,000 at the time of diagnosis

2.   ACUTE MYELOGENOUS LEUKEMIA (AML)

AML is the most common leukemia in adults 15-39 years of age. AML is divided into eight types, M0 – M7

Si/Sx: fever, fatigue, weight loss, bruising, petechia, bone pain, infection, lymphadenopathy and hepatosplenomegaly

Diagnosis:
- Best initial test is CBC with peripheral smear, which shows anemia, thrombocytopenia, and leukocytosis
- Bone marrow biopsy shows myeloblasts that are **Auer rods, myeloperoxidase and sudan black**

Treatment:
- Best initial treatment for AML is chemotherapy with daunorubicin, cytosine and arabinoside. Chemotherapy in AML consists of two phases: induction, and consolidation

---

Other *high-yield* **AML related points are:**

- If the patient has AML type M3 (promyelocytic leukemia), then add **all trans retinoic acid (ATRA) to the chemotherapy**
- M3, promyelocytic leukemia can cause disseminated intravascular coagulation (DIC)

---

3. CHRONIC LYMPHOBLASTIC LEUKEMIA (CLL)
CLL is the most common leukemia in adults 40-59 years of age. It affects B cell lymphocytes

Si/Sx: Most of the patients with CLL are asymptomatic, but some patients may have fatigue, lymphadenopathy and splenomegaly

Diagnosis:
- CBC shows isolated lymphocytosis (lymphocyte count > 5000/μL)
- Peripheral blood smear shows **smudge cell** (leukocytes that are partially lysed during the blood smear preparation)

Stages:
- Stage 0: Isolated lymphocytosis
- Stage 1: Enlarged lymph nodes
- Stage 2: Splenomegaly
- Stage 3: Anemia
- Stage 4: Thrombocytopenia

Treatment:

- **Supportive treatment** for patients with **stage 0** and **stage 1 CLL**
- **Fludarabine plus rituximab** for patient with **stage 2, stage 3 or stage 4 CLL**
- Cyclophosphamide is for refractory cases

4. CHRONIC MYELOGENOUS LEUKEMIA (CML)

CML is characterized by clonal bone marrow stem cell disorder in which proliferation of granulocytes (neutrophils, eosinophils, basophils), is seen
Cause: 90 % of the cases are associated with Philadelphia chromosome
t (9; 22), fusion **of BCR-ABL protein** with strong **tyrosine kinase activity**
Si/Sx: fatigue, night sweats, low-grade fever, abdominal fullness and splenomegaly
Diagnosis:

- CBC with peripheral smear shows elevated WBCs, **predominantly neutrophils**
- Best initial diagnostic test is **leukocyte alkaline phosphate (LAP)** score, which is **low** in CML
- Most accurate test is chromosomal translocation (9; 22), which can be done by PCR or FISH

Treatment:

- **Best initial treatment** is a **tyrosine kinase inhibitor** such as imatinib, dasatinib, or nilotinib.
- If tyrosine kinase inhibitor is ineffective, then do bone **marrow transplant (BMT)**

MYELODYSPLASTIC SYNDROME

Myelodysplastic syndrome is a cancer in which bone marrow does not make enough new blood cells and cells that are made are abnormal cells. It is most common in adults 60 -75 years of age.
Cause: there is no known specific cause, but risk factors are 5q- syndrome (deletion in the long arm of chromosome 5), radiation, benzene, acquired aplastic anemia, Fanconi anemia
Si/Sx: fever, fatigue, weight loss, bruising, petechia, bone pain, infection, lymphadenopathy and hepatosplenomegaly

Diagnosis:
- CBC shows low RBCs, WBCs, and platelet counts, **MCV> 100**
- Peripheral smear shows hypogranular neutrophil with pseudo-Pelger-Huet nucleus (**2 lobes neutrophils**)
- Blood chemistry shows **normal vitamin B 12 and folate level**
- Most **accurate test is bone marrow biopsy** that shows hypercellular to normocellular marrow. In 10% of the patients, marrow may be hypocellular
- Karyotyping is performed to check for 5q- syndrome

Treatment:
- Blood products transfusion, as needed
- Erythropoietin injection, as needed
- **Bone marrow transplant** for patients **younger than 60 years of age**
- Azacitidine is a specific treatment for myelodysplasia; it **reduces the need for blood transfusion**
- **Lenalidomide** is effective in reducing blood transfusion requirement in patients with the **5q- syndrome**

Note: it is easy to confuse myelodysplastic syndrome with vitamin B12 deficiency. To distinguish them look at the peripheral smear and vitamin B 12 level: **myelodysplastic syndrome shows bi-lobe neutrophil and normal vitamin B12,** whereas, vitamin B 12 deficiency shows multi-nucleated neutrophil and may have low vitamin B 12.

HAIRY CELL LEUKEMIA
Hairy cell leukemia is a cancer of B lymphocyte. It mostly affects the men over the 55 years of age.

Cause: There is no known cause

Si/Sx: Fatigue, night sweat, low-grade fever, abdominal fullness, recurrent infection, easy bruising or bleeding, **splenomegaly**

Diagnosis:
- CBC shows low RBCs, WBCs, and platelets
- Blood smear and a bone marrow biopsy show **hairy cell** (hair-like projection of cytoplasm of B-lymphocytes)
- **Most accurate test** is tartrate-resistant acid phosphatase (TRAP)

Treatment:
- **Best initial treatment is cladribine or pentostatin**
- Splenectomy is reserved for refractory case

LYMPHOMA

Lymphoma is cancer of the lymphatic system (lymph nodes, lymphatic channels and lymph nodes such as spleen and thymus)

Types: Hodgkin's lymphoma and Non-Hodgkin's lymphoma

1. HODGKIN'S LYMPHOMA

Hodgkin's lymphoma is cancer of the lymphatic system. It has bi-modal distribution, seen between 15-35 years of age and over 55 years old.

Risk factors: Epstein-Barr virus, family history, HIV,

Si/Sx: painless, enlarged, nonerythematous, nontender lymph nodes (cervical, supraclavicular and axillary). Some patients may have "B" symptoms (fever, soaking night sweats, and unexplained weight loss)

Diagnosis:
- CBC
- **Best initial test is excisional lymph node biopsy**
- Chest X-ray, CT head, chest, abdomen, pelvis and bone marrow biopsy are also performed to do the staging of the lymphoma

Variants of Hodgkin Lymphoma

Type	Characteristics
Lymphocytes predominance	**Predominant lymphocytes**, few RS cells, variable number of histiocytes, little fibrosis
Lymphocytes depletion	**Few lymphocytes**, many RS cells, diffuse fibrosis may be seen
Mixed cellularity	**Mixture** of neutrophils, lymphocytes, plasma cells, eosinophil, histiocytes and a **large number of RS cells**
Nodular sclerosis	**Collagen bands create nodular pattern**; RS cells are lacunar cells. Mixture of neutrophils, lymphocytes, plasma cells, eosinophils and histiocytes. Mediastinal, supraclavicular and cervical lymph nodes

Treatment: depends on the following:

Characteristics	Treatment
• If "B" symptoms are present (fever, weight loss and night sweats) • Stage 3 lymphoma (lymph node affected on **both sides** of the diaphragm) • Stage 4 lymphoma (**disseminated disease)**	**Mnemonic: ABVD** Adriamycin, Bleomycin, Vinblastine, and Dacarbazine
• B symptoms are absent • Stage 1 lymphoma (Single lymph node affected) • Stage 2 lymphoma (2 more lymph node affected on the **same side of the diaphragm)**	**Radiation**

2. NON-HODGKIN'S LYMPHOMA

Signs and symptoms are same as Hodgkin's lymphoma, but
Non-Hodgkin's lymphoma more likely to involve extralymphatic sites and
it looks similar to CLL.

Diagnosis:
- CBC
- **Best initial test is excisional lymph node biopsy**
- Chest X-ray, CT head, chest, abdomen, pelvis and bone marrow biopsy are also performed to do the staging of the lymphoma
- Cytometry and cytogenesis is also performed to check if **CD20 antigen** is present

Treatment: depends on the following:

Characteristics	Treatment
• If "B" symptoms are present (fever, weight loss, and night sweats) • Stage 3 lymphoma (Lymph node affected on **both sides** of the diaphragm) • Stage 4 lymphoma (**disseminated disease**)	**Mnemonic: CHOP** Chemotherapy, Hydroxy-Adriamycin, Oncovin and **Prednisone**
• B symptoms are absent • Stage 1 lymphoma (Single lymph node affected) • Stage 2 lymphoma (2 more lymph node affected on the **same side of the diaphragm**)	**Radiation**
• If CD 20 antigen is present	**Add rituximab to the treatment**

Key steps of management of Hodgkin's lymphoma and Non-Hodgkin's lymphoma

- Best initial test is excisional lymph node biopsy, then do staging
- For Non-Hodgkin's lymphoma also perform cytometry and cytogenesis to check if CD20 antigen is present
- If the patient has stage 1 or stage 2 lymphoma, then treat the patient with radiation
- If the patient has B symptoms, stage 3 or stage 4 lymphoma, then treat the patient with chemotherapy
- If the patient with Non-Hodgkin's lymphoma has CD 20 antigen, then add rituximab is to the treatment

PLASMA CELL DISORDERS

1. MULTIPLE MYELOMA
Multiple myeloma is a cancer of plasma cell in the bone marrow. It is characterized by **overproduction of IgG antibodies**. As the cancer grows it affects the production of normal blood cells, and causes bone pain, bone lesions,

Si/Sx: bone pain, multiple fractures, repeated infections, weight loss, weakness

Diagnosis:
- Initial test diagnostics test:
    o Labs: **hypercalcemia**, decreased anion-gap channel, elevated BUN and creatinine
    o Peripheral smear shows **blood rouleaux formation**
    o X-ray of affected bone shows punched out lytic lesion
    o **Serum protein** electrophoresis shows **IgG or IgA spike**
    o **Urine protein** electrophoresis shows **Bence-Jones protein**
- Diagnosis is **confirmed with bone marrow biopsy**, which shows >10 % plasma cell

Treatment:
- **Best initial treatment** for patients **< 70 years age** is thalidomide and dexamethasone.
- Most effective therapy is for patients < 70 years of age is **bone marrow transplant (BMT)**
- **Melphalan and prednisone** are for patients **> 70 years of age** or those who **cannot tolerate thalidomide and dexamethasone**

Differential diagnosis of multiple myeloma

Condition	Characteristics
Smoldering myeloma	• Patient have **isolated IgG spike > 3g/dl** • Usually **no treatment** is required
Monoclonal Gammopathy of Unknown Significance (MGUS)	• **Asymptomatic patients with IgG spike < 3g/dl.** • Usually **no treatment** is required. • **It may progress to multiple myeloma**

Complications:

- Common causes of cause of death are:
  - Infection from encapsulated organism such as N.meningitidis, H. influenza and pneumococcus
  - Renal failure

2. WALDENSTROM'S MACROGLOBULINEMIA

Waldenstrom's macroglobulinemia is cancer of B-lymphocytes. It is characterized by **overproduction of IgM antibodies** from B-lymphocytes. Uncontrolled production of IgM leads to hyperviscosity and interferes with RBCs and platelet production.

Si/Sx: Blurred vision, fatigue, headache, change in mental status, bleeding gums

Diagnosis:

- CBC shows increased lymphocytes and decreased RBCs and platelets
- **Best initial diagnostics test** is serum viscosity
- Serum protein electrophoresis shows **IgM spike**

Treatment: Plasmapheresis

BLEEDING DISORDERS

1. IDIOPATHIC THROMBOCYTOPENIC PURPURA (ITP)

Idiopathic thrombocytopenic purpura is characterized by isolated low platelet count (thrombocytopenia)

Cause: there is no specific known cause. Some known causes include viral illness (such as mumps, measles or flu), leukemia, lymphoma, anti-platelet antibody

Si/Sx: petechiae, purpura, prolong bleeding from cuts, epistaxis, bleeding gums, heavy menstrual flow in women and **normal size spleen**

Note: enlarged spleen size suggests possible other causes of thrombocytopenia

Diagnosis:

- Idiopathic thrombocytopenic purpura is a diagnosis of exclusion. It is important to rule out other cause of thrombocytopenia
- CBC shows low platelet count, and normal RBCs and WBCs

- Normal clotting factors with prolong bleeding time

Treatment:

- **No treatment is required** if the patient has no active bleeding and platelet count> 50,000. Check **platelets count at regular intervals**
- If platelet count is **<30,000,** start treatment with **corticosteroids.** Stop NSAIDs to improve platelet count, if applicable
- If platelet count is **< 10,000,** then treat patient with **IVIG or Anti-Rho**
- If platelet count **remains low after 4-6 weeks of treatment** or recurrent bleeding, then do **splenectomy**
- Thrombopoietin receptor agonist (Romiplostim, eltrombopag) may be used if steroids or splenectomy is ineffective. These **stimulate platelet production in the bone marrow.**
- **IVIG is the quickest way to increase the platelet count**

Note: If splenectomy is planned, make sure to vaccinate patient against encapsulated bacteria (N. meningitides, H. influenza and pneumococcus) 2 weeks prior to the procedure

2. VON WILLEBRAND DISEASE (VWD)

Von Willebrand disease is the most common heredity bleeding disorder. It is an autosomal dominant disorder caused by a deficiency of von Willebrand factor (vWF). vWF is required for platelet adhesion
Si/Sx: Platelet type bleeding: petechia, purpura, epistaxis, bleeding form gums, and heavy menstrual flow in women
Diagnosis:

- CBC shows normal platelet count
- Bleeding time shows **increased aPTT**
- Factor VIII level
- **Most accurate test is VWF level and ristocetin cofactor test** (detects VWF function)

Treatment:

- **Best initial treatment is desmopressin (DDAVP),** which releases the vWF from endothelial cells.
- If it is ineffective, then give factor **VIII replacement.**
- During emergency or for major surgery, VIII replacement is the best treatment

3. UREMIA INDUCED PLATELET DYSFUNCTION

In this condition platelets are working properly, but there is a defect in **platelet degranulation**

Si/Sx: **platelet type bleeding** with **normal bleeding time**

Boards possible scenario: look for a patient with platelet type bleeding with normal bleeding time and history of renal failure

Diagnosis: **VWF levels** and **ristocetin test** are both **normal**
Treatment: **Desmopressin**

Note: Patients with VWD and uremia induced platelet dysfunction present with similar symptoms. To distinguish them look at VWF levels and ristocetin test, which are normal in uremia induced platelet dysfunction

4. HEPARIN INDUCED THROMBOCYTOPENIA (HIT)

In this condition platelets count goes down soon after infusion of **regular heparin**

Si/Sx: decreased platelet count after starting heparin

Boards possible scenario: look for a patient with decreased platelet count soon after starting heparin

Treatment: **Immediately stop the heparin** and **give argatroban or lepirudin**
Important: Do not switch regular heparin to low molecular weight heparin if the patient develops HIT

Other *high-yield* HIT related point
- HIT could be prevented if low molecular weight heparin is used instead of regular heparin

---

4. HEMOPHILIA

Hemophilia is a rare **X-linked recessive disorder**, in which blood does not clot properly. It is more common in males and females are asymptomatic carriers

Types: Hemophilia A (Factor VIII deficiency), Hemophilia B (Factor IX deficiency)

Si/Sx: signs and symptoms depend on the level of the deficient factor. Patient with very low level of factor may experience spontaneous bleeding, whereas, patients with slight deficiency may only bleed after trauma or surgery.

Diagnosis:

- Normal bleeding time and PT, **increased PTT**
- **Mixing study:** if this study corrects the PTT time, then it means that the patient has factor deficiency. However, if mixing study does not fix corrects the PTT, then that patient may other condition (discussed in the table below)
- **Most accurate** test is **specific factor assay,** this test is performed if mixing study corrects the PTT

Treatment: discussed below

Hemophilia treatment

Condition	Treatment
Hemophilia A	• Vasopressin for mild bleeding • Factor VIII replacement for severe bleeding
Hemophilia B	• Factor IX replacement

MIXING STUDIES EVALUATION

- If prolongation is **corrected-** Dx. Clotting **factor deficiency**
- If prolongation is **not corrected** or **partially corrected-**Dx. Coagulation factor **inhibitor** is present
- If prolongation is **increased -**Dx. **Antibody** is present
- If prolongation is **increased,** as well as **PTT-**Dx. **Lupus anticoagulant**

4. VITAMIN K DEFICIENCY

Vitamin K plays an important role in the synthesis of coagulation factor. Its deficiency can lead to **decreased production of factors 2,7,9 and 10**

Si/Sx: oozing at venipuncture site. Bleeding is similar to the bleeding of hemophilia and may occur at any site

Diagnosis:
- **Both PT and PTT are elevated**
- PT and PTT **normalizes after vitamin K infusion**

Treatment:
- Mild bleeding is treated with vitamin K
- Severe bleeding is treated with fresh frozen plasma and vitamin K

5. LIVER DISEASE

Almost all clotting factors are made in the liver, except for factor VIII and vWF

Si/Sx: similar to vitamin K deficiency

Diagnosis:
- Both PT and PTT are elevated
- PT and PTT **does not normalize** after Vitamin K infusion

Treatment: Fresh frozen plasma and vitamin K replacement

Note: Patients with vitamin K deficiency and liver disease have similar symptoms. To distinguish them look at the PT and PTT time after infusion of vitamin K, which normalizes in vitamin K deficiency, but remains elevated in liver disease.

Other *high-yield* questions related to warfarin and supratherapeutic INR (2-3)

1. Patient is taking warfarin and his INR **is 5**, but there is **no active bleeding,** what is the next step in management?
   Answer: **omit 1 dose of warfarin**

2. Patient is taking warfarin and his INR **is between 5-9**, but there is **no active bleeding,** what is the next step in management?
   Answer: **omit 2 doses of warfarin**

3. Patient is taking warfarin and his INR **is INR is 7**, but he is at **increased risk of active bleeding or has peptic** ulcers. What is the next step in management?
   Answer: **give oral 2.5 mg of vitamin K**

4. Patient is taking warfarin and his INR is 7 and he is **going under elective surgery.** What is the next step in management?
Answer: **5 mg of Vitamin K**

5. Patient is taking warfarin and his INR is 9, but there is **no active bleeding.** What is the next step in management?
Answer: **hold the warfarin dose** and give **10 mg** of **oral vitamin K**

6. Patient is taking warfarin and is **actively bleeding** now. What is the next step in management?
Answer: give **fresh frozen plasma and vitamin K**

7. Patient is taking warfarin and now has **life-threatening bleeding.** What is the next step in management?
Answer: Give **prothrombin concentrate**

TRANSFUSION REACTION

1. ACUTE HEMOLYTIC REACTION
Acute hemolytic reaction occurs due to destruction of RBCs by preformed recipient antibodies
Cause: clerical error is the most common cause
Si/Sx: fever, chill chest pain, back pain, hemorrhage, shortness of breath, hypotension
Treatment: Stop transfusion, IV fluids and mannitol to prevent renal failure

2. FEBRILE NONHEMOLYTIC REACTION
Si/Sx: Fever, chills, temperature rises 1.0 F - 1.8 F from the baseline
Cause: recipient's antibodies to donor WBCs
Treatment: Leukoreduction – filtration of donor white cell from red blood cells products

3. TRANSFUSION-ASSOCIATED ACUTE LUNG INJURY
Si/Sx: Abrupt onset of fever, hypotension, non-cardiogenic pulmonary edema
Cause: donor's plasma antibodies

Treatment: most cases resolve within 72 hours

4. ALLERGIC REACTION
Occurs when the recipient has preformed antibodies to certain chemical in the donor blood
Si/Sx: urticaria, pruritus, may lead to anaphylactic shock
Cause: antibodies in donor blood
Treatment: antihistamines such as diphenhydramine

5. ALLERGIC ANAPHYLAXIS
Si/Sx: hypotension, tachycardia, loss of consciousness, shock, cardiac arrhythmia, cardiac arrest
Cause: IgA deficiency
Treatment: stop transfusion, maintain ABCs and give IgA washed blood products

---

Other *high-yield* transfusion related points

- If a patient requires emergency blood transfusion, and patient blood group is not known, then give patient **O negative blood**
- If during the blood transfusion, the patient experiences hypotensive, tachycardia, and shortness of breath, then immediately stop the blood transfusion, and **check LDH and bilirubin levels**:
  - LDH and bilirubin levels are **normal in allergic anaphylaxis reaction due to IgA deficiency**
  - LDH and bilirubin levels are **increased in ABO incompatibility**

TRANSPLANT REJECTION

1. HYPERACUTE REJECTION
Hyperacute rejection occurs within minutes of transplant. It occurs due to antibodies in organ recipient's blood that reacts to a transplanted organ
Cause: ABO incompatibility
Treatment: Remove the organ
Prevention: check ABO compatibility prior to transplantation

2. ACUTE REJECTION

Acute rejection occurs between 5 days to 3 months after transplant. It occurs due to cytotoxic T lymphocytes against foreign MHCs

Diagnosis: biopsy of organ shows T lymphocytes and antibody induced graft tissue injury

Treatment: Steroids and immunosuppressive drugs

3. CHRONIC REJECTION

Chronic rejection takes place over months to years after transplant

Diagnosis: biopsy of organ shows anti-body mediated vascular damage (fibrosis of blood vessels)

Treatment: chronic rejection is considered irreversible. There is no effective treatment

HEMATOLOGY CCS

CASE # 1

Case introduction
A 44-years old woman comes to the office because of fatigue, weakness, and loos of appetite.

Initial vitals signs
Temperature: 37.2 degrees
Pulse 85 beats/min, regular rhythm
Respiration rate: 21/ minutes

Blood pressure, systolic 119 mm Hg
Blood pressure, disystolic, 75 mm Hg

Height: 72.0 inches
Weight: 188.4 lbs.
Body mass index: 26.2 Kg/m2

History of present illness (HPI)
A 44-years old woman comes to the office because of fatigue, weakness, and loos of appetite. He has no fever, chills or weight loss. He denies breathing problem, cough, bleeding per rectum, and diarrhea. He does not smoke or use recreational drugs. He is been drinking 9-10 beers a day from last 15 years. He is sexually active with multiple partners and uses condoms whenever he engages in sexual activity. On a further question, he reveals that he is trying to lose weight and mainly on tea and toast diet. He denies any medical history.

Past medical history
Hospitalization: None
Other medical condition: None
Current medication: None
Allergies: penicillin, eggs
Vaccination: up to date

Family history
Father and mother are alive and well. Siblings are healthy

Social history
Marital history: Divorced; 2 children
Occupation: Bank teller
Recreational: football, golf
Personal habits: Drink 9-10 beers a day from last 15 years. Does not smoke, and use drugs

Review of system:
General: see HPI
Skin: see HPI
HEENT: see HPI
Musculoskeletal: see HPI
Cardiology: see HPI
Abdominal: see HPI
Genitourinary: see HPI

Please see pages 1-5 for general CCS cases approach

Step 1: None (patient is stable does not require any emergency measures)

Step 2: Order complete physical exam including rectal, and then move the
clock forward to get the results.

- Physical exam results shows:
    - Every thing is normal; no sign peripheral neuropathy,
      no loss of position and vibration sense

Step 3: Order following labs and move the clock forward to get the result

- CBC (under " stat' option)
- Folic acid level
- Vitamin B 12 level
- UA
- BMP
- FOBT (under " stat' option)
- Chest x-ray

Lab result shows:

- Blood smear shows hyper-segmented neutrophils.
- FOBT is negative
- Hb 9.2 g/dl
- MCV 120

Step 4: Medicine

- Multivitamin
- Thiamine
- Folic acid
- Vitamin B 12

Step 5: Location
> • Do the following counseling, and then move the patient home and make follow up appointment in a week
>> o No smoking, drinking, illegal drug use
>> o Safe sex
>> o Drive with seat belts
>> o Medicine compliance

Step 6: Move the clock forward to get folic acid/vitamin b 12 results
> • Folic acid: 3.4 ng/ml (Normal 6.0- 15.0 ng/ml
> • Vitamin B 12 is WNL

Step 7: Move the clock forward to the appointment day.
> • Patient feels better
> • Check reticulocyte count

Step 8: None (no consultation needed for this patient)

Step 9: Make a followup appointment in a month and move the patient home

Case should end here end.

Step 10: Counseling
> • Since most the basic counseling was already on step 5 so order
>> o Age and gender specific screening

Diagnosis: Folic acid deficiency

CASE # 2

Case introduction
A 32-years old African-American male come to ER with sudden onset of back pain, dark urine and jaundice

Initial vitals signs
Temperature: 38.2 degrees
Pulse 91 beats/min, regular rhythm
Respiration rate: 18/ minutes

Blood pressure, systolic 114 mm Hg
Blood pressure, disystolic, 74 mm Hg

Height: 68.0 inches
Weight: 166.4 lbs.
Body mass index: 26.2 Kg/m2

History of present illness (HPI)
A 32-years old African-American male come to ER with sudden onset of back pain, dark urine and jaundice. He denies breathing problem, cough, bleeding per rectum and constipation. He does not smoke or use recreational drugs. He is sexually active with his girl friend and uses condoms most of the time. He has no medical history except for diarrhea few days ago for which he took TMP-SMZ.

Past medical history
Hospitalization: None
Other medical condition: None
Current medication: None
Allergies: peanuts
Vaccination: up to date

Family history
Father and mother are alive and well. Siblings are healthy

Social history
Marital history: not married
Occupation: none
Recreational: football, tennis
Personal habits: Does not drink, smoke or drugs

Review of system:
General: see HPI
Skin: Pallor,
HEENT: icterus
Musculoskeletal: see HPI
Cardiology: see HPI
Abdominal: see HPI
Genitourinary: dark urine, no dysuria

Please see pages 1-5 for general CCS cases approach

Step 1: None (patient is stable does not require any emergency measures)

Step 2: Order complete physical exam including rectal, and then move the clock forward to get the results.
- Physical exam results shows
  - Patient has mild jaundice, pallor and scleral icterus
  - Rest of the physical exam is normal

Step 3: Order the following labs, and then move the clock forward to get the results
- CBC with blood smear
- UA
- BMP
- PT/INR
- PTT
- LDH
- LFT

Lab result shows
- Blood smear shows fragmented RBC with bite cells
- CBC shows Hb 9 g/dl, Hct 35%. MCV 96 fL.
- LDH: 1010
- LFT: total bilirubin; 4.5 mg/dl, direct bilirubin: .07mg/dl. Alkaline phosphate 109)
- PTT 28 sec
- PT/INR 13 sec/L

Step 4: Discontinue sulfa or offending drugs, if applicable

Step 5: Move the patient in wards

Step 6: Order the followings
- IV access
- IV normal saline
- NPO
- Monitor urine output

- Vitals every 8 hours

Step 7. Order the following labs, and the move the clock forward to get the results
- Haptoglobin
- Hematocrit
- Blood type and Rh
- Reticulocytes count
- G6PD assay

Labs show
- Blood type: O negative
- G6PD: Positive
- Haptoglobin: 23
- Reticulocytes count: 23%

Step 7. Order blood transfusion

Step 8. Order Hematologist consultation

Step 9: Check Hct/Hb level every 8 -12 hours
- After couple of 8-12 hours checks- patient will feel better, Hct/Hb are improving and case will end

Step 10: Counseling
- Age and case specific counseling
- Safe sex, wear seat belt, no smoking, no drinking, no drugs,
- Avoid sulfa drugs, fava beans

Diagnosis: G6PD deficiency

ENDOCRINOLOGY

DIABETES

Diabetes is a metabolic condition, which can be caused by too little insulin, insulin resistance or both

Type of diabetes: there are two types of diabetes: type 1 and type 2 diabetes (discussed in details below)

Diabetes screening: all patients with HTN should be screened for diabetes mellitus

TYPE-1 DIABETES

Cause: autoimmune destruction of pancreatic β –cell, which leads to insulin deficiency

Si/Sx: Polyuria, polydipsia, polyphagia and weight loss

Diagnosis: Any one of the following can be used to diagnose diabetes

- Fasting blood sugar > 125 mg/dl on two separate occasions
- One random blood sugar > 200 mg/dl, with polyuria, polydipsia, polyphagia
- Glucose > 200 mg/dl, after 2-hours postprandial test with 75 mg oral glucose
- Hemoglobin A1c > 6.5%

Treatment: type 1 diabetes is treated with **insulin**

Insulin profile

Type of insulin	Onset	Peak effect	Duration
Rapid-Acting insulin (Aspart, lispro, & glulisine)	10- 30 minutes	0.5 – 3 hours	3-5 hours
Short- Acting insulin (Regular insulin)	30- 60 minutes	2-5 hours	5- 8 hours
Intermediate-Acting insulin (NPH insulin)	2-4 hours	6-7 hours	Up to 12 hours
Long-Acting insulin (Detemir, glargine)	1-2 hours	1-2 hour	Up to 24 hours

Note: Oral hypoglycemics such as metformin or sulfonylurea, do not work in type 1 diabetes because they work by stimulating insulin release from the pancreatic beta-cells, which are destroyed in type 1 diabetes

NPH insulin and regular insulin's dose adjustment

1. **Regular insulin:** It is **usually given before a meal** to **prevent postprandial hyperglycemia** (2-4 hours after a meal). If a patient develops postprandial hypoglycemia, it means high dose of regular insulin was prescribed. It is managed by **lowering the dose of regular insulin before** a meal, and vice versa.

2. **NPH insulin:** It is given **to control the blood sugar between meals, overnight, and while fasting.** If a patient develops hypoglycemia around 7AM or 5 PM, it means high dose of NPH insulin was prescribed. It is managed by **lowering the dose of NPH insulin** in the evenings or mornings, and vice versa.

Dawn phenomenon and Somogyi effect

- **Dawn phenomenon** is characterized by early morning (≅ 3AM) **euglycemia.** It is caused by normal secretion of growth hormone and **decreased insulin effectiveness.** Patient is hyperglycemic around 7AM. It is **managed by increasing NPH insulin dose at dinnertime.**

- **Somogyi effect** is characterized by early morning (≅ 3AM) **hypoglycemia.** It is caused by **high dose of NPH insulin at the dinnertime.** Body responds to this by releasing epinephrine, which causes hyperglycemia around 7AM. Somogyi effect is **managed by lowering the dose of NPH insulin at dinnertime.**

Bottom line is if a patient have hyperglycemia around 7AM, and then have the patient check his glucose level at 3AM to distinguish between Dawn phenomenon and Somogyi effect

DIABETIC KETOACIDOSIS (DKA)

Diabetic ketoacidosis is an **acute life-threating** complication of diabetes mellitus. It mostly occurs in type 1 diabetes, and **blood sugar is > 250**
Cause: infection (UTI, influenza, gastroenteritis, pneumonia), missed treatment, stress, trauma, illegal drugs, alcohol

Si/Sx: Kussmaul hyperpnea, abdominal pain, dehydration, vomiting, fruity odor, increased anion gap metabolic acidosis, hyperkalemia. In severe condition patients may altered mental status

Management of **DKA is as follow:**

1. **IV normal saline** + **IV insulin**
    ↓
2. When blood **sugar drops to 250,** then **switch the normal saline** to **D5W**
    ↓
3. Keep the patient on **D5W** and IV **insulin until anion gap channel closes.** (Anion gap channel is calculated by: [Na- (CL+HCO3)] and value 8-12 is normal).
    ↓
4. Once Anion gap channel closes (between 8-12)
    ↓
5. Add **subcutaneous insulin + D5W + IV insulin + give patient something to eat**
    ↓
6. **Stop IV insulin approximately an hour later**

Other important management points of DKA

*   Make sure to **monitor K+** and give **KCL when K+ is < 4**
*   Patients should be **monitored in ICU**
*   Serum bicarbonate **is measured to** determine the **severity of diabetic ketoacidosis**

TYPE 2 DIABETES

Insulin resistance causes type 2 diabetes

Si/Sx: polyuria, polydipsia, polyphagia, weight loss, fatigue

Diagnosis: same as Type 1 diabetes

Treatment: is as follow

*   Best initial treatment is **lifestyle modification** (diet, weight loss and exercise) and **metformin,** if it is ineffective, then **add GLP-1 agonist or DDP-4 inhibitor,** and if dual is ineffective, then **add sulfonylurea or thiazolidinedione's.** If even triple therapy is ineffective, then **add long-acting insulin.**

- If a patient with Type-2 DM has **end stage renal failure**, then start the patient on **insulin**

Oral hypoglycemics profile

Medicine	Mechanism	Side effects
Metformin	Blocks hepatic gluconeogenesis	Lactic acidosis, renal insufficiency
Sulfonylurea (Glipizide, glyburide, glimepiride)	Increases the insulin release from the pancreas	Hypoglycemia, SIADH, weight gain
Thiazolidinedione's (Rosiglitazone, Pioglitazone)	Improves peripheral insulin sensitivity	Acute CHF exacerbation
Alpha-glucosidase inhibitor (Acarbose, miglitol)	Inhibits alpha-glucosidase enzyme in the small intestine	Bloating, abdominal cramps
GLP-1 agonist (Exenatide)	Increases insulin decreases glucagon and slows the gastric emptying	Pancreatitis
DDP-4 inhibitors (Sitagliptin, saxagliptin)	Inhibits the enzyme that metabolizes GLP-1 agonists	Sitagliptin-**pancreatitis, allergic reaction** Saxagliptin-**allergic reaction**

Other important points about metformin
- Contraindications for metformin are renal failure, CHF, COPD, alcoholics, and liver failure
- Stop metformin at least 24 hours prior to administration of contrast material to prevent renal failure

HYPEROSMOLAR DIABETIC COMA
Hyperosmolar diabetic coma is an acute complication of diabetes mellitus. It mostly occurs in **type-2 diabetes. Blood sugar is usually > 1000** mg/dl
Cause: illness, stress, dehydration, infection, and non-compliance with medicine

Si/Sx: high blood sugar level >1,000 mg/dl **without acidosis,** excessive thirst, change in mental status, vision loss

Management of hyperosmolar diabetic coma is as follow:

1. **Give IV fluids + IV Insulin**
   ⬇
2. When blood sugar drops to **300**
   ⬇
3. **Give IV fluids +**IV insulin + **sub Q insulin**
   ⬇
4. Hour later, stop **IV insulin +** add **short acting insulin +** give patient **some thing to eat**

Other important points of hyperosmolar diabetic coma
- Adjusting the blood sugar too fast can lead to **cerebral edema**
- Patient can be managed in hospital wards

CHRONIC COMPLICATIONS OF DIABETES (TYPE 1 AND TYPE 2)

1. **Cardiovascular**
   - Patient with diabetes is at increased risk of MI. Every 1% decrease in HbA1C decreases the risk of MI by 14 %. Patient should be instructed to be compliant with diabetic medication.
   - Blood pressure should be kept **< 130/80 mmHg.** Treat **high BP with ACE inhibitors,**
   - LDLs **< 100** in a patient with DM alone or LDL **< 70** in a patient with **DM plus CAD.** Treat **high LDLs with statins.**
   - Diabetes patients **>30 years of age** should be started on **low-dose aspirin.**

2. **Eye exam**
   - Patients with **DM 2** should have an **annual eye exam** after they are diagnosed with DM2
   - Patients with **DM1** should have their **first eye exam 5 years after they are diagnosed with DM1, then annually thereafter.**

Management: If proliferative retinopathy is seen anytime during eye exam, then treat it with **photocoagulation.**

3. **Nephropathy**
    - Patients are at risk of developing diabetic nephropathy. Patients should be annually screened for microalbuminuria (normal urine albumin are 30- 300mg in 24 hours).

    Treatment: Even a small increase above normal limits of microalbuminuria is treated with **ACE inhibitors or ARBs** to prevent further renal damage.

4. **Gastroparesis**
    - Gastroparesis develops years after DM, in which stomach takes a long time to empty its content. Food may turn into a hard mass, which may cause early satiety, nausea, vomiting, abdominal pain and constipation.

    Treatment:
    - **Best initial treatment** is diet modification: **high protein, low fiber and low fats.**
    - If **diet modification is ineffective**, then give metoclopramide **or erythromycin.**

5. **Neuropathy:**
    - High blood sugar can injure nerve fibers throughout the body, but nerves in legs and feet are most commonly affected first.
    - Late complications of neuropathy include impotence, orthostatic hypotension and mononeuropathy. Mononeuropathy involves damage to specific nerve, it can lead to wrist drop, foot drop, isolated cranial nerve palsies, mainly CN III or CN IV

    Treatment:
    - All patients with DM should be instructed to do **regular self-feet exam.**
    - Gabapentin is given to the patient, who has the burning sensation in hands or feet.

HYPOGLYCEMIA

Hypoglycemia is a medical emergency; it is characterized by low blood sugar

Cause: Insulinoma, exogenous insulin abuse, sulfonylurea, alcohol abuse

Si/Sx: dizziness, change in mental status, loss of consciousness, palpitations, shakiness, anxiety, sweating

Diagnosis:

- Fingerstick usually shows blood glucose < 70mg/dl
- Blood test to check the level of insulin, c-peptide, proinsulin (see table below)
- UA to check for urine sulfa (see table below)
- Abdomen CT, if Insulinoma is suspected
- In alcohol abuse cases glucose levels is usually < 45 mg/dl

Differential diagnosis of hypoglycemia

	Insulinoma	Exogenous insulin abuse	Sulfonylurea medicine
Insulin	High	High	High
C-Peptide	Increased	Low or nml	Increased
Proinsulin	Increased	Low or nml	Nml
Urine sulfa	Absent	Absent	Present

Treatment: raise the blood sugar

- Fruit juice, glucose tablet or candy usually treats mild symptoms.
- Patients with severe symptoms may need injection of glucagon or IV glucose.

THYROID DISORDER

Thyroid gland secretes hormones that are essential to regulate the rate of metabolism, growth and development. Over production of the thyroid hormones leads to hyperthyroidism, and underproduction of thyroid hormones leads to hypothyroidism.

Si/Sx: Usually all forms of hypo/hyperthyroidism have similar symptoms. (Discussed below)

Symptoms of hyperthyroidism and hypothyroidism

Hyperthyroidism	Hypothyroidism
Heat intolerance	Cold intolerance
Weight loss	Weight gain
Warm skin	Cold and pale skin
Nervousness	Weakness
Irritability	Lethargy, fatigue
Emotional liability	Memory impairment, dementia
Tachycardia, atrial fibrillation	Bradycardia

Causes and types: There are lots of conditions that can lead to over or underproduction of thyroid hormones. Level of thyroid hormones (T3, free T4 (fT4), TSH), and Radioiodine uptake scan (**RAIU**) help determine the cause or type hyperthyroidism. (Discussed below)

Hyperthyroidism differential diagnosis

Condition	T3	Free T4 (fT4)	TSH	RAIU
Grave's disease	High	High	Low	Increased **diffuse** uptake
Pituitary tumor	High	High	**High**	Increased **diffuse** uptake
Subacute thyroiditis	High	High	Low	Decreased uptake
Silent thyroiditis	High	High	Low	Decreased uptake
Exogenous thyroid hormone abuse	High	High	Low	Decreased uptake
Plummer's disease (Toxic multinodular goiter)	High	High	Low	Increased uptake in hot nodules with cold background

SPECIFIC CAUSES AND CHARACTERISTIC OF HYPERTHYROIDISM

1. SUBACUTE THYROIDITIS
Subacute thyroiditis is caused by **viral infection** such as influenza or mumps. Most obvious symptoms are **neck pain, and jaw pain**
Diagnosis:
- Physical examination may show **tender thyroid gland**
- Labs show:
  - o **Increased T3, T4, and ESR**
  - o **Decreased TSH** and **RIAU**

Treatment: Aspirin is given to relieve pain

2. EXOGENOUS THYROID HORMONE ABUSE

It is commonly seen in health care workers or someone with access to exogenous thyroid hormones.

Diagnosis:

- Physical exam may show **atrophy of thyroid gland**
- Labs show:
  - **Increased fT4**
  - **Decreased TSH** and **thyroxine-binding globulin (TBG)**

3. SILENT THYROIDITS

Silent thyroiditis **is autoimmune, self-limited condition,** in which the person alternate clinical course between hyperthyroidism, hypothyroidism, and return to normal thyroid function.

Diagnosis:

- Labs during hyperthyroidism phase shows:
  - **Increased fT4**
  - **Decreased TSH** and **RAIU**
  - **Anti-thyroid peroxidase and anti-thyroglobulin antibodies may be present**

Treatment:

- Symptomatic **treatment**
- **Propranolol,** non-selective beta-blocker is helpful in hyperthyroidism phase to **control adrenergic symptoms** (tachycardia, palpitations, tremors, and anxiety)

4. PITUITARY ADENOMA

Pituitary adenoma can cause hyperthyroidism by excessive production of TSH. It is the only hyperthyroidism condition in which TSH is increased.

Diagnosis:

- Labs show **increased TSH, fT4** and **diffuse uptake of RIAU**
- **Diagnosis is confirmed with MRI** of head

Treatment: surgical resection of adenoma

5. PLUMMER'S DISEASE

Plummer's disease also known a **toxic multinodular goiter is** common in elderly; it is caused by multiple foci of thyroid tissues that stop responding to T4 feedback inhibition.

Diagnosis:

- Labs shows
    - Increased fT4, increased RIAU uptake in toxic nodules with low uptake in rest of the gland
    - Low TSH

Treatment: Same as Grave's disease

6. GRAVES' DISEASE

Graves' disease is the most common cause of hyperthyroidism.

Diagnosis:

- Physical exam shows ophthalmology, onycholysis, and dermopathy.
- Labs show:
    - Increased, fT4, diffuse uptake of RIAU
    - Decreased TSH
    - Antimicrosomal and antithyroglobulin antibodies

Treatment:

- Propranolol, non-selective beta-blocker, is the best initial treatment to control adrenergic symptoms (tachycardia, palpitations, tremors, and anxiety); it also blocks the peripheral conversion of T4 to T3.
- Propylthiouracil (PTU) or methimazole is given to control gland before the definitive treatment. These decrease the peripheral conversion of T4 to T3.
- Definitive treatment for Graves's disease is subtotal thyroidectomy or radioactive iodine ablation.
    - Subtotal thyroidectomy is performed, if goiter is causing neck compression, dysphagia or if the patient do not want to have iodine ablation
    - Radioactive iodine ablation is preferred. Reproductive age women should be advised to not to get pregnant for a year following radioactive iodine ablation
- Following radioactive iodine ablation or subtotal thyroidectomy, patient should be placed on levothyroxine
    - Check TSH levels every 3-4 weeks and adjust the dose of levothyroxine accordingly (If THS is low, then decrease the dose. On the other hand, if TSH is high, then increase the dose)

Graves' disease management during pregnancy

- **PTU is given during the first trimester,** and **subtotal thyroidectomy is performed** during 2nd **trimester.** Methimazole should not be given to a pregnant woman because it causes congenital aplasia cutis.

6. THYROID STORM

Thyroid storm is a life-threatening condition of hyperthyroidism, which is caused by sudden **release of large amount of thyroid hormones**

Cause: severe infection or illness, severe stress, recent treatment with radioiodine, over-dose of thyroid hormones

Si/Sx: fever, tachycardia, decreased mental status, nausea, vomiting, dehydration

Treatment is given in the following order:

- IV fluids, steroids, beta-blockers are given initially to stabilize the patient
- Then, PTU to bring the thyroid gland under control
- Lastly, use iodine to block the iodine uptake by thyroid gland

7. SICK-THYROID SYNDROME

Sick-thyroid syndrome also known as euthyroid sick syndrome or non-thyroidal illness syndrome is **dysregulation of thyrotropic feedback control.**

Cause: it usually occurs after **acute or chronic non-thyroid condition** such pneumonia, fasting, MI, chronic renal failure, cirrhosis

Diagnosis:

- **Labs show the following:**
  - During acute stage - **increased reverse T3, decreased T4, and TSH is low, but never lower than 0.4, in other words TSH is in low normal vale range** (normal TSH range 0.4 – 6.0)
  - During recovery phase - **TSH is above 6.0**

Treatment: no treatment is required, patient usually recover spontaneously

Other high- yield hyperthyroidism related points

Remember during pregnancy, TIBG and total T4 are increased, **but** free T4 and TSH are normal
- If a pregnant woman presents with symptoms of hyperthyroidism, then check **free T4** (fT4):
    - If fT4 is **increased,** then the diagnosis is **hyperthyroidism**
    - If fT4 is within **normal range,** then the diagnosis is **anxiety**

HYPOTHYROIDISM
Hypothyroidism is caused by decreased production of thyroid hormones
Si/Sx: weight gain, cold intolerance, dry skin, depressed mood, fatigue, menstrual change, diminished reflexes
Causes: Hashimoto's disease, pituitary adenoma, post-ablative surgery or radioiodine, iodine deficiency, drugs such as lithium, amiodarone, interferons, sulfonamide

SPECIFIC CAUSES AND CHARACTERISTIC OF HYPOTHYROIDISM

1. HASHIMOTO'S DISEASE
Hashimoto's disease is an autoimmune disease; it is the most common cause of hypothyroidism. Women are affected more than men, with female to male ratio (8:1).
Diagnosis:
- Labs show **low T3, low T4 and high TSH**
- Diagnose **is confirmed with antithyroid peroxidase antibodies (TPO), and anti-microsomal antibodies.**
Treatment: Levothyroxine

Note: Antacids, calcium supplements, iron supplements and fiber **can decrease the absorption of levothyroxine.** Advise the patient to take levothyroxine empty stomach, and then take any of these products approximately 4 hours after the taking levothyroxine.

2. SUBCLINICAL HYPOTHYROIDISM

Subclinical hypothyroidism is a mild form of hypothyroidism. It is diagnosed when **T4 is within normal range,** but TSH levels are **mildly elevated.**

Treatment: Usually **no treatment is required.** However, **levothyroxine is given** if the patient has any of followings:

- TSH >10
- Thyroperoxidase (TPO) >1000
- Hyperlipidemia
- Menstrual change

3. PITUITARY TUMOR

Pituitary tumor can cause hypothyroidism by **suppressing the production of TSH.** This is the only hypothyroidism condition in which TSH is decreased

Diagnosis:

- Labs show **decreased TSH and T4**
- **Diagnosis is confirmed with MRI** of the head

Treatment: surgical resection of adenoma

4. MYXEDEMA COMA

Myxedema coma is a life-threatening form of hypothyroidism

Cause: severe infection or illness, severe stress, untreated hypothyroidism, trauma

Si/Sx: altered mental status, respiratory depression, hypothermia

Treatment: IV hydrocortisone and IV levothyroxine

Other *high-yield* **hypothyroidism related points**

- If a patient has hyperlipemia secondary to hypothyroidism, then the best initial treatment is **levothyroxine,** but if it is ineffective, then use **statins**
- **Levothyroxine** dose may need to be **increased** in **pregnant woman** or if woman is taking **oral contraceptive containing estrogen** because in these condtions thyroxine-binding globulin (TBG) is increased, which reduces the absorption of **levothyroxine**

THYROID NODULES

Majority of the thyroid nodules are discovered incidentally during physical exam.

Management of thyroid nodule is as follow:

1. Initial step is to **check TSH Level,** and then the further management is as follow:
2. If TSH is **low,** then get a **radionuclide uptake scan (RAUI)**
    2.a If radionuclides scan shows **hot nodule** (increased uptake), then treat the patient with **PTU**
    2.b If a radionuclide scan shows **cold nodule** (decreased uptake), then do **ultrasound-guided fine-needle aspiration (FNA)** (discussed below)

3. If TSH is **normal or high,** then the management is as follow:
    3a. **Nodule ≤ 1cm** and patient has **no risk factors for thyroid cancer,** then do **regular follow-up.** However, if patient **has risk factors for thyroid cancer,** then do FNA (discussed below)
    3b. **Nodule > 1cm** then do **FNA** (discussed below)

FNA results and treatment options:
- If FNA shows **malignancy,** then do **surgery or radioiodine ablation**
- If FNA shows **benign cytology,** then treat the patient with **levothyroxine** and **follow-up.**
    o If tumor is **regressing,** then **continue the treatment**
    o If t tumor is **still the same,** then **repeat the FNA or surgical excision**
- IF FNA shows **non-functioning or cold nodule,** then **repeat RAUI**
    o If scan shows **increased uptake,** then treat the patient with **PTU**
    o If scan shows **decreased uptake,** then **do surgery or radioiodine ablation**

THYROID CANCERS

1. PAPILLARY CARCINOMA
Papillary carcinoma is the **most common thyroid cancer**. It is a slow growing tumor, and **spreads via lymph node**
Cause: It is associated with radiation exposure to head and neck area
Diagnosis: Histopathology of biopsy shows **ground-glass orphan Annie nucleus & psammoma bodies**
Treatment: **Near total thyroidectomy,** and patient should be placed on levothyroxine after surgery

2. FOLLICULAR CARCINOMA
Follicular carcinoma is the **second most common** thyroid cancer. It **metastasizes to lungs and bones via blood**
Treatment: same as papillary cancer

3. ANAPLASTIC CARCINOMA
Anaplastic carcinoma is a highly malignant carcinoma. It **spreads by direct extension.**
Anaplastic carcinoma has worst prognosis, almost all patients die within 5 year after developing
Treatment: surgery, but it **does not prolong patient's life**

4. MEDULLARY CARCINOMA
Medullary carcinoma arises from parafollicular cells of the thyroid. It produces **calcitonin.**
It is a component of MEN type IIa, and MEN type IIb

MULTIPLE ENDOCRINE NEOPLASIA (MEN) SYNDROMES
Multiple endocrine neoplasia syndromes is group of disorders that affects the multiple endocrine glands

Types: discussed below

Types	Associated disorders
MEN Type 1 (Wermer's syndrome)	• Pituitary • Pancreases • Parathyroid tumor
MEN Type IIa (Sipple syndrome)	• Pheochromocytoma • Medullary thyroid cancer • Parathyroid hyperplasia
MEN Type IIb	• Pheochromocytoma • Medullary thyroid cancer • Neuroma

HYPERPARATHYROIDISM

Hyperparathyroidism is characterized by overactivity of the parathyroid gland, which leads to increased production of parathyroid hormone (PTH). PTH is the main hormone that regulates the calcium and phosphate level.

Types and causes: hyperthyroidism is of two types:

- **Primary hyperparathyroidism** is caused by dysfunction in the parathyroid **gland itself.**
    - o Most common cause is the **solitary adenoma** (80%)
    - o 2nd common cause is **four-gland hyperplasia** (19%)
    - o Least common cause is **parathyroid cancer** (1%)
- **Secondary hyperparathyroidism** is caused by chronic kidney failure, severe vitamin D deficiency and severe calcium deficiency

Si/Sx: there are no specific symptoms of hyperparathyroidism. Most of the cases are asymptomatic, **but some patient may have symptoms similar to symptoms hypercalcemia** such as bone pain, kidney stone, constipation, and psychiatry problems

Diagnosis:

- In **primary hyperparathyroidism,** both PTH and **ionized serum calcium** levels are **elevated,** but **phosphate levels are decreased, usually** <2.5 mg/dL
- In **secondary hyperparathyroidism,** PTH is elevated and **ionized calcium level is low-to-normal.** Phosphate level may vary;
    - o Phosphate level is **low in vitamin D deficiency**
    - o Phosphate level is **high in renal failure**

Management:

- Secondary hyperparathyroidism - **Treat the underlying cause**

- Primary hyperparathyroidism is treated as follow:
  - **Medical therapy** (Calcimimetic or bisphosphonates) is given, when any of the followings is present:
    - Serum calcium ≤ 11.5 mg/dl
    - Asymptomatic patient
    - Contradiction for surgery

  - **Surgery** (Parathyroidectomy) is performed, when any of the followings is present:
    - Serum **calcium >12.5**
    - Urine calcium> **400mg/dl in 24 hours**
    - Pregnant woman
    - Any degree of renal insufficiency
    - Any symptomatic disease, "stones, GI groans, psychiatry moans or bone disease"

ADRENAL GLAND DIEASES

1. HYPOADRENALISM

Hypoadrenalism also referred as adrenal insufficiency, is a condition in which adrenal glands **do not produce sufficient steroid hormones** (mainly cortisol) and aldosterone. Aldosterone is the main hormone that regulates sodium, potassium and water retention.

Cause:

- Primary adrenal insufficiency is caused by destruction of all three layers of the adrenal gland, due to conditions such as **Addison's disease (the most common cause)**, Tuberculosis, fungal infection, AIDS, and metastatic cancer
- Secondary adrenal insufficiency is caused by pituitary and hypothalamic failure

Si/Sx:

- General symptoms include weakness, fatigue, **anorexia, weight loss, nausea,** vomiting, hypotension, and **sparse body hair.**

- Patients with **primary adrenal insufficiency** also have **increased skin pigmentation**, which is due to high POMC, a precursor of ACTH

Diagnosis:

- **Lab shows hyponatremia, hyperkalemia, metabolic acidosis, hypoglycemia**, and ACTH
  - ACTH is **high in primary** adrenal insufficiency but **low** in **secondary** adrenal insufficiency.

- **Most accurate** test is **cosyntropin stimulation test:** Cortisol levels are measured before and after the administration of cosyntropin
  - **Cortisol will remain low** in **primary adrenal** insufficiency
  - **Cortisol will be increased** in **secondary** adrenal insufficiency
- **CT scan of adrenal gland** is usually **done, if** primary adrenal insufficiency **is suspected after cosyntropin stimulation test**

Treatment:

- **Primary adrenal insufficiency** is treated with glucocorticoids and mineralocorticoid
- **Secondary adrenal insufficiency** is treated with glucocorticoids alone

---

Other *high-yield* hypoaldosteronism related question

ACUTE ADRENAL CRISIS

Acute adrenal crisis is a life-threatening that occurs when a patient is **suddenly removed from long-term (>3 weeks) steroid therapy.** Patient present with altered mental status, profound hypotension and fever. It is managed as follow: draw blood cortisol level, and then give IV fluids and **100mg hydrocortisone**

Note:

- Patients with acute **adrenal crisis and septic shock** present with **similar symptoms** such as sudden onset of hypotension or altered mental status. Only way to distinguish them quickly is to look at **blood glucose level**, which is **low in adrenal crisis** and high in **septic shock**

- Patient on prolonged dose of prednisone treatment needs stress dose of corticosteroid before the surgery and every 6 hours after the surgery to prevent adrenal insufficiency

2. HYPERALDOSTERON

Hyperaldosteronism is characterized by **overproduction** of aldosterone
Cause:

- Primary hyperaldosteronism is caused by Conn syndrome (unilateral adrenal adenoma), adrenocortical carcinoma, and bilateral carcinoma
- Secondary hyperaldosteronism is caused by renal artery stenosis, adrenal tumor

Si/Sx: Muscle weakness, hypertension, polyuria, polydipsia
Diagnosis:

- Both primary and secondary hyperaldosteronism show **low potassium and metabolic acidosis**
- Aldosterone and plasma renin level help **distinguish primary and secondary hyperaldosteronism.** (See table below)

TYPE	Aldosterone	Plasma renin level
Primary hyperaldosteronism	High	Low
Secondary hyperaldosteronism	High	High

- **Primary hyperaldosteronism:** after checking aldosterone and plasma renin levels, **perform CT scan of adrenal glands**
- **Secondary hyperaldosteronism** is usually confirmed with high salt diet test, in which aldosterone remains elevated after high salt loading with normal saline
- Once the cause if known, then the further test are done as follow:
  - CT scan of adrenal glands to check tumor
  - If **renal stenosis** is suspected (physical exam shows **abdominal bruit**), then perform **ultrasound doppler,** and then confirm the diagnosis with **renal angiography**

Treatment:
- Unilateral adrenal tumors are **removed surgically**
- Bilateral adrenal hyperplasia or unresectable adrenal tumors are treated with **oral potassium sparing** medicines such as **spironolactone or eplerenone**
- Renal stenosis is treated with **angioplasty**

3. PHEOCHROMOCYTOMA

Pheochromocytoma is a neuroendocrine tumor of adrenal medulla; it secretes high levels of catecholamines, norepinephrine and epinephrine

Si/Sx: Episodic hypertension, palpitation, headaches, sweating, tremors, flushing, nausea, vomiting, diarrhea

Diagnosis:
- Best initial test is 24-hour urinary metanephrines (VMA and HVA).
- Diagnosis is confirmed with CT or MRI of adrenal glands

Note: 10 % of the pheochromocytoma is extra-adrenal. If CT or MRI does not identify a tumor, **then do MIBG scan**. MIBG scan is a nuclear isotope scan, which detects the extra adrenal pheochromocytoma.

Treatment: Treat the patient in the following order:
- Initial treatment is to give **IV fluids** and control the hypertension with **alpha-blocker** such as phenoxybenzamine or phentolamine
- Second, give **beta-blockers (propranolol) or calcium channel** blockers to control the hypertension and prevent reflex tachycardia
- Third, surgical removal of the tumor, it is usually performed after 2 weeks

CUSHING'S SYNDROME

Cushing's syndrome is a condition in which high levels of cortisol is secreted.

Cause: pituitary tumor (also referred as Cushing disease), small cell cancer of lungs, and adrenal tumor/hyperplasia

Si/Sx: discussed in table below

Symptoms of Cushing's syndrome

Physical findings	Moon faces, buffalo hump, truncal obesity, osteoporosis, purple striae
Psychological	Depression, psychosis
Metabolic changes	Hyperglycemia, hyperlipidemia
Lab. Abnormalities	Low potassium, high aldosterone, metabolic alkalosis
Reproductive organs abnormalities	Menstrual abnormality in women Impotence in men

Diagnosis: diagnostic tests are performed as follow:
1. Best initial test is **24 hours urine cortisol or 1mg overnight** dexamethasone suppression test
   1a. Elevated **24-hour cortisol** level **confirms** the Cushing syndrome.
   1b. **1 mg overnight dexamethasone** is usually done, when 24-hours urine cortisol is not an option. **Normal person** should have **suppressed cortisol levels** after 1mg overnight dexamethasone test. Cortisol suppression excludes the Cushing syndrome.

> **Important:** Dexamethasone is metabolized faster with drugs (phenytoin, rifampin) or physical stress (depression, anorexia, or depression). So it is necessary to check if patient's 1mg overnight dexamethasone test was **false negative** due to any of theses.

2. If 1 mg overnight dexamethasone suppression test does not suppress **cortisol levels, then 8 mg dexamethasone** is given and **cortisol levels are measured again**
   2.a If cortisol levels are suppressed after the test– Dx. **Pituitary tumor** (Cushing's disease)
   2.b If cortisol levels are not suppressed after the test, then measure ACTH levels:
   - If ACTH level is > 20 pg/mL–Dx. **Small cell cancer**
   - If ACTH level is < 8 pg/mL–Dx. **Adrenal tumor or hyperplasia**

3. **Confirm** the diagnosis as following:
   - Pituitary tumor is confirmed with **MRI of the head**. If MRI does not identify any tumor, **then do inferior petrosal venous sinus sampling**
   - Small cell cancer of lungs is confirmed with **CT chest**
   - Adrenal tumor or hyperplasia is confirmed with **CT abdomen**

Treatment:
   - Pituitary tumor, small cell cancer of lungs and adrenal tumor or hyperplasia are **surgically resected**
   - If tumor is unresectable, then give oral **ketoconazole or metyrapone**

PITUITARY GANLD DISEASES

1. PROLACTINOMA

Prolactinoma is characterized by **increased prolactin level**

Cause: Pituitary tumor, drugs (methyldopa, metoclopramide, Tricyclic antidepressants), pregnancy, lactation, hypothyroidism (high TRH levels stimulates prolactin secretion), seizures, nipple stimulation, and chronic renal failure

Si/Sx: Headaches, diplopia, CN III palsy, other gender specific symptoms are as follow:

Men	Impotence, gynecomastia, decreased libido
Women	Amenorrhea, galactorrhea, infertility

Diagnosis:
   - Prolactin level (usually > 200 mg/ml in prolactinoma)
   - **After measuring the prolactin level** and **before doing MRI of the head,** rule out other causes such as pregnancy medicine, hypothyroidism
   - Most accurate test is MRI of the head, it is performed to confirm the diagnosis, if pituitary tumor is suspected

Treatment: Treatment of prolactinoma **depends on the cause**

- If a prolactinoma is caused by pituitary tumor, then treat it with **dopamine agonist** (cabergoline or bromocriptine), but if dopamine agonist is ineffective, then do **transsphenoidal surgery.**
- Radiation is for a nonresectable pituitary tumor
- If a prolactinoma is caused by other causes such as dopamine antagonist, or hypothyroidism, then treat the underlying cause such as:
  - o If it is due to dopamine antagonists - Tx. **switch the medicine**
  - o If it is due to hypothyroidism - Tx. **Levothyroxine**
  - o If it is due to pregnancy - Tx. **Bromocriptine**

2. ACROMEGALY

Acromegaly is characterized by **excess secretion of growth hormone**
Cause: Acromegaly is almost always caused by **pituitary adenoma**
Si/Sx: are discussed below

Symptoms of acromegaly

Physical	Deep voice, coarse facial feature, thick skinfold, increase in shoes size, hat size, gloves size, ring size
Cardiovascular	CHF, Cardiomegaly, HTN
Metabolic	Glucose intolerance or diabetes
Reproductive organs	Amenorrhea in women, and impotence in men
Others	Carpel tunnel syndrome, colonic polyps

Boards possible scenario: look for someone with deep voice, coarse facial feature, thick skinfold, increase in shoes size, hat size, gloves size, ring size

Diagnosis:

- **Best initial diagnostic test** is insulin-like growth factor-1 (IGF-1)
- **Most accurate test is glucose intolerance test:** 100 mg glucose is given to a patient, normal person shows suppressed growth hormone, but a **patient with acromegaly shows growth hormone levels > 5ng/ml**
- **MRI of the head** is done after glucose tolerance test to locate the tumor

Management:
- **Best initial treatment is transsphenoidal surgery, and follow IGF-1:**
  - **If IGF-1 is still high after the surgery, then treat the patient with octreotide** (somatostatin analog)
  - **If IGF-1 is still high after octreotide treatment, then give pegvisomant** (growth hormone receptor antagonist)

Complication: **Heart disease is the most common cause of death** in acromegaly

3. HYPOPITUITARISM

Hypopituitarism is a condition in which pituitary gland does not produce some or all of its hormones.
Pituitary gland produces ADH, ACTH, LH, FSH, GH, TSH, oxytocin, and prolactin
Cause: Head trauma, brain surgery, radiation, stroke, infection
Si/Sx: depends on which hormone is lacking
Diagnosis: hormone levels
Treatment: Pituitary hormone replacement therapy

4. EMPTY SELLA SYNDROME

Pituitary gland resides in sella turcica, when pituitary gland shrinks or becomes flatted, then **sella turcica appears empty on imaging,** and this condition is known as empty sella syndrome.
Risk factors: intracranial hypertension, injury, surgery, radiation
Si/Sx: most of the patients are **asymptomatic**, but symptoms may include headaches, low libido, erectile dysfunction
Diagnosis: CT or MRI of head shows empty sella
Treatment: symptomatic treatment

Boards tip:
- Question often tries to confuse empty sella syndrome with pseudotumor cerebri. To differentiate between them **get a CT or MRI of the head**: CT of empty sella syndrome shows empty sella, whereas CT of pseudotumor cerebri shows enlarge ventricles and pituitary gland in sella turcica

5. SHEEHAN SYNDROME

Sheehan syndrome also known as postpartum hypopituitarism, occurs in a woman who **bleeds severely during childbirth**, which causes the ischemic necrosis of the pituitary gland

Si/Sx: most common presentation is inability to lactate after delivery. Others symptoms may not develop for years after delivery, which may include loss of pubic and axillary hair, lack of menstrual bleeding, fatigue

Diagnosis:
- Blood pituitary hormone levels
- MRI of the head is usually performed to rule out pituitary tumor

Treatment:
- Pituitary hormone replacement therapy
- Estrogen and progesterone hormone replacement therapy until the normal age of menopause

6. PITUITARY APOPLEXY

Pituitary apoplexy is an endocrine emergency that occurs due to infarction or hemorrhage of pituitary gland

Si/Sx: sudden onset of headaches, visual deficits, altered mental status

Diagnosis: CT or MRI of the head

Treatment: Emergency surgery

SIADH

Inappropriate secretion of antidiuretic hormone (**SIADH**) is characterized by excess release of antidiuretic hormone. It causes euvolemic hyponatremia

Cause: SSRI, sulfonylureas, small cell cancer, **CNS** abnormality

Si/Sx: confusion, convulsion, fatigue, irritability, coma, headache, vomiting

Diagnosis:
- Urine osmolality > 20 mEq/L
- Plasma osmolality < 100 mOsm/kg
- Low serum osmolality < 290 mEq/L
- Urine Na > 20
- Normal BUN, creatinine, and bicarbonate

Treatment:

- Water restriction to 1L/day, which may increase the sodium by decreasing the total body water
- Vasopressin receptors antagonist (Tolvaptan or conivaptan) are used in emergency situation, to raise the sodium in euvolemic hyponatremia
- Demeclocycline is used in chronic SIADH, it works by inhibiting the ADHs action on the collecting ducts of the kidneys
- Treat the underlying cause

DIABETES INSIPIDUS

Diabetes insipidus is characterized by excessive thirst and excretion of diluted urine

Type and cause: two types of diabetes insipidus are:

- **Central diabetes** insipidus, it is caused by lack of ADH secretion from the pituitary gland.
    - o Risk factors include brain tumor, head injury, infection, ischemia and autoimmune disease
- **Nephrogenic diabetes** insipidus is caused by kidney's resistance to circulating ADH.
    - o Risk factors include kidney disease, hypercalcemia, hypokalemia, and drugs such as lithium, amphotericin B, and demeclocycline

Si/Sx: polyuria, polydipsia, excessive thirst, lethargy, irritability, muscle pain

Diagnosis:

- Water deprivation test: patient excretes dilute urine after restricted water intake
- **Vasopressin test:** patient's **urine osmolality is checked after the dose of ADH:**
    - o Patient with central **diabetes insipidus** shows increased urine osmolality after the test.
    - o Patient with **nephrogenic diabetes insipidus** shows no change in urine osmolality after the test.

Treatment:

- **Central diabetes insipidus** is treated with **vasopressin** (IM, IV, or spray, but oral)
- **Nephrogenic diabetes** is treated with salt restriction, increasing the water intake and correct underlying cause such as hypercalcemia or hypokalemia. Diuretics (hydrochlorothiazide or amiloride) or NSAIDs may be used in refractory cases.
- Treat the underlying cause

ENDOCIRNEOLOGY CCS

CASE # 1

Case introduction
A 39-years old white female comes to the office because of progressive weight loss, palpitations and diarrhea

Initial vitals signs
Temperature: 37.2 degrees
Pulse: 105 beats/min, regular rhythm
Respiration rate: 21/ minutes

Blood pressure, systolic 134 mm Hg
Blood pressure, disystolic, 85 mm Hg

Height: 68.0 inches
Weight: 122.0 lbs.
Body mass index: 18.6 Kg/m2

History of present illness (HPI)
A 39-years old white female comes to the office because of progressive weight loss, palpitations and diarrhea. She says the palpitations occur without any warning and resolve spontaneously. She has 2-3 bowel movements a day and has lost 15 lbs. in last three months despite good appetite. She also reports decreased menstruation duration. She denies any chest pain, shortness of breath and dizziness. She is sexually active with her husband. She denies any medical history

Past medical history
Hospitalization: None
Other medical condition: None
Current medication: None
Allergies: latex
Vaccination: up to date

Family history
Father has DM, and mother is healthy. Sister has hypothyroidism

Social history
Marital history: Married; 2 children
Occupation: Cashier
Recreational: Cooking, travel
Personal habits: Does not drink smoke, or use drugs

Review of system:
General: see HPI
Skin: see HPI
HEENT: see HPI
Musculoskeletal: see HPI
Cardiology: see HPI
Abdominal: see HPI
Genitourinary: see HPI

Please see pages 1-5 for general CCS cases approach

Step 1. None (patient is stable does not require any emergency measures)

Step 2. Order the complete physical exam (avoid rectal, genital and breast exam, unless it is needed). And move the clock forward
- Results shows:
- o HEENT exam shows nontender, enlarge thyroid.
- o Rest of the physical exam is normal

Step 3. Order following labs under" stat" options, and move the clock forward
- CBC
- UA
- BMP
- TSH
- T3, T4
- EKG

- Results shows:
- o CBC, BMP is WNL
- o EKG shows sinus tachycardia
- o TSH -0.076 µU/mL
- o T3 & T4 are elevated

Step 4. Propranolol + Methimazole

Step 5. Office

Step 6. None

Step 7. Move the clock forward to next appointment date. Patient comes back to the clinic. Order following labs and move the clock forward
- 24-hour radioiodine uptake (RAIU)
- LFTs

- Results shows:
  o RAIU shows increased uptake
  o LFTs are normal

Step 8. None

Step 9. Move the patient home and make a follow up appointment after 4 weeks

- Stop methimazole 4 days before the next follow up appointment.
- Give Radioiodine
- Make an another follow-up appointment after 4- 6weeks
- Move the clock forward to next appointment date
- Case should end here
-

Step 10. Counseling and screening

- No Smoking, drinking, illegal drug, safe sex
- Medicine compliance
- Age and gender specific screening

Case # 2

Case introduction
A 39-years old white female comes to the office because of fatigue, constipation, weight gain, and constipation

Initial vitals signs
Temperature: 37.2 degrees
Pulse: 68 beats/min, regular rhythm
Respiration rate: 18/ minutes

Blood pressure, systolic 123 mm Hg
Blood pressure, disystolic, 75 mm Hg

Height: 62.0 inches
Weight: 135.0 lbs.
Body mass index: 24.7 Kg/m2

History of present illness (HPI)
A 39-years old white female comes to the office because of fatigue, constipation, weight gain, and constipation. She has 1 bowel movement in a week and has gained 15 lbs. in last three months. She also reports decreased menstruation duration., dry skin and losing hair. She denies any chest pain, shortness of breath and dizziness. She is sexually active with her husband. She denies any medical history

Past medical history
Hospitalization: None
Other medical condition: None
Current medication: None
Allergies: latex
Vaccination: up to date

Family history
Father has DM, and mother has hypothyroidism. Sister is healthy

Social history
Marital history: Married; 2 children
Occupation: Cashier
Recreational: Cooking, travel
Personal habits: Does not drink smoke, or use drugs

Review of system:
General: see HPI
Skin: see HPI
HEENT: see HPI
Musculoskeletal: see HPI
Cardiology: see HPI
Abdominal: see HPI
Genitourinary: see HPI

Please see pages 1-5 for general CCS cases approach

Step 1. None (patient is stable does not require any emergency measures)

Step 2. Order the complete physical exam (avoid rectal, genital and breast exam, unless it is needed). And move the clock forward
- Results shows:
- o Obese patient
- o Skin is cool and dry
- o Neurology exam shows delayed knee reflex

Step 3. Order following labs and move the clock forward to get EKG results
- CBC
- UA
- BMP
- TSH routine
- T3, T4 routine
- EKG " stat"

- EKG shows:
- o Sinus Bradycardia

Step 4. None

Step 5. Schedule next appointment when thyroid labs will be available, and move the patient home

Step 6. None

Step 7. Move the clock forward to get the labs results, and then move it forward to next appointment date
- Labs show
- o TSH is 26 μU/ml
- o T3 & T4 are within normal limit

Step 8. None

Step 9. Order lipid panel and make a follow up appointment after 6 weeks

Step 10. Counsel and screening
- No smoking, drinking and illegal drugs
- Safe sex
- Medicine compliance
- Seat belts use
- Age and gender specific counseling

Diagnosis: **Hypothyroidism**

ELECTROLYTES

SODIUM
Normal range of sodium (Na^+) is 135 - 145 mEq/L

HYPERNATREMIA
Hypernatremia refers to the condition in which body's sodium is >145mEq/L
Si/Sx: weakness, lethargy, and neurologic abnormalities such as seizure, irritability, confusion, or coma
Causes
- Central diabetes insipidus
- Nephrogenic diabetes insipidus
- Diuretic, DKA
- Infection

Diagnosis: sodium levels, urine osmolality
Treatment of hypernatremia: depends on patient's condition
- If the patient has **acute hypernatremia** or **low blood pressure, then** give **IV normal saline** to expand the volume and correct the blood pressure
- If the patient is **unstable** or has **neurologic abnormalities**, then give **IV D5W or ½ normal saline**, with maximum correction 1 mEq/hour, otherwise, patient may develop cerebral edema
- If the patient is **stable and has normal blood pressure, then give oral water and treat underlying cause**

HYPONATREMIA
Hyponatremia refers to the condition in which body's sodium is <135mEq/L
Si/Sx: confusion, convulsion, fatigue, irritability, coma, headache, vomiting
Cause:
- **Pseudohyponatremia:** Every 100 mg/dl glucose above the normal limit, decrease sodium by 1.6 mEq/L
- **Hypervolemia:** CHF, cirrhosis, nephrotic syndrome
- **Hypovolemia:** diarrhea, vomiting, sweating, renal insufficiency, low aldosterone

- **Euvolemic**: hypothyroidism, psychogenic, polydipsia, SIADH, oxytocin

Treatment:

- If the patient is **stable,** then **restrict the water intake to 1 L/day**
- If the patient is **confused** or has **mild symptoms,** then give **normal saline and loop diuretics**
- If the patient has **severe symptoms** (seizure, coma), then give **3 % hypertonic saline, but** do not exceed > 0.5mEq/ hour or 12mEq in a day otherwise patient may develop **central pontine myelinolysis**
- A stable patient with pseudohyponatremia is treated by **correcting the glucose level**

POTASSIUM

Normal range of potassium (K^+) is 3.5 - 5.5 mEq/L

HYPERKALEMIA

Hyperkalemia refers to the condition in which body's potassium is >5.5 mEq/L

Si/Sx: weakness, muscle weakness and palpitation. High potassium may cause cardiac arrhythmias or sudden cardiac death

Causes of hyperkalemia include:

- Acidosis, aldosterone deficiency, ACE inhibitors, ARBS
- Beta-blockers
- Crush injury
- Digitalis, insulin deficiency
- Renal, RTA type IV

Diagnosis:

- Blood potassium level
- EKG, which usually shows **peaked T wave, absent P wave and prolong PR** interval in hyperkalemia

Treatment:

- If EKG shows **arrhythmias, then** give **calcium gluconate** (stabilizes the cardiac cell membrane) followed by **IV Insulin** (drives K^+ into the cell), **glucose** (given to prevent hypoglycemia), IV **sodium bicarbonate** (shifts K^+ into the cell) and **kayexalate** (removes potassium from the body)

- If **EKG** is normal, then give **IV insulin, glucose,** sodium **bicarbonate** and **kayexalate**
- If patient has a renal failure or medicines are ineffective, then do **dialysis**

Note: beta-blockers also drive potassium into the cell, and may be given when other options are not available

---

Key to approach hyperkalemia case

Initial step is to look at EKG if the patient has any EKG abnormalities, then give IV calcium gluconate. Rest of the treatment for hyperkalemia, with or without any EKG changes is the same: IV Insulin, glucose, sodium bicarbonate and kayexalate

---

Pseudohyperkalemia refers to a condition in which potassium is >5.5 mEq/L, but patient has **no symptoms** of hyperkalemia. It is commonly caused by hemolysis that occurs during venipuncture. No treatment is required; just repeat the blood potassium level.

HYPOKALEMIA
Hypokalemia refers to the condition in which body potassium is < 3.5mEq/L
Si/Sx: muscle weakness, spasm, constipation, fatigue, palpitations
Causes of hypokalemia include:
- Amphotericin, Hyperaldosterone
- Batters syndrome
- Diuretics, Distal RTA
- Proximal RTA

Diagnosis:
- Blood potassium level
- EKG usually shows U wave

Treatment:

- If the patient is **unstable, has arrhythmia or ileus, then** give **IV K⁺**. However, do not exceed IV K⁺ > 0 .5 mEq /hour and make sure that the patient is attached to the EKG, to monitor the EKG changes
- If the patient is **stable,** then give **oral potassium replacement.** There is no maximum or minimum limit for oral K⁺ replacement

Complication: Rhabdomyolysis

Note: Avoid giving dextrose-containing fluids to a patient with hypokalemia because dextrose drives K⁺ into the cell and may worsen the hypokalemia

---

Key to distinguish sodium from potassium imbalance is to look at cardiac and neurology abnormalities:

- **Sodium** imbalance **does not cause** any **cardiac abnormalities,** and **potassium does not cause** any **neurologic abnormalities**

CALCIUM

Normal calcium (ca²⁺) range is 8.5- 10.5 mEq/L

HYPERCALCEMIA

Hypercalcemia is the condition in which body's calcium is > 10.5 mEq/L
Cause:

- **Primary hyperparathyroidism** (most common cause)
- Familial **hypocalciuric** hypercalcemia
- Malignancy: **squamous cell carcinoma (PTH-like protein)**
- Granulomatous disease (Sarcoidosis)
- **TB, berylliosis, histoplasmosis**
- Thiazide, **vitamin D intoxication**

Si/Sx: symptoms includes:

- Neurologic: **decreased mental activity**
- GI: **constipation, anorexia**
- Renal: nephrogenic **diabetes** insipidus, **kidney stone**

Diagnosis:
- Check serum calcium levels, serum PTH levels, serum vitamin D level, and urine calcium
- EKG shows **decreased QT interval**

Treatment: depends on the followings:
- If the patient is **unstable, symptomatic or calcium is >14 mg/dl,** then give **IV hydration,** followed by **furosemide.** If this is ineffective, or there is a need to lower the calcium promptly, then give **calcitonin**
- If the patient is **stable patient or asymptomatic,** then give **oral bisphosphonates** (pamidronate)
- **If a stable** patient has a **granulomatous disease,** then give **steroids**

Important: In **familial hypocalciuric hypercalcemia** urine calcium is < 200mg/day or spot urine calcium is < 0.01 mg

HYPOCALCEMIA
Hypocalcemia refers to the condition in which calcium is <8.5mEq/L
Cause
- Parathyroidectomy
- Hypomagnesemia
- Hyperphosphatemia
- Pseudohypoparathyroidism (kidney resistance to parathyroid - patients have short 4th figure, mental retardation)
- Renal failure
- Vitamin D deficiency

Symptoms: symptoms include:
- Seizure, depression
- Cramping, Tetany (Chvostek sign, Trousseau sign)

Diagnosis:
- Calcium level, calcium levels bound to albumin
- EKG shows **increased QT interval**

Management:
- **Oral** calcium replacement
- If hypocalcemia is due to **vitamin D deficiency, then treat the patient with** vitamin D and **calcium** replacement

- If hypocalcemia is due to **hyperphosphatemia, then** treat the patient with **phosphate binders (calcium carbonate, calcium acetate) and calcium replacement**

Note: Hypocalcemia caused by renal failure shows low ca^{2+} and high phosphate, whereas hypocalcemia caused by vitamin D deficiency shows low ca^{2+} and low phosphate

MAGNESIUM
Normal magnesium range is 1.5 -2.5 mEq/L

HYPOMAGNESEMIA
Hypomagnesemia is the condition in which body's magnesium is < 1.5 mEq/L
Symptoms: abnormal eye movement, fatigue, convulsion, muscle spasm, muscle weakness, numbness
Cause: causes include:
- Alcohol withdrawal
- Drugs: loop diuretics, gentamicin, cisplatin

Treatment: magnesium replacement

Complications: hypocalcemia, torsades de pointes

HYPERMAGNESEMIA
Hypermagnesemia is the condition in which body's magnesium is >2.5 mEq/L
Symptoms: muscle weakness, loss of deep tendon reflexes (DTR), hypotension, hypocalcemia, arrhythmia, bradycardia
Cause:
- Magnesium containing laxative
- **MgSo₄ (seizure prophylaxis given during labor and delivery)**
- **Real failure**
- DKA, adrenal insufficiency

Management:
- ABCs and intubate the patient, if needed
- IV saline
- Last resort is dialysis

HEAT DISORDERS

1. HEAT CRAMPS
Heat cramps is a mild heat disorder that occurs due to loss of large amount of water and salt during exercise
Si/Sx: painful, involuntary muscle contraction, muscle tenderness. **Normal body temperature**, patient is able to **sweat and has no neurological** abnormalities
Treatment: rest, oral hydration and electrolyte replacement

2. HEAT EXHAUSTION
Heat exhaustion is a severe heat disorder
Si/Sx: muscle and abdominal cramps, weakness, fatigue and dizziness. Body temperature may be **slightly elevated**; patient is able to sweat and may have **mild neurological abnormalities** such as headaches, anxiety
Treatment: rest, oral hydration and electrolyte replacement. Patients with severe weakness may require IV fluids

3. HEAT STROKE
Heat stroke is a life-threatening condition
Si/Sx: body temperature is **elevated (>104 F), patient has lost his ability to sweat, severe neurological abnormalities** such as confusion, disorientation, and blurry vision
Diagnosis: clinical diagnosis, but labs show increased BUN/Cr, increased WBCs, hemoconcentration
Treatment: IV fluids, rapid cooling, place the patient in a cool environment, spray water and fanned to evaporate the fluids. Chlorpromazine or diazepam may be used to control shivering.

Note: Do not immerse the patient in ice water because that can result in overcooling and hypothermia

HYPOTHERMIA
Hypothermia is a medical emergency in which body's core temperature falls below the required temperature (95.0 F) for normal metabolism and body function
Cause: alcohol, water immersion

Si/Sx: mild hypothermia can cause shivering, HTN, tachycardia, and tachypnea. **Moderate hypothermia** causes violent shivering, muscle incoordination and mild confusion. **Severe hyperthermia** causes altered consciousness and arrhythmia, which can lead to death.

Diagnosis:
- Core body temperature
- EKG usually shows arrhythmia, most characteristic feature of hypothermia is an elevation of **J point**, also knows as Osborn J wave, which can be mistaken for ST elevation MI

Treatment: Rewarming measures such as warm bed, warm bath or covering patient in a warm blanket. Warm IV fluids can be used in severe hypothermia. CPR should be continued during rewarming.

SHOCK

Shock is a life-threating condition that occurs due to inadequate blood flow and perfusion.

Causes and symptoms
1. **Cardiogenic shock** is usually caused by heart condition such as MI, CHF. Patient usually presents with **JVD, pale and cold skin**
2. **Hypovolemic shock** is caused by fluid loss, in conditions such vomiting, diarrhea, use of diuretics. Patients usually present with **cold and pale skin**
3. **Septic shock** is caused by infections such as E.coli, S. aureus. Patients usually have **fever, and warm skin**
4. **Neurogenic shock** is caused by damage to the nervous system. Patients usually have **warm skin.**

Differential diagnosis of shock

Type of shock	HR	CO	PCWP	SVR
Septic shock	Increased	**Increased**	Decreased	Decreased
Cardiogenic shock	Increased	Decreased	**Increased**	**Increased**
Hypovolemia shock	Increased	Decreased	Decreased	**Increased**
Neurogenic shock	Increased	Decreased	Decreased	Decreased

HR = heart rate, CO= cardiac output, PCWP= pulmonary capillary wedge pressure, SVR= Systemic vascular resistance

Treatment: maintaining ABCs (airway, breathing and circulation) is the primary goal. Give bolus of fluids and reassess the patient. If fluids does not increase the blood pressure, then vasopressor may be required. Vasopressors and their mechanism is as follow:

- Norepinephrine increases the peripheral vascular resistance and maintains the organ perfusion
- Dopamine at low dose keep the kidneys perfused, at high dose it increases the heart contractility, and at the highest dose it causes vasoconstriction
- Dobutamine increases the heart contractility

ANAPHYLAXIS

Anaphylaxis is a life-threatening allergic reaction that occur within seconds or minutes after exposure of allergen, such as bee stings, medicines or peanuts

Si/Sx: **wheezing, difficulty breathing, hypotension, weak rapid pulses**

Treatment: Immediately secure the airway, subcutaneous epinephrine, corticosteroids and H1 antihistamine

NEPHROLOGY

ACUTE RENAL FAILURE

Acute renal failure is characterized by sudden decline in kidney's function, which leads to abnormal clearance of waste products, fluids and electrolytes.

Cause: three main causes of acute renal failure are:

- Prerenal failure
- Intrarenal failure
- Postrenal failure

Differential diagnosis of acute renal failure

Test	Prerenal failure	Intrarenal failure	Postrenal failure
BUN/Cr ratio	> 20	< 15	> 15
Urine Na	< 20	> 20	> 40
Urine fractional Na excretion	< 1%	> 2%	> 4%
Urine osmolality	> 500	< 350	< 350
Urine analysis	Hyaline cast	Muddy brown cast, RBC cast, or eosinophils	White cell casts

PRERENAL FAILURE

Prerenal failure is an abrupt loss of renal function that is caused by decreased blood flow to the kidneys

DIFFERENTIAL DIAGNOSIS AND TREATMENT OF PRERENAL FAILURE

1. **Dehydration** is the most common cause of prerenal failure. Treatment: IV fluids and electrolytes replacement. Diuretics are also given to prevent the fluid overload

2. **Congestive heart failure (CHF):** it is treated with IV hydration, diuretics and other treatment as per CHF

3. **Cirrhosis:** it is treated with IV hydration, diuretics and other treatment as per cirrhosis

4. **Shock:** two most commonly tested shocks are toxic shock and adrenal shock
   - **Toxic shock** syndrome is treated with **IV fluids, antibiotics and dopamine**
   - **Adrenal shock** is treated with **IV fluids and prednisone**

5. **Renal artery stenosis:** it is treated with angioplasty

6. **Hepatorenal renal syndrome**
   Look for a patient with prerenal failure and preexisting liver disease. It is usually diagnosed as follow:
   - Urine osmolality is measured before and after giving 1.5 L normal saline. Patient with hepatorenal renal syndrome shows **no change in urine osmolality after receiving 1.5 L saline**

   Treatment: Liver transplant

7. **ACE inhibitors (ACEIs)**
   - Mechanism: ACEIs work by **dilating the efferent arterioles.** However, patient with preexisting renal failure has **constricted efferent arterioles to maintain the glomerular perfusion.** When a patient takes ACEIs, **it dilates the efferent arterioles, which decreases the renal perfusion and leads to pre-renal failure or exacerbation of pre-existing pre-renal failure**

   - Management: **depends on creatinine levels**
     - If creatinine **is increased ≥ 30 %**, then stop **ACEIs**
     - If creatinine **is increased**, but is **≤ 30 %**, then **continue ACEIs** because the benefits of keeping patient in ACEIs outweighs the risks

POSTRENAL FALIURE

Postrenal failure occurs when an obstruction in the urinary tract system below the kidneys interrupts the urine flow and wastes build up in the kidneys.

Cause: causes of postrenal failure are:

- Obstruction of ureters by stones, stricture, or blood clots
- Benign prostatic hyperplasia
- Cervical cancer
- Retroperitoneal fibrosis
- Neurogenic bladder (multiple sclerosis, spinal cord injury)

Diagnosis:

- Physical exam **shows distended bladder**
- BUN/Cr ratio **>15:1**
- Urine **Na >40**
- Urine fractional excretion of **Na > 4%**
- Urine osmolality **< 350**
- **Urinalysis (UA) shows white cell cast**
- **CT or ultrasound** shows **bilateral hydronephrosis**
- **Post residual** volume **> 50 ml**

Management:

- **Best initial management is to** relieve the obstruction with foley **catheter,** then give fluid **and replace electrolytes,** and treat the underlying cause, such as
  - If patient has **BPH,** then give **prazosin or terazosin**
  - If patient has **neurogenic bladder,** then give **bethanechol**
  - If patient has **kidney stone,** then **treat as per stone management**
- Dialysis, if needed

INTRARENAL FAILURE

Intrarenal failure is caused by **direct damage to the kidneys** due to accumulation of the **toxic metabolites**

Diagnosis

- BUN/Cr ratio **close to 10:1**
- Urine sodium **>20**
- Urine fractional excretion Na **>2%**

- Urine osmolality **<350**

Differential diagnosis of intrarenal failure

1. ACUTE PAPILLARY NECROSIS

Acute papillary necrosis is characterized by necrosis of some or all of renal medullary pyramids and papillae

Cause: most common cause is NSAIDs, but other causes may include sickle cell anemia, kidney transplant rejection

Si/Sx: are **similar to pyelonephritis** such as **fever, flank pain, CVA tenderness**

Diagnosis:

- Best initial test is UA, which shows **WBCs, but no bacteria**
- **Most accurate test is CT scan,** which shows **irregular renal contours**

Treatment:

- Treat the underlying cause, and stop NSAIDs, if applicable

Exam tip:

- Question often tries to confuse acute papillary necrosis with pyelonephritis. Best way to distinguish them is to get abdominal CT scan, which shows irregular renal contours in acute papillary necrosis

---

2. RHABDOMYOLYSIS

Rhabdomyolysis is a condition in which damaged muscle cell release **toxic metabolites** such as myoglobin, which affects the kidneys and leads to kidney failure

Cause: muscle damage is caused by strenuous exercise, prolong immobility, statins, hypokalemia, crush injury, seizure

Diagnosis:

- **Best initial test is UA, which shows RBCs on urine dipstick,** but **no RBCs are seen on microscopy urine analysis**
- **Most accurate test** is **urine myoglobin**
- **Creatine phosphokinase (cpk)** levels are elevated
- **Potassium** may be elevated

Management:

- **Most urgent step** is to get an **EKG** because rhabdomyolysis causes **hyperkalemia**, which can lead to arrhythmia (EKG in hyperkalemia shows peaked T, loss of P-wave and widened QRS)

  - If EKG shows **arrhythmia**, then give **IV calcium gluconate, insulin, glucose sodium bicarbonate and kayexalate**
  - If EKG shows **no arrhythmia** or after treating arrhythmia, then give bolus of IV fluids, and then mannitol, and diuretic.

- If urine pH is acidic, then also give sodium bicarbonate to alkalinize the urine and decrease precipitation of myoglobin in renal tubules

Complication: increased creatine phosphokinase (cpk) increases the risk of developing compartment syndrome

3. CHOLESTEROL EMBOLIZATION

Cholesterol embolization refers to embolization of cholesterol usually from atherosclerotic plaque, which can travel to kidney via blood and causes intrarenal failure

Risk factors: medical procedures such as **vascular surgery, angiography**

Si/Sx: most common symptoms are **bluish discoloration of fingers and or toes**

Diagnosis:

- Best initial test is **UA with Wright-Hansel stain** that shows **increased eosinophils**
- **Most accurate test is skin biopsy**, which shows **cholesterol crystals**

Treatment: supportive care

4. ACUTE INTERSTITIAL NEPHRITIS (AIN)

Acute interstitial nephropathy is characterized by inflammatory infiltrate and edema in the renal interstitium.

Cause: infections, or reaction to the medicine, but reaction to medicine accounts for 71-92% cases. Medicines that cause this reaction are:

- Penicillin
- Sulfonamide
- Diuretics

- NSAIDs
- Phenytoin
- Rifampin
- Allopurinol
- H2 blockers

Si/Sx: Fever, **maculopapular rash**, flank pain, swelling of the body, change in mental status

Diagnosis:
- Best initial test is **UA with Wright-Hansel stain** that shows **increased eosinophils**
- To **distinguish if AIN is caused by NSAIDs or from other drugs**, check **urine protein:**
  - If urine protein is **> 3.5 grams, then it is NSAIDs** induced AIN
  - If urine protein is **< 3.5 grams, then it is** other drugs induced AIN such as **sulfa, allopurinol, H2 blockers**

Treatment:
- Most of the AIN **spontaneously resolve** after removing the offending drug or treating the underlying infection.
- If the patient continues to have renal failure, then give **steroids**

5. ETHYLENE GLYCOL POISONING

Ethylene glycol poisoning is caused by ingestion of ethylene, usually automotive **antifreeze** and hydraulic brake fluid. It is extremely toxic and can lead to intrarenal failure

Diagnosis:
- Best initial test is UA, which shows **envelop shaped crystals**
- Labs show **high anion gap metabolic acidosis**

Treatment: Best initial treatment is **IV fomepizole**, which prevents the formation of crystals by inhibiting dehydrogenase, and then do **dialysis**

Exam tip:
Question often try to confuse ethylene glycol poisoning with methanol glycol poisoning. Remember:
- **Methanol glycol poising affects eye and CNS, whereas ethylene glycol poisoning affects kidneys**
- Treatment for both types of poisoning is the same

---

6. CONTRAST INDUCED RENAL FAILURE

Contrast induced renal failure refers to renal failure that occurs after exposure of contrast material such as angiography, contrast CT

Diagnosis:
- Best initial test is UA, which shows **muddy brown casts**

Treatment: IV hydration

Prevention:

Contrast induced renal failure can be prevented by the following:
- Give IV normal saline and bicarbonate or N-acetyl cysteine, or both before performing contrast imaging
- In **DM patients** stop oral hypoglycemic medicines at least 48 hours in advance, and give IV normal and bicarbonate or N-acetylcysteine before performing contrast imaging

7. TUMOR LYSIS SYNDROME

Tumor lysis syndrome is a **compilation of chemotherapy** that causes severe electrolytes abnormalities and leads to renal failure

Diagnosis:
- Best initial test is microscopic UA, which shows **urate crystal**

Treatment: IV fluids and sodium bicarbonate

Prevention:
- Tumor lysis syndrome can be prevented by giving IV hydration and allopurinol before chemotherapy

---

Boards tips to solve renal cases:
- Best initial test is UA, then check BUN/Cr to check for pre-, intra- or post-renal case
- Then go back to the case and check the recent history to see what contributed to the symptoms
- Treat the underlying cause
- Dialysis is for refractory case

Indications for dialysis are:	Mnemonic: **AEIOU**
• Acid-base disorder	
• Electrolyte abnormality	
• Intoxication	
• Volume overload	
• Uremia (uremic encephalopathy, uremic pericarditis)	

MAIN DIFFERENCESES IN NEPHROTIC AND NEPHRITIC SYNDROME

	Nephrotic syndrome	**Nephritic syndrome**
Si/Sx	Hematuria, hypertension, oliguria, azotemia	Protein urea, hypoalbuminemia, hyperlipidemia, generalized edema
UA	Fatty casts in urine	RBC and granular casts in urine

NEPHRITIS SYNDROME

Nephritis syndrome is a group of conditions, which causes inflammation of the internal structures of the kidney.

1. **POSTSTREPTOCOCCAL (POSTINFECTIOUS) GLOMERULONEPHRITIS (PSGN/PIGN)**

   PSGN/PIGN is a nephritis syndrome that can occur after any infection, but commonly occurs after infection with **Group A-hemolytic streptococcus bacteria:**
   - **1-2 weeks after pharyngitis**
   - **3-6 weeks after impetigo**

   Si/Sx: **triad of periorbital edema, smoky-brown urine, and hypertension**
   Diagnosis:
   - Urinalysis shows RBCs casts, **smoky-brown urine**
   - Best initial test is **low serum C3 complement level, anti-DNase antibodies, and increased antistreptolysin O (ASO)**
   - **Most accurate** test is **renal biopsy**, which shows **lumpy-bumpy** granular deposits of IgG and C3 in the basement membrane

Note: Biopsy is rarely required to diagnose PSGN; blood tests are sufficient to make diagnosis

Treatment: there is no specific treatment for PSGN/PIGN. **Treatment is directed towards symptoms**, which is as follow:
- Antibiotics such as penicillin, is given for streptococcal bacteria
- Anti-hypertensive medicines such as calcium channel blockers or ACE inhibitors, may be needed for hypertension
- Diuretics to prevent fluid overload

2. GOODPASTURE SYNDROME
Goodpasture syndrome is an **autoimmune disorder** that affects the **kidneys and lungs**
Si/Sx: hematuria, hemoptysis, shortness of breath
Diagnosis
- CBC shows iron deficiency anemia
- Best initial test is blood test, which shows anti-basement membrane antibodies
- **Most accurate test is a biopsy of lungs or kidney**; do the lung biopsy first if it is inconclusive, then do kidney biopsy
  - Biopsy of lungs show hemosiderin-laden macrophage
  - Biopsy of kidney shows smooth linear deposits of IgG

Treatment: Plasmapheresis

3. IgA NEPHROPATHY
IgA nephropathy is also known as Berger disease is the most common cause of glomerulonephritis in the world.
Si/Sx: Episodic hematuria that occurs **1-2 days after infection** such as upper respiratory infection, urinary tract infection
Diagnosis:
- Blood test shows normal C3
- **Best initial test** is **urine immunoelectrophoresis** to measure IgA, but IgA levels are increased only in half of the patients
- **Most accurate test** is kidney biopsy, which shows proliferation of the mesangium with IgA deposit on immunofluorescence or electron microscope.

Treatment: There is no specific treatment to cure IgA nephropathy. Approximately 50% of the patient will progress to end-stage renal failure. Treatment is given to slow the progression to chronic renal failure, which is as follow:

- **Fish oil** can be given to a stable person, it **slows the disease progression**
- **Angiotensin-converting enzyme (ACE) inhibitors** are given to patients with **severe proteinuria**
- **Steroids** are given to patient with **acute flares or if the condition is worsening,** these works by suppressing the immune system

---

Boards tip:
Question often tries to trick IgA nephropathy with post-streptococcal glomerulonephritis (PSGN). Remember, **IgA** nephropathy occurs 1-2 **days** after infection, whereas PSGN occurs 1-6 **weeks** after the infection

---

4. WEGNER'S GRANULOMATOSIS

Wegner's granulomatosis is a systemic vasculitis (causes inflammation of the blood vessels) of small and medium sized vessels in many organs. It mainly affects the **kidney, upper and lower respiratory tract**, but it can also affect other organs such as skin, eyes, GI, joints and CNS.

Cause: unknown etiology

Si/Sx: fever, cough, **sinusitis, hemoptysis, hematuria,** joint ache

Diagnosis:

- Chest X-ray shows cavities in lung
- **Best initial test is** anti-neutrophil cytoplasmic autoantibodies **(ANCA),** which is also known as **anti-proteinase-3 antibody**
- **Most accurate test** is a **biopsy of the affected organ** such as kidney, lungs or skin; always do biopsy of **least invasive site first**, if it is inconclusive then move to next less invasive site. For example, start with skin, then lungs and then kidney
  - Biopsy of the kidney shows segmental necrotizing glomerulonephritis.

Treatment: prednisone plus immunosuppressive (azathioprine, methotrexate, or cyclophosphamide)

5. CHURG-STRAUSS SYNDROME

Churg-Strauss syndrome is similar to Wegner's granulomatosis and is also known as **eosinophilic granulomatosis**. It affects the small and medium size blood vessels in may organs in a person with **asthma, eosinophilia and atopy**

Si/Sx: fever, cough **asthma, hemoptysis, hematuria**
Diagnosis:

- **Best initial test is elevated eosinophils and positive P-ANCA or anti-myeloperoxidase**
- **Most accurate test is biopsy of lungs or kidneys;** do the biopsy of lungs first, if it is inconclusive, then do biopsy of kidneys

Treatment: prednisone and cyclophosphamide

6. POLYARTERITIS NODOSA

Polyarteritis nodosa is a systemic vasculitis (causes inflammation of the blood vessels) of small-and medium sized vessels in many organs. It mainly affects the kidney; it can also affect any other organ such as skin, eyes, GI, joints and CNS, **but it spare lungs**

Cause: unknown etiology, but it can be **associated with hepatitis B or C**

Si/Sx: Fever, hematuria, abdominal pain, abdominal pain, decreased appetite

Diagnosis:

- Initial test is blood test, which **shows increased WBCs, ESR, and C-reactive protein**
- **Angiography** shows aneurysm or narrowing of affected blood vessels
- **Most accurate test** is biopsy of the **kidney or sural nerve**

Treatment: prednisone plus immunosuppressive (Azathioprine, methotrexate, or cyclophosphamide)

Other important points about Polyarteritis nodosa

- If angiography is already performed, then there is no need to do biopsy of kidney or sural never
- All patient with Polyarteritis nodosa should also be **tested for Hepatitis B and C** because it is associated with hepatitis B or C infection

Boards tips:

- Wegner's granulomatosis - look for a patient with **sinusitis, hemoptysis, hematuria**
- Churg-Strauss syndrome- look for a patient with **asthma, hemoptysis, hematuria**
- Polyarteritis nodosa- looks for a patient with **hematuria and motor and sensory pain** from all organs, but **no respiratory complaints**

7. CRYOGLOBULINEMIA

Cryoglobulinemia is a condition in which cryoglobulin proteins, mostly immunoglobulins, become **insoluble** and builds up the body

Cause: in 90 % of the cases it is caused by **hepatitis C**, but other causes my include HIV infection, autoimmune disease

Si/Sx: **hematuria, joint pain, purpuric skin lesions**

Diagnosis:
- **Best initial test is serum cryoglobulins components** -monoclonal immunoglobulin, usually **IgM, and light chains**
- Most accurate test is **biopsy**

Treatment :Interferon and ribavirin

Boards tip for Cryoglobulinemia
- Look for **hepatitis C patient or IV drug user** (look for needle tracks on arms) with **hematuria**

8. ALPORT SYNDROME

Alport syndrome is a genetic defect of type IV collagen; it causes glomerulonephritis, hearing and visual disturbance

Si/Sx: hematuria, hearing loss, decreased vision or vision loss

Diagnosis: renal biopsy: electron microscope shows glomerular **basement membrane splitting**

Treatment: There no specific treatment for Alport syndrome, treatment is directed towards symptoms

NEPHROTIC SYNDROME

- All nephrotic syndromes show the followings:
  - o **Edema**
  - o Hyperlipidemia
  - o Hypoproteinemia
  - o Proteinuria > 3.5 g in 24 hours

- Most accurate test of nephrotic is renal biopsy

- Patients with nephrotic syndrome are at increased risk of thromboembolism because protein C and protein S are lost in the urine

Differential diagnosis of nephrotic syndrome

1. MINIMAL CHANGE DISEASE
Minimal change disease is the most common cause of nephrotic syndrome in children
Cause: unknown etiology, but risk factors include NSAIDs, tumors, vaccinations, and viral infections
Diagnosis: kidney biopsy shows electron microscope shows **fusion of foot process**
Treatment:
- If patient has **respiratory compromise**, then admit the patient and treat with albumin infusion and furosemide
- If patient has **normal respiratory** function, then treat as follow:
  - o Best Initial therapy is **steroids and ACE inhibitors or ARBs**
  - o If that is **ineffective**, then give cyclophosphamide or cyclosporine

2. FOCAL SEGMENTAL GLOMERULOSCLEROSIS
Focal segmental glomerulosclerosis is kidney disease in which some parts ("segmental") of the glomerulus are sclerosed
Cause: idiopathic, **heroin, HIV, diabetes, sickle cell disease, diabetes**
Diagnosis: kidney biopsy shows **sclerosis in capillary tufts**
Treatment: Prednisone and cyclophosphamide
Prognosis: More than half of the patients progress to end stage renal disease

3. MEMBRANOUS GLOMERULONEPHRITIS

Membranous glomerulonephritis is the most common cause of nephrotic syndrome in adults. It is characterized by basement membrane thickening
Cause: causes include:
- Cancers, specially lung and colon cancer
- Infection: HBV, HCV, syphilis, malaria
- Medicines: gold salts, penicillamine
- Autoimmune disease: SLE, rheumatoid arthritis, Graves' disease

Diagnosis:
- o Kidney biopsy; electron microscopy shows **"spike and dome"** appearance, which is due to IgG and C3 immune, complex in a basement membrane

Treatment: Prednisone and cyclophosphamide
Prognosis: 50% of the patients progress to end-stage kidney failure
Complication: this condition is associated with occult malignancies, therefore it important to do **age and gender appropriated cancer screening**

4. MEMBRANOPROLIFERATIVE GLOMERULONEPHRITIS (MPGN)

MPGN is characterized by deposits in the glomerular mesangium, and glomerular basement membrane thickening. It can present with **nephritis or nephrotic features**
Cause: HBV, HCV, CLL, SLE
Type: two types of MPGN are:
- Type 1 MPGN is characterized by subendothelial and mesangial immune deposits
- Type 2 MPGN is less common than type 1. It is associated with autoantibodies against C3 nephritic factor (C3 convertase)

Diagnosis: diagnosis is confirmed with **kidney biopsy**
- Type 1 MPGN shows **immune complex deposits** and abnormal mesangial cell proliferation between glomeruli basement membrane and endothelial cells, which gives **" tram-track "** appearance of the capillary wall
- Type 2 MPGN shows **dense deposits** along glomeruli basement membrane

Treatment: There is no cure for MPGN. Treatment is given to control the symptoms and slow the disease progression:

- Steroids and cyclophosphamide
- Anti-hypertensive medicine and diuretics are given for HTN

Screening: Screen all patients for **HBV and HCV infection**

Prognosis: MPGN has a poor prognosis. It often slowly progresses to kidney failure

5. DIABETIC NEPHROPATHY

Diabetic nephropathy also known as Kimmelstiel-Wilson syndrome is the most common cause of ERSD in United States. It is generally caused by long-standing **poorly controlled diabetes**

Diagnosis:

- UA shows microalbuminuria
- Kidney biopsy with light microscopy shows **mesangial expansion but sometimes is may show nodules, mesangial hypercellularity, and glomerular basement membrane thickening.**

Treatment: Strict glucose control, and ACE inhibitors to slow the renal progression to ESRD

6. RENAL AMYLOIDOSIS

Amyloidosis is a group of conditions in which abnormal proteins are deposited in the extracellular space of organs. Renal amyloidosis is result of **amyloidosis deposits in the renal.**

Association: it is associated with immune cell disorder such as multiple myeloma, inflammatory diseases

Diagnosis: biopsy of affected organ or fat pad; stain biopsied tissue with Congo red; stain shows **apple-green birefringence**

Treatment:

- Prednisone and melphalan
- Renal transplant is reserved for refractory disease

7. LUPUS NEPHRITIS

Systemic lupus erythematosus (SLE) is an autoimmune disease that can affect any organ. Lupus nephritis is a **complication of SLE**

Diagnosis:

- Blood test shows **antinuclear antibody and anti-double stranded DNA**
- Most accurate test is **renal biopsy**. World health organization (WHO) has classified lupus nephritis in 5 types based on the biopsy findings.

Treatment: treatment depends on the biopsy findings (see table below)

Lupus nephritis stages and treatment

Type	Biopsy finding	Treatment
Type I	**Normal appearing kidney**	None
Type II	**Mesangial proliferation**	Symptomatic treatment only
Type III	**Focal segmental proliferation**	Prednisone and mycophenolate
Type IV	**Diffuse proliferative** • May present with combination of nephrotic and nephritic disease • Light microscope shows **wire-loop abnormality**	Prednisone and mycophenolate
Type V	**Membranous disease**	There is no clear beneficial treatment. Prednisone may help

END-STAGE RENAL DISEASE (ESRD)

End-stage renal failure defined as a complete kidney failure; that they no longer able to work at the level required to for day-to-day life. People often need dialysis or kidney transplant

Cause: Two most common causes are diabetes and high blood pressure; other causes may include glomerulonephritis, polycystic kidney disease, pyelonephritis, renal artery stenosis, long-term NSAIDs use

Si/Sx: Headaches, anorexia, fatigue, convulsion, pericarditis, bruising

Treatment for ESRD:
- Salt and water restriction, protein restriction
- Dialysis to correct the acid-base or electrolytes abnormalities,
- Treat the other complications (discussed below)

Complication of ESRD

Complication	Cause/ characteristic	Treatment
Anemia	Normochromic normocytic anemia, due to **decreased** production of **erythropoietin**	Erythropoietin
Coagulopathy	Platelet count is normal, but bleeding is prolonged because of **defect in platelet degranulation**	DDAVP
Osteomalacia	Decreased conversion of **25hydroxycholecalciferaol** to **1,25-dihydroxy** leads to hypokalemia and hyperphosphatemia	Vitamin D replacement and calcium carbonate
Hyperphosphatemia/ hypocalcemia	Due to decreased active of vitamin D and renal failure	Oral phosphate binder such as calcium carbonate or calcium acetate
Hypermagnesemia	Due to decreased clearance from the kidney	Restrict food high in magnesium, laxatives
High circulating insulin	Insulin is high because its **clearance is decreased**	Decrease the dose of oral hypoglycemics in diabetics
Decreased libido and impotence in men	Decreased testosterone	Testosterone replacement

Note: Vitamin D deficiency causes ⬇ phosphate & ⬇ calcium, whereas kidney pathology causes ⬆ phosphate and ⬇ calcium

- Most common cause of death in ESRD is CAD, followed by infection

> **Indications for dialysis are:**   Mnemonic: **AEIOU**
> - Acid-base disorder
> - Electrolyte abnormality
> - Intoxication
> - Volume overload
> - Uremia (uremic encephalopathy, uremic pericarditis)

DIALYSIS

Dialysis is a way to filter blood when kidneys are not functioning properly

Types: there are two types of dialysis
- **Hemodialysis**, it is most **commonly performed**
- **Peritoneal dialysis**, it is not commonly performed and causes peritonitis

Urgent dialysis vs. Refractory dialysis

- **Urgent dialysis is done when a patient has any of the followings:**
  o Uremia encephalopathy
  o Uremia pericarditis
  o BUN> 80

- **Refractory dialysis means that treat the condition as you would normally treat. If it is ineffective, then perform dialysis.** Example of conditions that are treated with refractory dialysis are:
  o Acidosis
  o Hyperkalemia
  o Fluid overload

NEPHROLITHIASIS

Nephrolithiasis also known as kidney stones or renal calculi is a solid mass that is made up of tiny crystals.

Types: Calcium oxalate stones are the most common kidney stones, but other less stones include calcium phosphate, struvite, uric acid and cystine stones

Si/Sx: sudden colicky flank pain that may radiate to ipsilateral tests or labia, nausea, vomiting

Diagnosis:

- UA shows gross or microscopic hematuria. However, absence of microhematuria does not exclude kidney stone because 10-15% of the patients do not have hematuria
- Urinary pH (normal urine pH is 5.85)
- Abdominal x-ray to look for stone (use renal **ultrasound in pregnant women)**
- Renal ultrasound to check for any obstruction

Differential diagnosis of kidney stones

Type	Association	Treatment
Calcium oxalate or calcium phosphate stones	• Calcium oxalate is the **common cause of kidney stones** (80- 85%) • Most common cause is idiopathic hypercalciuria. Other causes include increased absorption, decreased clearance • Abdominal X-ray shows **radiopaque stones**	Hydration, thiazide diuretics
Struvite stones	• 2nd most common cause of kidney stones (9%) • **Large staghorn or struvite calculus** • Associated with **urease-producing organisms** such as Proteus, pseudomonas, Klebsiella, or staphylococcus • Urine pH > 7.2 • Abdominal X-ray shows **radiopaque stones**	Hydration, treat the underlying infection
Uric acid stones	• 3rd most common causes of kidney stones (7%) • Associated with gout, hyperuricemia, myeloproliferative disease, • Urine pH is < 5.5 (acidic) • Abdominal X-ray shows **radiolucent stone**	Hydration, alkalinization of urine, treat the underlying cause
Cystine stones	• Least common type of kidney stones (1%) • Associated with abnormal renal excretion of cystine, ornithine, lysine and arginine • **Hexagonal** shaped kidney stones • Abdominal X-ray shows **radiopaque stone**	Hydration, alkalinization of urine

Treatment:
- **Stone < 3 mm is treated with hydration, pain relievers, and a particular treatment depend on the stones** (as mentioned in the table on the previous page).
- Stone 5-10mm is removed with **extra-corporeal shock wave lithotripsy**
- Stone >10mm is removed with **laser lithotripsy or basket extraction.**

Note: if a patient with kidney stone or patient who is allowed to pass kidney stones spontaneously develops high fever, chills and flank pain, then give the patient IV antibiotics and perform percutaneous nephrostomy

RENAL ARTERY STENOSIS
Renal artery stenosis is narrowing of an artery that carries blood to the kidney

Cause: the most common in young patient (<30 years) is **fibromuscular dysplasia**, and in old patient (>50 years) **atherosclerosis**

Si/Sx: refractory hypertension, deterioration of kidney function when treatment with ACE inhibitors is initiated

Physical exam may show audible abdominal bruit on the affected side

Diagnosis:
- Labs: same as pre-renal failure plus **low potassium**
- Best **initial test is** Doppler ultrasound or Magnetic resonance angiogram (MRA)
- Most **accurate test** is angiography

Treatment: Angioplasty

POLYCYSTIC KIDNEY DISEASE (PKD)
Polycystic kidney disease is an inherited disease. It is characterized by presence of **fluid-filled cysts in the kidney.**

Type: two types of PKD are:
- **Autosomal dominant PKD (ADPKD):** This is the most common type PKD. Symptoms usually develop **after 30 years** of age.

- **Autosomal recessive PKD (ARPKD):** This is less common, but severe form of PKD. Most of the patients are **infants or young children.**

Associations: PKD is associated with the following conditions:

- Aortic aneurysm
- Cysts in liver, pancreas, spleen (**Liver cysts are most common cysts outside the kidney**)
- Diverticula
- Mitral valve prolapse

Si/Sx: Pain, hematuria, kidney stones, UTI, hypertension

Diagnosis: Abdominal CT or ultrasound

Treatment:

- There is no specific treatment for PKD. Treatment is directed towards symptoms such as, treat HTN, UTI and kidney stones.

Prognosis: it slowly progresses to ESRD, and renal failure is the most common cause of death

BENIGN PROSTATE HYPERTROPHY (BPH)

Benign prostate hypertrophy is a hyperplasia of prostate cells. It is a normal condition in males over 50 years of age.

Si/Sx: weak urine stream, incomplete emptying of bladder, dribbling at the end of urinating,

Diagnosis:

- Urinalysis and urine culture, to rule out infection
- Creatinine level, to check kidney function
- Digital rectal exam
- Prostate–specific antigen (PSA) level to screen for prostate cancer

Treatment:

- **Mild symptoms** are treated with **reassurance and lifestyle modifications** such as avoiding fluids within 2 hours of bedtime, pelvic muscle strengthening exercises, avoid decongestants or antihistamines because these drugs increase the BPH symptoms.
- **Mild to moderate symptoms** are treated with **alpha 1-blockers** (terazosin, prazosin) or **5-alpha reductase** (Finasteride)
- **Moderate to severe symptoms** can be treated with **surgical procedures** such as Transurethral resection of the prostate (TURP), or simple prostatectomy

ERECTILE DYSFUNCTION

Erectile dysfunction is a sexual dysfunction that is characterized by an inability to keep or maintain erection that is firm enough to have intercourse.

Cause: Psychological, marital problems, medications (beta-blockers, digoxin, antidepressant), disease (diabetes, HTN, thyroid disorder, multiple sclerosis, Parkinson's disease), nerve damage, low testosterone

Diagnosis:
- Clinical diagnosis
- Check testosterone and gonadotropin levels
- Rule out endocrine abnormalities such as prolactin level

Treatment:
- **Best initial management** is to **rule out psychological or marital problems**
- Treat the underlying condition, if applicable
- Phosphodiesterase -5 (PDE5) inhibitors such as Sildenafil (Viagra), Vardenafil (Levitra) or tadalafil (Cialis) – these medications increase the blood flow to corpora cavernous.
- If PDE5 inhibitors are ineffective, then any of the following may be used; Penis pumps, penile implants or intercavernous Injection
- Testosterone replacement may be used in patients with low testosterone levels

ANION GAP

Anion gap is the difference in the measured cations and anion in serum, plasma or urine. It is measured to **determine the cause of metabolic acidosis.**

It is calculated with the equation = $[Na^+] - ([Cl^-] + [HCO_3^-])$, and normal anion gap is 4-12 mEq/L.

- **Normal anion** gap metabolic acidosis is seen in conditions such renal tubular acidosis **(RTA) or diarrhea.**
- **High anion gap** (> 12 mEq/L) metabolic acidosis is seen in conditions **such as uremia, ethanol toxicity**

1. **Normal anion** gap metabolic acidosis is seen in **RTA and diarrhea.** To distinguish between them **urine anion gap (UAG) is calculated.**

   UAG = urine Na^+ − urine Cl^-
   - A **positive** UAG suggest **RTA**
   - A **negative** UAG **suggests diarrhea**

Usually the most important unmeasured ion is NH_4^+. It is difficult to measure NH_4^+ directly, but its excretion is usually accompanied by chloride $NH4^+CL$

1a. RENAL TUBULAR ACIDOSIS (RTA)

Renal tubular acidosis is a medical condition, which is caused by kidney's insufficiency to reabsorb bicarbonate or excrete H+ that results in non-anion metabolic acidosis

Type: Three main types of RTA are type I, II and IV.

Differential diagnosis of RTA

Type	Type I (Distal)	Type II (Proximal)	Type IV
Defect	Distal tubule defect	Proximal tubule defect	Decreased aldosterone or decreased aldosterone **effect on the kidney**
Cause	• Autoimmune disease • Sickle cell anemia • Amphotericin • Analgesics • Lithium	• Multiple myeloma • Amyloidosis • Fanconi syndrome • Carbonic anhydrase inhibitors	• Diabetes • Hypertension • HIV • Hyporeninemic hypoaldosteronism
Blood K+	Low	Low	High
Urine pH	> 5.4	> 5.4 in early; <5.5 as acidosis worsens	< 5.4
Test	Ammonium chloride	Sodium bicarbonate	Urine sodium (which will be high)
Treatment	Oral bicarbonate plus oral potassium citrate	Bicarbonate plus thiazide	Oral fludrocortisone
Complications	Kidney stones	Rickets, Osteomalacia	Hyperkalemia

2. HIGH ANION GAP METABOLIC ACIDOSIS

High anion gap metabolic acidosis (> 12 mEq/L) occurs due to increased production of anions such as lactate or acetate, and secondary loss of bicarbonate. Classic mnemonic to remember the causes is **MUD PILES**

2a. Methanol glycol poising
Patient presents with eye and CNS defects
Treatment: Initial treatment is IV Fomepizole; it prevents crystal formation by inhibiting ADH dehydrogenase, and then perform dialysis

2b. Uremia
Treatment: Dialysis

2c. Diabetic ketoacidosis (DKA)
It is usually seen in patients with type 1 DM
Treatment: IV fluids + insulin

2d. Pyrazinamide
Treatment: Stop the drug

2e. INH
Treatment: Stop the drug

2f. Lactic acidosis
It is usually caused by hypoperfusion
Treatment: treat the underlying cause

2g. Ethanol glycol poising
Look for a patient, who tried to commit suicide by ingesting antifreeze
Diagnosis: UA shows envelope crystals
Treatment: Initial treatment is IV Fomepizole, it prevent crystal formation by inhibiting ADH dehydrogenase), and then perform dialysis

2h. Salicylic acids (aspirin)
Clue often given on the boards is **tinnitus**
Management: Initial treatment is alkalization of urine with D5W, 3 amps of bicarbonate, charcoal, and then perform dialysis

INFECTIOUS DISEASES

URINARY TRACT INFECTION (UTI)

Urinary tract infection is the infection of urinary tract (kidney, ureters, bladder or urethra). Infection of the bladder is called **cystitis,** infection of the kidney is called **pyelonephritis,** and infection of urethra is called **urethritis.**

Cause: E. coli is the most common cause of UTI, but other causes may include Enterobacter, Serratia, Klebsiella pneumonia, S. saprophytes, Pseudomonas, and proteus mirabilis.

Risk factor: female gender (women tend to get more UTIs than men because they have shorter urethra), diabetes, having a urinary catheter, surgery or instrumentation of urinary tract, kidney stones, enlarged prostate, pregnancy

Si/Sx, diagnosis, and treatment: discussed under cystitis, pyelonephritis and urethritis.

CYSTITIS

Cystitis is inflammation of the bladder

Cause: discussed in UTI section

Si/Sx: urgency, frequency, burning, suprapubic tenderness, hematuria

Diagnosis:

- **Initial test is urine analysis** that shows increased urinary nitrites, increased leukocyte esterase, pyuria, bacteriuria
- **Most accurate test is urine culture:** positive for offending bacteria with colony count exceeding 10 x 5/ml

Treatment:

- Women with uncomplicated UTI are treated with TMP/SMX for 1-3 days
- Complicated UTIs are treated with TMP/SMX for 7 days. Complicated UTIs means; male with UTIs, diabetics, urinary obstruction, renal transplant, immunosuppressed, pregnancy

Note:

- A patient with a **complication UTIs, or UTIs secondary to obstruction** should have abdominal CT or ultrasound, before starting medication

- Urine culture is usually not needed for a woman with single UTI. Patient can be directly started on the treatment based on UTIs symptoms. Urine culture is performed if a woman gets recurrent UTIs, which means ≥ 2 UTIs in 6 months or ≥ 3 UTIs in 1 year

Prophylactic antibiotic:
- If a woman gets **UTIs after** every **intercourse**
  - o Tx. advise her to **void and** take a **double strength TMP/SMX** after every intercourse
- If a woman gets recurrent **UTIs without** any **correlations with intercourse**
  - o Tx. Single dose **TMP/SMX** everyday

PYELONEPHRITIS
Pyelonephritis is inflammation of the kidney
Causes: discussed in UTI section
Si/Sx: urgency, frequency, dysuria, fever, chills, flank pain, costovertebral angle (CVA) tenderness
Diagnosis:
- **Best initial test is urine analysis,** which is same as cystitis **plus** presence of **white cell casts**
- **Most accurate test is urine culture,** which is same as cystitis
- Renal ultrasound or CT, it is done to check for stones or other source of obstruction

Treatment:
- **Outpatient** treatment with **oral ciprofloxacin**
- **Inpatient** treatment with **IV ampicillin and gentamicin.** Inpatient treatment is given, if the patient has any of the followings:
  - o **Pregnant women**
  - o **Unstable**
  - o **Cannot take oral medicine** due to nausea vomiting

- If patient is **not responding to treatment** after **5-7 days, then get CT or ultrasound:**
  - o If imaging shows **obstruction** (stricture or stone), then do **ureteral stent** or **percutaneous nephrostomy**

- o If imaging shows **abscess, then** do **ultrasound guided biopsy** and treat the patient with **quinolone and oxacillin** or nafcillin, until culture and sensitivity is known

URETHRITIS

Urethritis is swelling and inflammation of the urethra.

Symptoms: purulent discharge, urgency, frequency, burning while urinating

Cause: two most common causes are **Neisseria gonorrhea and Chlamydia trachomatis**

Diagnosis:

- Best initial test is **urethral swab** to get gram stain and culture. Also, get culture **of all possible sites of sexual contact** such as oral, anus, vagina
- Most effective test is **nucleic acid amplification test**

Treatment:

- Neisseria gonorrhea urethritis is treated with **single** shot **IM ceftriaxone** or **single dose oral cefixime**
- Chlamydia trachomatis urethritis is treated with **single** dose of **oral azithromycin** or **7 days doxycycline**

Important:

- If Neisseria is found in the culture, then treat the patient for **Neisseria and chlamydia**
- If chlamydia is found in the culture, then treat the patient for **chlamydia** only

---

ASYMTOMATIC BACTERIURIA

Asymptomatic bacteriuria is characterized by presence of significant number **of bacteria (> 10,000 mL) in the urine,** but **no UTIs symptoms** are present

Treatment: no treatment is required. However, **amoxicillin is given if** patient has any of the followings:

- Pregnant women
- Kidney transplant recipient
- Going for a urinary tract surgery

BACTERIAL PROSTATITIS

Bacterial prostatitis is the inflammation of the prostate, which can be caused by any urinary tract infection. In **acute bacterial prostatitis** symptoms starts quickly. However, if symptoms or infection lasts for **3 or months**, then it is called **chronic bacterial prostatitis**.

Si/Sx: fever, chills, dysuria, low back pain, perineal pain

Treatment: TMP/SMX or ciprofloxacin (**4-6 weeks for acute prostatitis**, and **6-8 weeks for chronic prostatitis**)

EPIDIDYMITIS

Epididymitis is characterized by inflammation of epididymis. It is common in young men between 19-35 years of age

Causes: gonorrhea and chlamydia are the most common cause, but other causes may include regular use of a urethral catheter, recent surgery of urinary tract

Si/Sx: testicular pain with fever, pyuria, painful scrotal swelling

Diagnosis:

- Physical exam show **tests at the normal position**, tenderness around epididymis
- Urinalysis and urine culture

Treatment: bed rest and antibiotics

Boards tip:

- Question often tries to trick epididymitis with testicular torsion. To distinguish between look at testes position and cremasteric reflex
  - o In epididymitis testes are at **normal position** and **cremasteric reflex is present**
  - o In epididymitis testes are **high riding** and **cremasteric reflex is absent**

SEXUALLY TRANSMITTED DISEASES (STD) DIFFERENTIAL DIAGNOSIS

1. CHANCROID

Characteristics: Painful ulcer with **ragged edges**

Diagnosis:

- Best initial test is **urethral swab** for gram stain, culture
- Most accurate test is **culture** with Nairobi medium or Mueller-Hinton agar

Treatment: Single shot IM ceftriaxone or **single dose of oral azithromycin**

2. HERPES SIMPLEX VIRUS (HSV)

Characteristics: Multiple vesicles on genitals or mucous membrane

Diagnosis:

- Best initial test is **Tzanck test**
- Most accurate test is **culture**

Treatment

- Acyclovir or valacyclovir
- If patient is resistant to acyclovir or valacyclovir, then give **foscarnet**

3. LYMPHOGRANULOMA VENEREUM

Characteristics:

- Lesion that ulcerates and heals
- **Enlarged lymph nodes may develop draining sinuses tracts**

Cause: chlamydia trichromatic

Diagnosis: Serology of chlamydia trichromatic

Treatment:

- **Single dose of oral azithromycin** or **doxycycline** for 7 days

4. GRANULOMA INGUINALE

Characteristics: Red beefy genital lesion that **ulcerates**

Diagnosis: Biopsy

Treatment: **TMP/SMX or doxycycline**

5. SYPHILIS

Syphilis is a highly contagious STD, which progress in stages

5a. PRIMARY SYPHILIS

Characteristics: Painless chancres appear within 3 weeks after the exposure of infection and **disappear within 10-90 days**

Diagnosis:
- Best initial test is **VDRL or RPR**
  - VDRL and RPR are not positive in all patients with **primary syphilis.** If VDRL or RPR test is negative, then do darkfield exam
- Most accurate test is **darkfield exam**

Treatment:
- **Single shot** of **IM penicillin**
- **If patient is allergic to penicillin,** then give **doxycycline**

5b. SECONDARY SYPHILIS

Characteristics: pinkish or pale rash in **a white** person or **copper-colored** in **a black** person. Other symptoms includes alopecia areata, condylomata lata

Diagnosis:
- Best initial test is **VDRL or RPR**
- Confirmatory test is **FTA**

Treatment:
- **Single shot** of **IM penicillin**
- **If patient is allergic to penicillin,** then give **doxycycline**

5c. LATENT SYPHILIS

Latent syphilis is diagnosed when **VDRL or RPR is > 1:8, but patient has no symptoms of syphilis**

Treatment
- **3 shots** of **IM penicillin** (1 shot each week, total three weeks)
- **If patient is allergic to penicillin,** then give **doxycycline**

5d. TERTIARY SYPHILIS

Characteristics: neurosyphilis, symptoms such as **Tabes dorsalis, Argyll-Robertson pupil, gummas** (soft, on-cancerous growth of tissue)

Diagnosis:
- Best initial test is **VDRL or RPR**
- Confirmatory test is **FTA**
- **Lumbar puncture, it is** performed when a patient has any of the followings:
  - When a patient with syphilis develops neurologic or ocular symptoms
  - HIV positive patient with CD4 < 350, or RPR>1:32

Treatment:
- IV penicillin for 10-14 days
- If patient is allergic to penicillin, then do **penicillin desensitization,** and then **treat the patient with penicillin**

Other high-yield syphilis related point

- If the patient with a primary or secondary syphilis is **allergic to penicillin,** then treat the patient with **doxycycline.** However, if a pregnant woman is in any stage of syphilis or a patient with **tertiary syphilis** is allergic to penicillin, **then desensitize them** with penicillin, and still treat them with penicillin

6. GENITAL WARTS

Characteristics: Cauliflower type mass found on warm moist area in the genitals

Diagnosis: Clinical, but biopsy must be done to rule out cancer

Treatment:
- Best initial treatment is **trichloroacetic acid or sclerotherapy**
- **Imiquimod**
- **Podophyllin** (not used in pregnant woman)
- **Large mass is usually surgically removed**

NEPHROLOGY SURGERY

RENAL CELL CARCINOMA
Renal cell carcinoma is a kidney cancer that starts in the tubules of the
kidney.
Risk factors: smoking, polycystic kidney disease, family history,
Von Hippel-Lindau disease
Si/Sx: hematuria, flank pain, flanks mass, fever, secondary polycythemia
Diagnosis:
- Labs show **increased Ca^{2+}, RBCs, AST and ALT**
- Ultrasound or abdominal CT shows heterogenic solid mass
Treatment: Surgery

BLADDER CANCER
Bladder cancer is the second most common urologic cancer; usually
transitional cell carcinoma
Risk factor: male gender, cigarette smoking, aniline dye,
cyclophosphamide, schistosomiasis
Si/Sx: Painless gross hematuria is the most common finding, but most of
the patients are asymptotic in the early stages,
Diagnosis:
- UA often shows hematuria
- CT or ultrasound is performed to detect local invasion and
  distance metastases
- **Most accurate test is cystoscopy with biopsy**
Treatment: Surgery and **intravesical BCG**

PROSTATE CANCER
Prostate cancer is the most common cause of cancer in men, and the second
most common of cancer-related death in men
Si/Sx: prostate cancer is usually asymptomatic; **most of the tumors are
discovered incidentally on prostate digital rectal exam.** Some patient may
present with urinary hesitancy, weak stream, urinary retention
Diagnosis:
- Palpable hard nodule on digital rectal exam
- Increased PSA

- CT scan is performed to detect any malignancy
- **Most accurate test** is the biopsy of the prostate gland

Treatment:

- Surgery and radiation for localized cancer
- **Metastatic** cancers are treated as follow: **flutamide is given first because it** blocks the androgen flare up, and **then give leuprolide** a GnRH agonist

TESTICULAR CANCER

Testicular cancer is the cancer of testes that may affect one or both testes.
Risk factor: cryptosporidium, abnormal testicle development, Klinefelter syndrome, history of testicular cancer
Type: Two most common types of testicular cancers are seminoma and non-seminoma

- **Seminoma cancer** is slow growing cancer
- **Non-seminoma cancer** is fast growing cancer. It is made up of one or more types of cells and identified based on cell type: choriocarcinoma, teratoma, embryonal carcinoma, yolk sac tumor

Si/Sx: painless lump, pain or discomfort in testes, feeling of heaviness in the scrotum,
Diagnosis:

- **Best initial test** is testicular ultrasound
- **Most accurate test** is biopsy **with inguinal orchiectomy**
- Imaging such as X-ray or CT of abdomen and pelvis is performed to check for metastasis
- Tumor markers: AFP, LDH, beta-HCG
  - o In seminoma **AFP is increased, but beta-HCG is normal**
  - o In non-seminoma AFP and beta-HCG **both are increased**

Treatment:

- **Seminoma** cancer is treated with **orchiectomy and radiation**
- **Non-seminoma** cancer is treated with **orchiectomy and chemotherapy**

NEPHROLOGY CCS

Case # 1

Case introduction
A 33-years old female presented to the office because of frequent urination and a burning sensation when she urinates.

Initial vitals signs
Temperature: 37.2 degrees
Pulse: 68 beats/min, regular rhythm
Respiration rate: 19/ minutes

Blood pressure, systolic 124 mm Hg
Blood pressure, disystolic, 75 mm Hg

Height: 63.0 inches
Weight: 120.0 lbs.
Body mass index: 21.3 Kg/m2

History of present illness (HPI)
A 33-years old female presented to the office because of frequent urination and a burning sensation when she urinates. She says it started 3 days ago and she has been urinating 5-6 times a day. She denies fever, cough, vaginal discharge and change in urine color. She denies any medical history. She is sexually active with her boyfriend and uses condoms for birth control. Her menstrual period was 2 and half weeks ago.

Past medical history
Hospitalization: None
Other medical condition: None
Current medication: None
Allergies: none
Vaccination: up to date

Family history
Father, and mother are healthy. Sister has hypothyroidism

Social history

Marital history: not married- has a boyfriend

Occupation: wedding planner

Recreational: Cooking, travel

Personal habits: Does not drink smoke, or use drugs

Review of system:

General: see HPI

Skin: see HPI

HEENT: see HPI

Musculoskeletal: see HPI

Cardiology: see HPI

Abdominal: see HPI

Genitourinary: see HPI

Please see pages 1-5 for general CCS cases approach

Step 1. None (patient is stable does not require any emergency measures)

Step 2. Order complete physical exam and move the clock forward to get the results
- Results show:
    o Abdomen exam shows suprapubic discomfort
    o Rest of the physical exam is normal

Step 3. Order following labs, and then move the clock forward to get the results
- **Urine pregnancy test**
- CBC
- UA
- BMP
- Urine culture and sensitivity

- **Labs show:**
    o Negative pregnancy
    o UA shows positive nitrate, positive esterase, Bacteria > 20, WBC > 30

Step 4. Give TMP-SMZ for 3 days. However, if the patient was pregnant, then use Nitrofurantoin or Amoxicillin for 7 days.

Step 5. Send patient home and make a follow-up appointment after 5-7 days

Step 6. None

Step 7. Move the clock forward to get the culture and sensitivity results, and then move the clock forward to next appointment date.
- Change the medicine based on culture and sensitivity, if needed

Step 8. None

Step 9. Send patient home and make a follow-up appointment after 5-7
days

Step 10. Counsel and age and gender specific counseling
- PAP smear (now or schedule in a week)
- Safe sex
- Medicine compliance
- No smoking, drinking, drugs

Diagnosis: Cystitis

CASE # 2

Case introduction
An 83-years-old nursing home patient is brought to the ER because of because of altered mental status

Initial vitals signs
Temperature: 37.2 degrees
Pulse: 92 beats/min, regular rhythm
Respiration rate: 19/ minutes

Blood pressure, systolic 118 mm Hg
Blood pressure, disystolic, 75 mm Hg

Height: 63.0 inches
Weight: 120.0 lbs.
Body mass index: 21.3 Kg/m2

History of present illness (HPI)
An 83-years-old nursing home patient is brought to the ER because of because of altered mental status. Nursing home staff says that he has been having watery from the last 5 days, he vomited few time yesterday and has not urinated in the last 15 hours. Staff also tells that he has been drinking fruit juice and does not have the appetite for food.

Past medical history
Hospitalization: 2 hospitalizations for MI, and appendicitis
Other medical condition: DM
Current medication: insulin, aspirin, captopril, metoprolol
Allergies: penicillin
Vaccination: up to date

Family history
Father and mother are healthy. Sister has hypothyroidism

Social history

Marital history: widowed, 2 children

Occupation: retired

Recreational: none

Personal habits: Does not drink smoke, or use drugs

Review of system:

General: see HPI

Skin: see HPI

HEENT: see HPI

Musculoskeletal: see HPI

Cardiology: see HPI

Abdominal: see HPI

Genitourinary: see HPI

Please see pages 1-5 for general CCS cases approach

Step 1. Oder following emergency measures
- Pulse oximetry
- Oxygen
- IV access
- IV normal saline
- BP monitor
- EKG
- Vitals x 8 hrs.

Step 2. Order complete physical exam, and then move the clock forward to get the results
- Results show:
- o Patient looks sleepy, oriented to time and place
- o Skin exam shows dry mucosa
- o Abdominal exam shows epigastric tenderness, soft abdomen
- o Rectal exam shows mildly enlarged prostate

Step 3. Order labs, and then move the clock forward to get the results
- CBC
- UA
- BMP
- Chest X-ray
- Monitor urine output, Foley catheter
- UA
- Urine culture & sensitivity
- Urine Na
- Serum phosphate /magnesium
- ABG
- Glucose

- Labs result shows:
- o EKG is normal
- o BMP shows BUN 80 mg/ dl, Cr 2.3 mg/dl, K 5.0 mEq/L
- o UA shows RBC, urine osmolality 450 mOsm/L

- ○ ABG shows paCO2 45mm Hg, PaO2, pH 7.37
- ○ Glucose is 270 mg/dl

Step 4. Medicine
- Digoxin
- Furosemide
- Insulin
- KCL

Step 5. Admit in wards

Step 6. Order followings
- Complete bed rest
- Pneumatic compression
- Diabetic diet

Step 7: Order the followings, and then move the clock forward to get the results
- Ultrasound of kidney
- 24 hours urine protein
- HbA1c
- Echo

- Labs shows
- ○ Ultrasound shows normal kidney
- ○ 24 hour urine protein: 10 mg
- ○ HbA1c- 7.5%

Step 8. Order nephrology consults, and then move the clock forward to get consult result

Step 9. Follow-up every 4-8 hours until patient stabilize

Case should end here

Step 10. Counsel:

- Advance directive
- No smoking, drinking, illegal drugs
- Medicine compliance
- Foot care
- FOBT
- Colposcopy
- Influenza vaccine

Diagnosis: **Acute renal failure**

NEUROLOGY

STROKE

Stroke is a condition in which blood supply to a part of the brain is reduced or blocked. This interrupted blood supply and deprives brain cell of oxygen, and brain cells begin to die.

Type: Two types strokes are **hemorrhagic stroke** and **ischemic stroke**. Hemorrhagic stroke occurs when blood vessels in the brain leaks or ruptures. Ischemic stroke occurs when blood vessels in the brain are blocked or narrowed by thrombus or emboli. 85% of strokes are ischemic strokes.

Symptoms: headaches, difficulty walking, difficulty speaking and understanding, paralysis or numbness body parts, and trouble with seeing. Other symptoms depends on the site of artery occlusion (see table below)

Artery occlusion and symptoms

Artery occlusion	Symptoms
Anterior cerebral artery (ACA)	• Contralateral lower extremity weakness • Urinary incontinence
Middle cerebral artery (MCA)	• Contralateral hemiparesis • Contralateral sensory loss • Wernicke's aphasia • Broca's aphasia • Apraxia
Posterior cerebral artery (PCA)	• Agnosia • Hallucination • Contralateral homonymous • Hemianopia
Posterior inferior cerebral artery (PICA)	• Vertigo • Ataxia • Dysarthria • Ipsilateral face numbness • Contralateral body numbness
Basilar artery	• Locked- in syndrome • Only vertical eye movement is spared

How is a transient ischemic attack (TIA) different from a stroke?
Transient ischemic attack is caused by temporary decrease in blood supply
to the part of the brain, usually due to emboli or thrombosis. The patient
may have **symptoms similar to a stroke**, but symptoms **resolve within 24
hours.** Conversely, stroke causes a permanent neurological damage

Diagnosis:
- **Best initial test is CT head without contrast.** CT scan is done to
  see if patient had a hemorrhagic stroke or ischemic stroke
- Most **accurate test is MRI** of head

Initial management:

- **If a CT or MRI shows hemorrhagic stroke,** then check the **blood
  pressures (BP)**

    o **If BP is > 220/120 mmHg,** then give IV nitroprusside,
      labetalol or nicardipine, but do **not more than 25% or lower
      than 185/100, otherwise** patient will have cerebral ischemia

    o **If BP is < 220/ 120 mmHg, then lower the intracranial
      pressure to prevent further damage:** elevate head,
      hyperventilation to keep pCO2 between 25- 30 mmHG and
      mannitol and get surgical consult

- **If CT shows non–hemorrhagic stroke, then treat the patient** as
  follow:
    o If a patient presents **<4 hours** of initial stroke symptoms, then
      give tissue plasminogen activators (**tPAs**). However, make
      sure that the patient has no contraindications for tpAs
      (contraindications for tpAs are discussed on the next page)

    o If a patient has any **contraindications for tPAs** or patient
      presents **>4 hours** after the initial stroke symptoms, then give
      aspirin. However, if the patient is already on aspirin, then
      **add dipyridamole or stop the aspirin, and then give
      clopidogrel.**

Note:

- Aspirin and clopidogrel are not given together to a patient with TIA because combination of these may worsen TIA

- If tPAs was given, then transfer the patient in ICU and do periodic neurology checkups

Contraindication for tPAs

Absolute contraindication	Relative contraindication
• Previous intracranial bleeding at anytime • Closed head trauma within last 3 months • Ischemic stroke within last 3 months • Brain tumor • Active bleeding disorder • Blood pressure > 180 systolic, >100 diastolic	• Prolonged CPR (> 10 minutes) • Pregnancy • Active peptic ulcer • Invasive procedure in last 2 weeks

Further management: Once the patient has been stabilized, it is necessary to evaluate the patient to **determine the cause of stroke** to prevent future stroke(s):

1. Most common cause of stroke in **patients >50** years of age is **atrial fibrillation, thrombi emboli, or carotid stenosis.**

1a. **Carotids**
   - Check for carotids bruits by auscultating carotids
   - If carotid bruits is present, then do **carotid angiography** or **doppler**

Treatment: If carotid angiography shows **stenosis > 70%, but <100%,** then perform **carotid endarterectomy**

Note: Carotid endarterectomy is not performed if carotid artery is 100% stenosed

1b. EKG and Holter monitor
- EKG is done to check for atrial fibrillation. If EKG is normal, then get 24-48 hours Holter monitor
  - Atrial fibrillation can also be caused by hyperthyroidism, after EKG is performed check TSH, if hyperthyroidism is suspected

Management: **Warfarin and treat the cause of A-fibrillation**

1c. Echocardiogram
- **Echocardiogram is performed to check for:**
  - Valve vegetation
  - Valve defect (unrepaired VSD can cause systemic emboli)

Management:
- **Warfarin** is given for **clot(s)**
- If **valve vegetation** is present, then preform **surgery**
- If **VSD is** present, then do **percutaneous catheter repair**
-

2. Most common cause of stroke in **patients <50 years of age:**
- **Cocaine abuse**
- **SLE**
- **VDRL**
- **Hypercoagulable state:** most common cause is Factor V Leiden mutation (protein C resistance), but other causes may include protein S, antiphospholipid syndrome

Treatment: **treat the underlying cause**

Prevention: Reduce the risk of recurrent stroke by followings:
- Stop smoking
- Keep blood pressure < 130/70 mmHG
- Keep LDL < 100
- Control diabetes (keep HbA1C < 7 %)

MOVEMENT DISORDERS

1. PARKINSON'S DISEASE

Parkinson's disease is a neurological disorder that affects movement
Cause: depletion of dopamine. A lack of dopamine results in abnormal
nerve function, that results in loss of ability to control body movements. In
older patients (>50), it is usually caused **loss of dopamine** in substantia
nigra. Other things that can affect the dopamine levels are **antipsychotic
medicines, MTPT, stroke, encephalitis**

Si/Sx: Mnemonic: **TRAP**
- Resting tremor
- Rigidity
- Akinesia
- Postural instability

Diagnosis: Parkinson's disease is a clinical diagnosis

Treatment: depends on **age** and **severity** of impairment

Mild symptoms are treated as follow:
- **Anticholinergic medication** (benztropine, trihexyphenidyl) is
  used in **patients < 60 years of age**. Side effects of anticholinergic
  medicines are dry mouth, blurred vision, dry cough, worsening
  prostate hypertrophy and constipation. Anticholinergic medicines
  are not given to patients above 60 years of age due to their side
  effects.
- **Amantadine** is given to patients **> 60 years of age**

Severe symptoms are treated as follow:
- **Levodopa and carbidopa**: levodopa crosses the blood brain barrier
  and converts to dopamine. **Carbidopa prevents the peripheral
  breakdown of levodopa.** Side effects of levodopa and carbidopa
  include dyskinesia, akathisia and **on-off phenomena**, which can
  be **controlled by one of the followings:**
  o **Not eating any protein until nighttime**
  o **Adding adjunct therapy** of COMT inhibitors (Entacapone,
    tolcapone) or MAOI inhibitors (selegiline, rasagiline).

- If adding COMT inhibitors or MAOI inhibitor is ineffective, then **add antidepressant** such as SSRIs because there is a high incidence of depression in patients with Parkinson's disease.
- **Thalamotomy or deep brain stimulation** is reserved for refractory cases

Other medications for Parkinson's disease

- **Dopamine agonist** such as **Pramipexole, ropinirole, and cabergoline** can also be used to treat Parkinson's. These have high efficacy and low side effects.
  - o Side effects of dopamine agonist includes **increase libido and erection**

Other differential diagnosis of Parkinson's are:
- Parkinson's, ataxia and orthostatic hypotension - Dx **Shy-Drager syndrome**
- Parkinson's and dementia –Dx. **Lewy Body Dementia**

Other High-yield Parkinson's symptoms related question

- **Anti-psychotics** medicines can also induce **Parkinson's symptoms**. If a patient presents with Parkinson's symptoms after taking anti-psychotics, then treat it by **lowering the dose of anti-psychotic and add diphenhydramine (Benadryl), or benztropine.**

---

2. BENIGN ESSENTIAL TREMORS

Benign essential tremor is a movement disorder that is characterized by tremor of body parts, but hands are most commonly involved
Cause: there is no known clear cause
Si/Sx: action tremors, tremor gets worse with physical or mental stress, but **goes away with alcohol intake**
Diagnosis: clinical diagnosis
Treatment: Propranolol

3. CEREBELLAR TREMORS

Cerebellar tremors are also known as **intention tremors**, which appear at the end of purposeful movements

Cause: damage to cerebellum such as tumor, stroke, multiple sclerosis

Si/Sx: tremors at the **end of purposeful movements**

Treatment: Treat the underlying cause

4. RESTLESS LEG SYNDROME (RLS)

Restless leg syndrome is a disorder of nervous system in which patient gets **irresistible urge to move their legs** and moving relieves the discomfort

Causes: there is no specific known cause, but it associated with **uremia, diabetes, iron deficiency, and pregnancy**

Si/Sx: unpleasant sensation in legs that are often expressed **as crawling, creeping, and gnawing**

Diagnosis: clinical diagnosis

Treatment: treat the underlying cause. Dopamine agonist (Pramipexole or ropinirole) are used to control leg movements

5. HUNTINGTON DISEASE

Huntington disease is progressive neurodegenerative disorder that causes **movement, cognitive and psychiatric disorders.**

Cause: Autosomal dominant disorder; genetic defect in chromosome 4, which results CAG repeats

Si/Sx: **Choreiform movements**, unsteady gait, personality change, dementia, behavioral disturbance, **hallucinations, irritability**

Diagnosis:
- Huntington disease is a clinical diagnosis
- CT or MRI of the head may show cerebral atrophy (caudate and putamen)
- Genetic testing may also be done to determine the CAG repeats

Treatment: there is no treatment to cure Huntington disease
- **Tetrabenazine** is used to treat **involuntary movements** and **haloperidol** is used to treat **psychosis**

- Genetic testing should be offered to young family members

Prognosis: Most of the patients die within 15-20 years after the diagnosis

NEUROMUSCULAR DISORDERS

1. MYASTHENIA GRAVIS (MG)

Myasthenia gravis is a neuromuscular disorder that causes muscle weakness

Cause: Autoantibodies against **postsynaptic acetylcholine receptor**

Si/Sx: muscle weakness **after repetitive use**, dysphagia, diplopia, and ptosis (ptosis is pathognomonic for MG)

Diagnosis:

- **Best initial test is acetylcholine receptor antibody**
- Edrophonium test is performed **when other tests are inconclusive.** In this test patient shows sudden improvement in muscle strength after edrophonium injection
- **Electromyography (EMG) is the most accurate test.** In this test patient shows decreased muscle strength with repetitive nerve stimulation
- Chest CT is performed to check for thymoma and other abnormality in thymus
- Pulmonary function test (PFTs) to evaluate breathing

Treatment:

- If patient's **PFTs are affected**, then give **IVIG and plasmapheresis.** It is also the best treatment in **acute myasthenia crisis**
- Best **initial treatment is pyridostigmine or neostigmine.** If it is ineffective and the patient is a **postpubertal, but < 60 years** to age, then do **thymectomy.** However if patient is **> 60 years** of age, then give **oral prednisone**
- If symptoms still continue, then give
  - Azathioprine is 1st choice
  - Cyclosporine and cyclophosphamide is the 2nd choice

Board's Tip for Myasthenia gravis patient's

- Make sure to check PFT's before giving treatment for MG, if PFTs are affected, then give IVIG and plasmapheresis

---

2. LAMBERT-EATON SYNDROME

Lambert-Eaton syndrome is neuromuscular disorder that causes muscle weakness after **period of inactivity**, but patient **regains** the muscle **strength after the use of that muscle**

Cause: autoantibodies against presynaptic Calcium channel blocker, it is often seen in patients with small cell cancer of lungs

Si/Sx: muscle weakness with rest, dry mouth, impotence

Diagnosis:

- Blood test to check for antibodies against voltage-gated calcium channel blockers
- EMG shows increased muscle strength with repetitive stimulation
- Chest CT to identify tumor

Treatment:

- Treat the underlying cause
- Anticholinesterase (pyridostigmine) can be used to improve for muscle strength

DEMENTIA

Dementia is a term used to describe a group of symptoms affecting memory, thinking and social ability.

Cause: there is no specific cause of dementia, but it is seen in conditions such as Alzheimer disease vascular dementia, picks disease, normal pressure hydrocephalus, Lewy body dementia, Creutzfeldt-Jakob disease

Diagnosis:

- All **patients with dementia** should have following checked:
  - **T4, TSH, B12, VDRL, and head CT**

1. ALZHEIMER DISEASE

Alzheimer disease is the **most common cause of dementia** in patients over 70 years of age

Si/Sx: Slow progressive memory loss particularly short-term memory, mild personality change, but as the disease progress patients become irritated, quarrelsome, and may even experience hallucinations, delusions

Diagnosis:

- Clinical diagnosis
- CT head shows **diffuse atrophy of the brain**
- Definitive diagnosis is only possible at autopsy

Treatment:
- Supportive therapy for patient and family members
- **First-line treatment** is anticholinesterase inhibitors (Donepezil, rivastigmine, or galantamine), these can slow dementia progression
- **Memantine** is used in **advance cases**
- Antipsychotics and antidepressants, if needed
- **Vitamin E** (alpha–tocopherol) can also be given, it slows the cognitive decline
- **Ginkgo biloba** is herbal medicine that can be used to **enhance the memory.**
  - Ginkgo biloba **increases the bleeding time**. Therefore, it should not be given to patients with bleeding disorders, taking warfarin or aspirin

2. VASCULAR DEMENTIA
Vascular dementia is also known as multi-infarct dementia, which is caused by **impaired blood supply to the brain**
Risk factors: Atherosclerosis, hypertension, stroke, smoking, diabetes
Si/Sx: acute stepwise decline in memory loss, multiple focal deficits, personality change and cognitive changes
Diagnosis: CT head
Treatment: Treat the underlying cause

3. PICK'S DISEAE
Pick's disease is a neurodegenerative disease that causes **progressive dementia** that is similar to Alzheimer disease, except that it tends to affects **frontal and temporal lobes**
Si/Sx: Memory loss, aphasia, **abrupt mood swings**, **violent behavior**
Diagnosis: MRI of head shows **frontal and temporal lobe atrophy**
Treatment: There is not treatment for picks disease. Symptomatic treatment as **per Alzheimer's disease**

4. CREUTZFELDT-JAKOB DISEASE (CJD)
Creutzfeldt-Jakob disease is a progressive **neurodegenerative disease** that **causes dementia and, ultimately, death**
Si/Sx: progressive dementia, **jerky movements (myoclonus), seizure**, personality change, anxiety

Diagnosis:

- Best initial test is CT or MRI of head, which shows **brain lesion**
- EEG shows **3hz spike** in brain activity
- Lumbar puncture: CSF is drawn to check for **14-3-3 protein**
- **Brain biopsy** is the **most accurate test**. However, if MRI shows brain lesions and CSF shows 14-3-3 protein, then there is no need to do brain biopsy

Treatment:

- There is no treatment for CJD
- **Clonazepam and valproate may help relieve myoclonus seizures**

Prognosis: patients usually die within 6 months after the diagnosis

5.   LEWY BODY DEMENTIA

Lewy body dementia is neurodegenerative disease caused by abnormal clumps of alpha-synuclein. These clumps are called Lewy body, and are found throughout midbrain, cerebral cortex, and brain stem

Si/Sx: Memory loss, **hallucination, Parkinson's symptoms**

Diagnosis: CT or MRI

Treatment: anticholinesterase inhibitors – donepezil, rivastigmine or galantamine

6.   NORMAL PRESSURE HYDROCEPHALUS

Normal pressure hydrocephalus is a condition in which cerebrospinal fluid (CSF) in the brain is increased that affects the brain function. However, pressure of CSF is usually normal.

Si/Sx: Memory loss, **ataxia, urinary incontinence**

Diagnosis:

- **Best initial test is CT head**
- **Lumbar puncture (LP) shows:**
  - Normal pressure of CSF

Note: Patient's gait improves after LP

Treatment: LP shunt

7. OTHER *HIGH-YIELD* NON-NEUROLOGICAL CAUSES OF DEMENTIA

7a HYPOTHYROIDISM
Hypothyroidism can also cause dementia. Look for a patient with dementia and hypothyroidism symptoms such as weight gain, dry skin, constipation
Diagnosis: labs show decreased fT4 and increased TSH
Treatment: Levothyroxine

7b PSEUDODEMENTIA
Pseudodementia is a condition in which patient have symptoms **similar to dementia**, but actually **suffering from depression**

Key to distinguish Pseudodementia from dementia
- o   In Pseudodementia patient **looks withdrawn and usually makes no eye contact**
- o   In Pseudodementia patient often complain about memory loss, but careful testing shows **intact memory**
- o   Patient with Pseudodementia **makes no effort to answer hard question**, whereas patient with dementia do not give up easily

Management:
- Best step in management is to inquire about suicidal thoughts
- SSRIs

BOARDS TIP TO GET DEMENTIA DIAGNOSIS

- **Hypothyroidism:** Look for a patient with **memory loss** and symptoms of hypothyroidism such as **weight gain, dry skin, and constipation**

- **Alzheimer disease**: look for an elderly patient (> 70 years of age) with **slow progressive memory loss**

- **Vascular dementia:** look for a patient with **stepwise progressive memory loss**

- **Picks disease:** look for a patient with **memory loss, personality change behavior change**

- **Lewy body dementia:** look for a patient with memory loss, **hallucination, and Parkinson's symptoms**

- **Creutzfeldt-Jakob disease:** look for a patient with memory loss, **jerky movements (myoclonus), seizure**

- **Normal pressure hydrocephalus:** look for a patient with **memory loss, ataxia, urinary incontinence**

- **Pseudodementia:** look for a withdrawn patient

HEADACHE

Headache is a pain anywhere in the region of head or neck. Headache may be a sharp, throbbing, and dull. Headache may be on certain location or all overhead.

Important:
- Any patient presenting with a sudden onset of severe headache with or without focal neurologic deficits, **should have CT of the head** to rule out secondary cause such as subarachnoid hemorrhage (SAH)

1. MIGRAINE HEADACHE

Si/Sx: Mnemonic: **POUND**
- **P**ulsating
- **O**nset, it lasts between 4 -72 hours
- **U**nilateral
- **N**ausea
- **I**nterferes with **daily** activity

Triggers: Emotional stress, food (aged cheeses, alcoholic beverage), menstrual periods, tensions, tension and change in normal sleep pattern.
Diagnosis: clinical diagnosis

Treatment:
- Avoid known trigger
- **Mild migraine** is treated with **NSAIDs**
- **Acute migraine** attacks are treated with **abortive medications** - sumatriptan or ergotamine.
  - ○ If a patient has no **cardiovascular** disease, then give **sumatriptan** or **ergotamine**
  - ○ If a patient has **cardiovascular** disease, then give **ergotamine**
  - ○ If a patient has **nausea or vomiting**, then give **IV sumatriptan** and **IV Phenergan**

- **Prophylactic medicine:** is given to a patient, who **has 4 or more migraine headaches per month**
  - ○ 1st choice is propranolol
  - ○ 2nd choice is valproic acid
  - ○ 3rd choice is verapamil
  - ○ Last option is TCAs or SSRIs

Note: Prophylactics medicines are not used for acute attacks because these usually take 2-6 weeks to work

2. CLUSTER HEADACHE
Cluster headache is characterized by **unilateral headache mostly around eyes**
Si/Sx: Multiple recurrent unilateral headaches, **tearing or watering of the eye, rhinorrhea, stuffy nose, and changes in pupil size**
Diagnosis:
- Clinical diagnosis
- If diagnosis is not clear, then advice patient to keep a diary of headaches

Treatment:
- **Abortive therapy is 100% oxygen**
- **Adjunct treatment is sumatriptan**

Prophylactics medicine: none

3. TENSION HEADACHE

Tension headache is **the most common cause of headache**
Cause: Inadequate rest, anxiety, fatigue, hunger, emotional stress
Si/Sx: Vise-like bilateral headaches, tenderness on scalp, neck and shoulder muscles
Diagnosis: diagnosis of exclusion
Treatment:

- **Best initial therapy is relaxation techniques and hot baths**
- **NSIADs or acetaminophen is first-line abortive therapy**

4. PSEUDOTUMOR CEREBRI

Pseudotumor cerebri is characterized by **increased fluid pressure around the brain and spinal cord**
Si/Sx: headache **that gets worse** with increased intracranial pressure such as **during coughing, sneezing or leaning forward**. Other symptoms include blurred vision, double vision, nausea, vomiting
Cause: overweight, tetracyclines, vitamin A toxicity, oral contraceptives
Diagnosis:

- Best initial test is CT head, which is usually normal
- Most accurate test is lumber puncture, which shows **increased opening pressure**

Treatment:

- Best **initial treatment is to remove the offending agent, weight loss and acetazolamide**
- If it is ineffective, then do **recurrent lumber puncture** to lower the intracranial pressure
- If a patient continues to experience symptoms after repeated lumber puncture, then do **ventricular peritoneal shunt**

Boards tip:

- Always get CT or MRI of the head, before performing lumber puncture

---

5. TEMPORAL ARTERITIS
Temporal arteritis (TA) is a condition in which temporal arteries of the head become inflamed and damaged
Si/Sx: headache and tenderness in temple area, jaw claudication, fever, vision impairment
Diagnosis:
- Erythrocytes sedimentations rate (ESR) higher than 60mm/hour, but it is usually >100 mm/hour in TA
- Most accurate test is temporal artery biopsy

Treatment: high dose prednisone, which should be started immediately following ESR test results, otherwise patient may develop irreversible blindness

6. HEADACHES AFTER SPINAL TAP
This type of headache usually occurs after an hour or so after lumbar puncture or spinal anesthesia
Si/Sx: headaches that increase with leaning forward and gets better with lying horizontally
Treatment: advice the patient to lie horizontally, this type of headaches usually resolves spontaneously within 24 hours

7. ANALGESIC REBOUND HEADACHES
Analgesic rebound headaches also known as medication overuse headache, which usually occurs when multiple analgesics are taken frequently to relieve headaches
Si/Sx: headaches improve with analgesics but returns as analgesics wears-off
Treatment: stop all analgesics and use one specific medicine

8. SUBARACHNOID HEMORRAHGE
Subarachnoid hemorrhage (SAH) is a medical emergency in which blood buildup in the subarachnoid space, between the arachnoid membrane and pia mater.
Cause: bleeding from a cerebral aneurysm, bleeding from an arteriovenous malformation, head injury, and bleeding disorder
Si/Sx: sudden onset of the worst headache of life, vomiting, confusion, pupil size difference, stiff neck, altered consciousness

Diagnosis:
- Non-contrast head CT
- Non-contrast head CT is usually normal. In that case, get a **lumbar puncture (LP)**; CSF sample is collected, and then centrifuged and analyzed; CSF gives **yellow appearance** (xanthochromia) in **SAH**.
- Angiography is also done to locate the bleeding vessel

Note: Occasionally, there may be blood in the CSF sample that came from the spinal tap itself. If CSF sample remains **clear after centrifusion**, then it means the patient did not have SAH. Blood on the CSF sample was from the spinal tab (LP procedure)

Treatment:
- Initial management is surgical clipping of the bleeding blood vessel
- Calcium channel blocker (nimodipine) –is given to prevent ischemic stroke
- Seizure prophylaxis

VERTIGO

Vertigo is characterized by sudden sensation that a person is spinning

Differential diagnosis of vertigo

Condition	Hearing loss and tinnitus	Special characteristic	Treatment
Benign positional vertigo (BPV)	No hearing loss and tinnitus	Vertigo related to **head movement**	Meclizine
Vestibular neuritis	No hearing loss and tinnitus	Vertigo **not related** to head movement	Meclizine
Labyrinthitis	Hearing loss and tinnitus both are present	Symptoms (vertigo) started **following URI**	Meclizine
Meniere's disease	Hearing loss and tinnitus both are present	**Episodic vertigo**	Surgery

DEMYELINATING DISEASES

1. MULTIPLE SCLEROSIS (MS)

Multiple sclerosis is an autoimmune disease that affects the myelin sheath of white matter of central nervous system (brain and spinal cord)

Si/Sx:
- Patient often presents with CNS abnormalities such as visual problems, ataxia or diplopia that **resolved spontaneously but later return**
- **Optic neuritis is the common** initial presentation

Diagnosis:
- **MRI** is the **best initial and most accurate test**. MRI shows multiple, asymmetric, periventricular white matter plaque
- If MRI is inconclusive, then do **lumbar puncture (LP)**.
  - LP shows mild increase in proteins, WBCs< 100, increased IgG oligoclonal band (nonspecific for MS)

Treatment: discussed below

Conditions in MS	Treatment
Acute exacerbation	IV steroids, if steroids are ineffective do plasma exchange
Relapsing- remitting disease	Interferon-β1a, or Interferon-β1b, or Glatiramer
Secondary progression	Interferon-β1b
Muscle spasticity	**Baclofen** is for **daytime** **Tizanidine** is for **nighttime**. Tizanidine is not recommended for daytime use because it cause dizziness
Fatigue	Amantadine
Urinary retention	Bethanechol
Urinary incontinence	Oxybutynin

2. AMYOTROPHIC LATERAL SCLEROSIS

Amyotrophic lateral sclerosis (ALS) also known as Lou Gehrig's disease, is a progressive neurodegenerative disease that affects nerve cells in the brain and the spinal cord

Si/Sx:

- Asymmetric, slow progressive muscle weakens and coordination
- Breathing and swallowing muscles may be affected
- Upper motor neuron (UMN) signs and lower motor neuron (LMN) signs, are discussed below

Sign	UMN sign	LMN sign
Weakness	+	+
Atrophy	-	+
Fasciculation	-	+
Muscle Tone	Increased	Decreased
Muscle reflexes	Increased	Decreased

Note: sexual function are not affected in ALS

Diagnosis:

- Pulmonary functions tests (PFTs)
- EMG is **best initial diagnostic** test

Treatment:

- If patient's PFTs are affected, then do intubation and mechanical ventilation
- There **is no cure** for ALS. **Riluzole** is given **slowdown the symptoms**

3. GUILLAIN- BARRÉ SYNDOMRE

Guillain-barré syndrome is an autoimmune disorder that affects the peripheral nerves

Si/Sx: muscle weakness and paralysis that **starts in legs and spreads to upper body**, bladder or bowel incontinence, and autonomic symptoms

Cause: Recent infection with campylobacter jejuni, mycoplasma, or virus

Diagnosis:
- Pulmonary functions tests (PFTs)
- Best initial test is lumbar puncture (LP), which **shows increased protein and normal WBCs** (albuminocytologic dissociation)
- EMG is used to confirm the diagnosis. It shows diffuse demyelination

Treatment:
- If patient's PFTs are affected, then do intubation and mechanical ventilation.
- IVIG or plasmapheresis is the first-line of treatment

Boards tip for demyelinating diseases
- Always check PFTs before treating ordering disease specific labs or treatment. If PFTs are affected, then do intubation and mechanical ventilation

---

4. Other *high-yield* **non-demyelinating diseases, which may look like Guillain-barré syndrome**

4a. TRANSVERSE MYELITIS
Look for a patient with back pain, **ascending paralysis**, paresthesias, **band like tightness** in mid chest
Cause: inflammation of spinal nerves that is caused by infection, autoimmune disease or certain vaccination (MMR, DTP, and hepatitis B)
Diagnosis: **MRI**   (**Note**: Guillain-Barré is diagnosed with LP)
Treatment:
- IV steroids and treat the underlying cause
- If steroids are ineffective, then do plasmapheresis

4a. BOTULISM TOXIN
Look for a patient with **descending paralysis**, constipation, hypotonia, decreased gag & suck reflex, with **clear sensorium**
Cause: ingestion or inhalation of clostridium botulin spores
Diagnosis:
- Pulmonary functions tests (PFTs)
- Clinical diagnosis
- Diagnosis can be confirmed by serum botulinum toxin

Treatment:
- If PFTs are affected, then do intubation and mechanical ventilation
- If PFTs are normal then supportive management

SEIZURE
Seizure is a physical finding or change in behavior that occurs after disorganized and sudden electrical activity in the brain

Cause: Etiology includes: **Mnemonic: VITAMIN C**
    Vascular (stroke, bleed, AV malformation)
    Infection (meningitis, encephalitis)
    Trauma
    Autoimmune disease
    Metabolic (sodium, calcium, magnesium, glucose)
    Idiopathic
    Neoplasm
    PsyChiatric

Types: Seizures can be divided into two main types partial seizure also known as focal seizure and generalized seizure
- Partial seizure is generated and affects one part of the brain. Symptoms depends on that affected part of the brain
- General seizure is produced by disorganized electrical impulse throughout the brain

Diagnosis:
- Urgent CT Head
- Check sodium, calcium, magnesium, creatinine, glucose, oxygen and urine toxicology
- If diagnosis if still inconclusive, then get EEG

Note: potassium abnormalities does not cause neurological abnormalities

Management:
- Maintain ABCs
- Treat the underlying cause
- It is not necessary to start the patient on antiepileptic medicine after single episode of treatment. However, treatment should be started after single episode of seizure if:
    o Patient has family history of seizure
    o Patient has status epilepticus
    o Patient has abnormal neurological exam

- o   Abnormal EEG
- Treatment for specific type of seizure is discussed on the next page

DIFFERENTIAL DIAGNOSIS OF SEIZURES

Type	Characteristic	Treatment
Partial seizures		
Simple partial seizure	Consciousness is **maintained.** Symptoms depend on the affected brain area	Carbamazepine or phenytoin is the first choice. Valproic acid or lamotrigine is the 2nd choice
Complex partial seizure	Consciousness is **impaired.** Lip smacking, involuntary but coordinated movements	Same as simple partial seizure
Generalized seizures		
Tonic- clonic seizure	**Rhythmic sudden stiffness and violent jerking of muscles.** Marked by urinary incontinence and tongue biting. EEG shows 10-Hz	Valproic acid is the 1st choice. Lamotrigine, or Carbamazepine or phenytoin is 2nd choice.
Tonic seizures	**Stiffening of muscles**	Same as tonic-clonic seizure
Clonic seizures	**Repetitive, rhythmic jerks of both sides of the body at the same time**	Same as tonic-clonic seizure
Myoclonic seizures	**Isolated, jerking movements**	Valproic acid is 1st choice. Clonazepam is 2nd choice
Atonic seizures	**Sudden and generalized loss of muscle tone**	Same as tonic-clonic seizure
Absence seizure	**Short (5 -10 seconds) loss of consciousness** with few or no symptoms. A patient appears **daydreaming or staring blankly.** EEG shows 3-Hz spike-and-wave	Ethosuximide

STATUS EPILEPTICUS

Status epilepticus is a life-threatening conditioning in which patient have repeated epileptic seizures without gaining consciousness between them

Management is as follow

Step 1 – Maintain ABCs		
Step 2 - IV Lorazepam		
Step 3 –Patient is still seizing after 10-20 minutes, then give **phenytoin or fosphenytoin** Step 4 - Patient is still seizing after 10-20 minutes, then **add 5-10 mg/kg IV phenytoin or fosphenytoin** Step 5 - Patient is still seizing after 10-20 minutes, then **give IV Phenobarbital** Step 6 - Patient is still seizing after 10-20 minutes, then **add 5-10 mg/kg IV phenobarbital** Step 7 - Patient is still seizing, then **intubate the patient plus give propofol or midazolam**	OR	Step 3 - if patient develops status epilepticus in a ICU, has comorbid condition or seizure lasting > 60 minute, then **intubate the patient plus give propofol or midazolam**

BRAIN TUMOR

Brain tumors can be classified as primary brain tumor (originates within the brain) and secondary brain tumors (metastatic tumor)

Most **common types of brain** tumors are **secondary brain tumors** (metastatic tumor) that often arise from lungs, breast, kidney, and GI tract.

Si/Sx: headaches, nausea, vomiting, seizures, memory problem, mood and personality change

Diagnosis:

- Contrast CT or MRI to localize the tumor
- CT or MRI guided needle biopsy

Primary brain tumors differential diagnosis

Type	Characteristic	Treatment
Astrocytoma	• Arises from astrocytes • **Most occur in the cerebrum** • Grade III astrocytoma is called anaplastic astrocytoma • Grade IV astrocytoma is called glioblastoma multiforme	Grade III – surgical resection or radiation Grade IV – surgical resection, radiation and chemotherapy
Ependymomas	• Most common in children • **Arise from ependymoma cells** in ventricle or spinal cord and may lead to hydrocephalus	Surgical resection and Radiation
Medulloblastoma	• Most common in children • Arises **from the 4th ventricle** and leads to obstructive hydrocephalus	Radiation and chemotherapy
Meningioma	• Benign slow growing tumors • Arise **from meninges**	Surgical resection. Radiation for unresectable tumor
Schwannomas (Acoustic neuromas)	• Arises from Schwann cells • Affects women as twice as men • Cause **ipsilateral hearing loss**	Surgical resection

SPINE DISORDERS

1. BACK SPRAIN
Back sprain is the most common type of back injury
Cause: improper lifting, overstressing back muscles
Si/Sx: pain that worsens with movement, muscle cramping, decreased range of motion, difficulty walking, bending forwards or sideways and standing
Diagnosis: clinical diagnosis, spine X-ray may be required to rule out fracture
Treatment: NSAIDs and physical therapy

2. SYRINGOMYELIA
Syringomyelia is defined as development of a cavity in the spinal cord. It is mostly seen between T8- C1
Si/Sx: loss of **bilateral pain and temperature in a cape-like distribution across neck and arms**
Note: position, vibration and tactile sensation are spared
Diagnosis: Spine MRI
Treatment: Surgery

3. SPINAL STENOSIS
Spinal stenosis is an abnormal narrowing of spinal canal that can put pressure on spinal cord and nerves that travel through the spine
Cause: overgrowth of bone, herniated disks, thickened ligament, tumor and spinal injuries
Si/Sx: (pseudoclaudication) back pain that exacerbates when walking downhill and **relives with walking uphill, bending forward**
Diagnosis: Spine MRI
Treatment: surgery

4. CAUDA EQUINA SYNDROME

Cauda equina syndrome is a serious neurological condition in which nerve roots of cauda equina are damaged

Cause: trauma, tumors, lesions, spinal stenosis, and inflammatory conditions

Si/Sx: acute urinary retention, saddle anesthesia (loss of sensations in buttocks and perineum), decreased anal tone that leads to fecal incontinence, sexual dysfunction, weakness and loss of reflexes in lower extremity

Diagnosis: Spine MRI

Treatment: Corticosteroids and emergent surgical decompression

5. SPINAL TUMOR

Spinal tumor is a benign or malignant tumor that gowns near or within the spinal cord.

Si/Sx: Pain that is **worse at night or in supine position,** constitutional symptoms (Fever, chills, night sweat, weight loss)

Diagnosis: Spine MRI

Treatment: corticosteroids, surgery and/or radiation therapy

6. ANTERIOR SPINAL ARTERY SYNDROME

Anterior spinal artery syndrome is condition in which blood supply to the anterior part of the spine is interrupted

Si/Sx: Flaccid paralysis below the level of occlusion, loss of pain and temperature

Note: Proprioception and vibration are spared

Treatment: Supportive

7. BROWN-SÉQUARD SYNDORME

Brown-séquard syndrome is a condition that results from a lesion in lateral half of the spine

Cause: most common cause is traumatic penetrating injury such as stab or gunshot. Other causes includes tumor, disk herniation, radiation and cervical spondylosis

Si/Sx: Ipsilateral spastic paralysis, Ipsilateral loss of position, vibration and tactile discrimination, **contralateral loss of pain and temperature starting 2-3 segments below the lesion**

Diagnosis: Spine MRI

Treatment: treat the underlying cause

8.   SUBACUTE COMBINED DEGENERATION

Subacute combined degeneration is a neurological condition in which **dorsal and lateral corticospinal tracts** of spine are affected

Si/Sx: Distal paresthesia and weakness, loss of proprioception and vibration

Cause: Vitamin B12

Diagnosis: Serum Vitamin B 12 level, Spine MRI

Treatment: Vitamin B 12 replacement

9.   SPINAL EPIDURAL ABSCESS

Spinal epidural abscess is defined as an inflammation caused by pus between the dura and the bones of the spine

Cause: infection that usually occur during LP or epidural shot

Si/Sx: **back pain, tenderness, fever,** bowel or bladder incontinence

Diagnosis: **MRI**

Treatment: **Drain the abscess and give antibiotics**

NEUROLOGY INFECTIOUS DISEASES

MENINGITIS
Meningitis is an inflammation of meninges of brain and spinal cords
Cause: infection with bacteria, viral, fungus, HSV, TB
Si/Sx: Fever, nausea, vomiting, neck stiffness, photophobia, change in mental status, **positive Kernig's sign and Brudzinski's sign**

Note:
If a patient present with **symptoms of meningitis** and has **impaired consciousness**, then the diagnosis is subarachnoid hemorrhage (**SAH**)

Initial management:
- If a patient has any of the followings, **then** 1st step is to get a **blood culture**, 2nd give **empiric antibiotics**, 3rd get **CT of the head**, and then perform lumbar puncture (**LP**)
  - Focal neurologic deficit
  - Papilledema
  - Altered mental status
  - Seizures
  - If lumbar puncture is delayed

- If patient **does not** have any of the **above, then** proceed to do LP

Empiric treatment by age

Age	Most common cause	Empiric antibiotics
Neonate (≤ 1 month)	Group B. Strep E.coli Listeria	For neonates < 7 days of age neonate **ampicillin** and **gentamycin** **For neonates > 7 days of age neonate ampicillin and Cefotaxime**
Children, teens	N.meningitidis Pneumonia	**Cefotaxime and vancomycin**
Adults < 60 years of age	S.pneumonia	Cefotaxime and vancomycin
Adults > 60 years of age	S.pneumonia, Listeria, Meningococci, gram-negative bacilli	Ampicillin and cefotaxime and vancomycin

CSF findings and differential diagnosis of meningitis

Organism	Opening Pressure (Normal 50–180 mmH₂O)	WBCs cell type	Glucose (Normal 40–85 mg/dL)	Protein (Normal 15–45 mg/dL)	RBCs
Bacteria	High	Neutrophil	Low	High	None
Viral	Normal	Lymphocytes	Normal	Normal	**None**
Fungal	Normal	**Lymphocytes**	Low	**High**	None
HSV	Normal	Lymphocytes	Normal	Normal	**Present**
TB	Normal	**Monocytes**	Low	**High**	None

1. NEISSERIA MENINGITIS

Neisseria meningitis is caused by Neisseria meningitides

Transmission: it is transmitted from person-to person via respiratory droplets or throat secretions

Population at risk: infants, adolescents, college freshmen living in dorms, military recruits, asplenia and terminal complement pathway deficiency

Si/Sx: Fever, nausea, vomiting, neck stiffness, photophobia, change in mental status, positive Kernig's sign and Brudzinski's sign. Other less common signs are petechiae on trunk, and legs

Diagnosis:

- LP: as mentioned in bacterial section of CSF finding and differential diagnosis of meningitis table
- Diagnosis is confirmed with blood culture

Treatment: Respiratory isolation and IV ceftriaxone

Neisseria meningitis prophylaxes

A Neisseria meningitis prophylaxis is the primary method to prevent transmission of disease from infected person to **close contacts or health care workers**

- Close contacts are defined as household members and anyone exposed to **patient's saliva** (kissing, sharing utensil)

- **Health care workers,** who had **unprotected direct contact with patients' oral or nasal secretion or intubated** the patient

Prophylaxis medicine: Rifampin, ciprofloxacin or ceftriaxone
- **Rifampin** should be **avoided in women taking OCPs** because it increases the cytochrome p450 activity and can cause **OCPs failure**
- **Ciprofloxacin is not used in < 16 years** of age because it can cause cartilage destruction
- **Ceftriaxone** is safe for anyone

2. LISTERIA MENINGITIS

Listeria meningitis is seen in **neonates, elderly and immunocompromised patients**
Diagnosis:
- Blood culture shows **gram-positive bacilli**
- LP shows **elevated neutrophils**

Treatment: **Ampicillin**

3. FUNGAL MENINGITIS

Fungal meningitis is a rare form of meningitis; the most common cause of fungal meningitis is **Cryptococcus**
Risk factors: immunocompromised patients such as AIDS, cancer
Si/Sx: Fever, nausea, vomiting, neck stiffness, photophobia, change in mental status, positive Kernig's sign and Brudzinski's sign
Diagnosis: Lumber puncture's findings as follow:
- CSF finding as mentioned as mentioned in fungal section of CSF finding and differential diagnosis of meningitis table
- Cerebrospinal fluid (CSF) culture with **Indian ink** stain shows encapsulated yeast
- **Most accurate test is cryptococcal antigen test**

Treatment: Amphotericin B plus flucytosine

4. TUBERCULOSIS MENINGITIS

Tuberculosis meningitis is caused by mycobacterium tuberculosis
Si/Sx: Look for a patient with TB and symptoms of meningitis
Diagnosis: LP- as mentioned in TB section of CSF finding and differential diagnosis of meningitis table

Treatment: Same as **pulmonary TB medications plus steroids for 12 months**

ENCEPHALITIS

Encephalitis is an acute **irritation and inflammation** of the brain

Cause: most common causes of encephalitis are HSV and arbovirus. Other causes may include CMV, Toxoplasmosis, poliovirus, coxsackievirus, West-Nile virus, tick-borne viruses (Borrelia, rickettsia), Measles, mumps, and rubella

Si/Sx: confusion, altered consciousness, seizures, fever, headaches, and focal neurological deficits

Diagnosis and treatment: discussed below with the specific cause of encephalitis

1. HERPES SIMPLEX VIRUS (HSV) ENCEPHALITIS

HSV is the **most common cause of viral encephalitis**

Si/Sx: olfactory hallucination, confusion, altered consciousness, seizures, fever, headaches, and focal neurological deficits

Diagnosis:

- **Best initial test is CT head**
- Lumber puncture: normal opening pressure, glucose and protein, lymphocytes and RBC.
- Most **accurate test is CSF PCR-DNA**

Treatment: Acyclovir. If a patient is resistant to acyclovir, then give foscarnet

2. TOXOPLASMOSIS ENCEPHALITIS

Toxoplasmosis encephalitis is caused by toxoplasma gondii. It is the most common cause of encephalitis in **HIV-positive patient with CD 4 count < 200 cells/µL**

Si/Sx: confusion, altered consciousness, seizures, fever, headaches, and focal neurological deficits

Diagnosis:

- CT head shows **multiple ring enhancing lesions**
- Toxoplasmosis antibody test is **sensitive test**

Management:

- Standard care of toxoplasmosis encephalitis is **pyrimethamine plus sulfadiazine for 2 weeks, and then repeat CT of the head.**
  - o If CT head shows that ring-enhancing lesions are **resolving,** then **continue treating the patient** with pyrimethamine plus sulfadiazine.
  - o If CT head shows **no improvement** in ring-enhancing lesions, then **order brain biopsy**

Boards tip for ring enhancing lesions

Ring enhancing lesions in the head are caused by number of different things, but standard management for ring enhancing lesions is as follow:
- If the patient is **HIV-negative,** then order brain biopsy
- If the patient is **HIV-positive**, then manage the patient as per toxoplasmosis

---

BRAIN ABSCESS

Brain abscess is an abscess caused by inflammation and infection material, usually from bacterial or fungal infection

Cause: direct infection or germs that can reach brain via blood

Risk factors: weak immune system, infection, cancer, immunosuppressive medicines (corticosteroids or chemotherapy), and Right-to-left shunt.

Symptoms: headaches, fever, change in mental status, increased intracranial pressure, focal neurological findings

Diagnosis:
- Blood culture
- Best initial test is head CT or MRI
- Needle biopsy is usually performed to identify the cause of the infection

Treatment: surgical drainage and antibiotics

NEUROCYSTICERCOSIS

Neurocysticercosis is the most common parasitic disease of the nervous system

Cause: accidental ingestion of food contaminated with eggs of *Taenia solium* (pork tapeworm)

Si/Sx: signs and symptoms of encephalitis in Latin American is neurocysticercosis until proven otherwise.

Diagnosis:

- Best initial test is head CT, which shows multiple cystic lesions
- Diagnosis is confirmed with serology

Treatment: Albendazole plus steroids

NEUROSURGERY

SKULL FRACTURE
- **Closed** linear skull fracture requires **no surgical repair**
- **Open** fracture, **comminuted** fracture or **depressed** fracture requires **surgical repair**

HEAD TRAUMA MANAGEMENT
- Best initial test **is CT of the head**
- If CT of the head and neurological exam is normal, then patient can be sent home, as long as, he has someone at home to frequently wake him up, and watch for any signs of mental change

ACUTE EPIDURAL HEMATOMA
Acute epidural hematoma is a medical emergency in which traumatic injury to the head leads to blood buildup between the dura mater and the skull.

Blood vessel involved: middle meningeal artery

Si/Sx: lucid interval followed by unconsciousness, contralateral hemiparesis, fixed dilated headache, vomiting

Diagnosis: CT head shows **biconvex lens shaped hematoma**

Treatment: Surgical evacuation of hematoma

ACUTE SUBDURAL HEMATOMA
Acute epidural hematoma is a medical emergency in which traumatic injury to the head leads to blood buildup between the dura mater and the arachnoid mater.

Blood vessel involved: bridging vein

Si/Sx: Gradually increasing headache and confusion

Diagnosis: CT of the head shows **crescent-shaped hematoma with or without midline shift**

Treatment:
- If CT shows **midline shift, then** do **emergency craniotomy**
- If CT shows **no midline shift, then lower intracranial pressure to prevent further damage:** elevate head, hyperventilation to keep pCO_2 between 25- 30 mmHg and mannitol

PARENCHYMAL HEMORRHAGE

Parenchymal hemorrhage is accumulation of blood within brain parenchyma

Cause: hypertension, arteriovenous malformation, intracranial neoplasm, amyloid angiopathy, vasculitis, and trauma

Bleeding site: Internal capsule, basal ganglia or thalamus

Si/Sx: altered level of consciousness, nausea, vomiting, headache, seizures, and focal neurological deficits

Diagnosis: Non-contrast head CT shows focal edema

Treatment:

- **Lower intracranial pressure to prevent further damage:** elevate head, hyperventilation to keep pCO_2 between 25- 30 mmHg and mannitol.
- Surgical evacuation of hematoma is necessary, if signs of mass effect are present.

DIFFUSE AXONAL INJURY

Diffuse axonal injury occurs after severe acceleration/ declaration or rotational injuries

Diagnosis:

- CT of the head shows **diffuse blurring of gray–white matter**

Treatment:

- If CT of the head shows **blood,** then **surgical evacuation of the blood**
- If **CT of the head shows no blood, then lower the intracranial pressure to prevent further damage:** elevate head, hyperventilation to keep pCO_2 between 25- 30 mmHg and mannitol

NEUROLOGY CCS

CASE # 1

Case introduction
A 73-years-old white male is brought to the office by his son because of 2-year history of memory impairment

Initial vitals signs
Temperature: 37.2 degrees
Pulse: 68 beats/min, regular rhythm
Respiration rate: 19/ minutes

Blood pressure, systolic 124 mm Hg
Blood pressure, disystolic, 75 mm Hg

Height: 63.0 inches
Weight: 120.0 lbs.
Body mass index: 21.3 Kg/m2

History of present illness (HPI)
A 73-years-old white male is brought to the office by his son because of a 2-year history of memory impairment. He lives alone and takes care of his own home and financials since the death of his wife two years ago. Son noticed a gradual memory impairment and difficulty finding words. Lately, he has difficulty with recognizing family and friends. Two days ago he was got lost a block from his home.

Past medical history
Hospitalization: None
Other medical condition: None
Current medication: None
Allergies: none
Vaccination: up to date

Family history
Father died of MI, and mother had Alzheimer's disease

Social history
Marital history: Widowed
Occupation: retired
Recreational: gardening
Personal habits: Does not drink smoke, or use drugs

Review of system:
General: see HPI
Skin: see HPI
HEENT: see HPI
Musculoskeletal: see HPI
Cardiology: see HPI
Abdominal: see HPI
Genitourinary: see HPI

Please see pages 1-5 for general CCS cases approach

Step 1. None (patient is stable does not require any emergency measures)

Step 2. Order complete physical exam, and then move the clock forward to get the results
- Result shows:
- o Mini-mental exam: patient unable to recall objects, difficulty following commands
- o Rest of the is physical exam is normal

Step 3. Order the labs, and then move the clock forward to get the labs results
- CBC
- UA
- BMP
- Chest x-ray
- TSH
- LFT
- Vitamin B 12
- VDRL
- CT head

- Result shows:
- o CT head shows diffuse cortical atrophy
- o Rests of the testes are within normal limit

Step 4. Donepezil, Vitamin E

Step 5. Make a follow-up appointment after 2-3 months and send patient home

Step 6. None

Step 7. Move the clock forward to next follow-up appointment

Step 8. None

Step 9. Make another follow-up appointment in 2- 3months

Step 10. Counsel and age and gender specific screening

- Advance directive, living will
- No smoking, drinking, no illicit drugs
- Medicine compliance
- FBOT
- Colonoscopy
- Cholesterol
- Influenza and Pneumovax shot

Diagnosis: Alzheimer's disease

CASE # 2

Case introduction
A 65-years-old female is brought to ER by her husband because her husband noticed sudden slurring in her speech and her face was dropping on one side.

Initial vitals signs
Temperature: 37.2 degrees
Pulse: 68 beats/min, regular rhythm
Respiration rate: 19/ minutes

Blood pressure, systolic 149 mm Hg
Blood pressure, disystolic, 88 mm Hg

Height: 63.0 inches
Weight: 120.0 lbs.
Body mass index: 21.3 Kg/m2

History of present illness (HPI)

A 65-years-old female is brought to ER by her husband because her husband noticed sudden slurring in her speech and her face was dropping on one side. She says it approximately 2 hours ago she felt some numbness on the right side of her face and in her right arm, but thought it was due to fatigue. She never had similar symptoms before. She has had hypertension from last 10 years and taking hydrochlorothiazide.

Past medical history
Hospitalization: For C-section delivery at age 25
Other medical condition: HTN
Current medication: hydrochlorothiazide.
Allergies: none
Vaccination: up to date

Family history
Father died of MI, and mother died of lung cancer.

Social history
Marital history: married, 1 child
Occupation: retired; bank teller
Recreational: gardening, cooking, bingo
Personal habits: Does not drink smoke, or use drugs

Review of system:
General: see HPI
Skin: see HPI
HEENT: see HPI
Musculoskeletal: see HPI
Cardiology: see HPI
Abdominal: see HPI
Genitourinary: see HPI

Please see pages 1-5 for general CCS cases approach

Step 1. Give emergency management
- Pulse oxy
- Oxy
- IV access
- IV normal saline
- BP Monitor
- Vital

Step 2. Order complete physical exam, and then move the clock forward to get the results
- Results show:
- o HEENT: Right carotid bruits
- o Rest of the exam is within normal limit

Step 3. Order the labs, and then move the clock forward to get the results
- CBC
- UA
- BMP
- Chest X-ray
- CT head " stat"
- EKG " stat"

- Results show:
- o CBC shows 8000 WBC with 75% PMN
- o CT head shows no bleeding
- o EKG is normal

Step 4. Give aspirin

Step 5. Admit in wards

Step 6. Order the followings
- NPO
- Bed rest with bathroom privilege
- Pneumatic stocking

Step 7. Carotid Doppler and echocardiography

Step 8. Vascular surgeon consult and, then move the clock forward to get the labs results ordered in step 7 and, vascular surgeon consult
- Results show:
  o Carotid Doppler- 89 % right carotid stenosis, 45 % left carotid stenosis
  o Echocardiography- EF 57%

Step 9. Order pre-surgical labs and, and endarterectomy, and then move the clock forward to the results
- PTT
- PT/INR
- Blood type and cross-match
- Right carotid endarterectomy

- Results show:
  o Blood Type- O negative
  o Endarterectomy is performed

Case usually ends here

Step 10. Counsel and age and gender specific screening
- No smoking, alcohol, illegal drugs
- Seat belt, safe sex
- Medication compliance
- Influenza, Pneumovax vaccination
- Age and gender specific screening can be scheduled for later date

Diagnosis: Transient ischemia attack (TIA)

RHEUMATOLOGY

OSTEOARTHRITIS

Osteoarthritis (OA) is the most common form of arthritis around the world. It is a slowly progressive non-inflammatory, asymmetric arthritis that is **caused by destruction of cartilage due to wear-and-tear of joints.** Incidence of osteoarthritis increases with age. Most commonly affected joints are weight bearing joint such as hip and knee.

Si/Sx: Joint pain, crepitations with joint motion, **stiffness lasting less than 20 minutes,** which **increases with exercise and relieves with rest.**

Diagnosis:

- Physical exam may show **Heberden's nodes** (swelling on DIP joints of hands), **Bouchard's nodes** (swelling on PIP joints of hands)
- X-ray of affected joints shows **osteophytes (bony spurs) and unequal joint space loss.**
- Aspiration of synovial fluid shows straw colored fluid, WBCs < 2000 cell/μL, PMNs < 25%.

Treatment:

- **Best initial management** is **weight loss and muscle strengthening exercises**
- **Acetaminophen is the first-line treatment.** NSAIDs are 2nd line. NSAIDs are not used as a primary treatment because of their toxicity
- If a patient presents with **severe pain or if the treatment is ineffective,** then give **interarticular steroids**
- Joint replacement is reserved for refractory disease

RHEUMATOID ARTHRITIS

Rheumatoid arthritis (RA) is a chronic inflammatory arthritis that mainly affects the synovium of joints. It involves symmetric joints. **Inflammatory reaction** can lead to **synovial hypertrophy and a pannus formation** that can cause cartilage destruction, bone erosion and joint deformity. It is more common in women than men.

Physical findings:

- **Boutonnière deformity**: Flexion of PIP and hyperextension of DIP
- **Swan neck deformity**: Extension of PIP and flexion of PIP
- Most **common finding is rheumatoid skin nodule**

Labs:

- **Best initial test is** rheumatoid factor (RF) - IgM antibodies against Fc portion of IgG. However, **RF is not specific** for RA because it is present in 70- 80% of the patients with RA
- **Anti-cyclic Citrullinated peptide** (anti-CCP) is more **sensitive** and **specific** for RA, but its presence signifies **worst prognosis**
- ESR is elevated
- Aspiration of synovial fluid shows cloudy fluid, WBCs between 200- 50,000 ml, PMNs > 50%
- Joint X-ray shows joint erosion

Note: If RF is **negative, then** check **anti-CCP**, it appears **earlier than RF**

Other findings may includes

- Heart: Pericarditis, valvular disease
- Blood: Normocytic anemia
- Lungs: Bilateral pleural effusion, decreased glucose in pleural effusion

Diagnosis: Require 4 or more symptoms of the following:

- **Morning pain and stiffness** lasting > 1 hour for > 6 weeks.
- **MCP and PIP** joints of fingers and wrist for > 6 weeks.
- **Swelling of ≥ 3 joint** for > 6 weeks.
- **Symmetric** joint for > 6 weeks.
- **Rheumatoid nodules**
- **RF factor**

Boards Tip:

- If a patient presents with RA like symptoms that are present for **< 6 weeks**, then the diagnosis is a viral infection, most likely **Parvovirus**. It is treated with **NSAIDs**

Treatment:

- Prednisone is used in acute RA flare-ups
- NSAIDs or prednisone can be given to control the pain
  - If **a patient has mild** RA and has **renal** insufficiency or **CAD,** then give **prednisone**
  - If **a patient has mild** RA and **has no renal** insufficiency or **CAD, then give NSAIDs. If NSAIDs are ineffective,** then give **methotrexate**
- Disease modifying antirheumatic drugs (DMARDs) should be started early to **slow the disease progression.**
  - **Methotrexate** is the first-line treatment for RA or **if the x-ray shows joint erosion.**
  - **Hydroxychloroquine** can be used for **mild RA.** Its most common side effect is macular damage. Therefore, patient should have a regular eye exam
  - **TNF inhibitors:** Infliximab, adalimumab or etanercept, can be added **to methotrexate,** if methotrexate fails
    - TNF inhibitors can reactivate TB granuloma. Patient should have **PPD test prior to starting TNF inhibitors.**(If PPD induration is > 5mm, then give isoniazid (INH) and vitamin B 6).

Summary of DMARDs

Medicine	Indications	Side effects
Methotrexate	First-line treatment for RA, **X-ray shows joint erosion.**	Megaloblastic anemia, bone marrow suppression, pneumonitis, rheumatoid skin nodule flare, elevated LFTs
TNF inhibitor (Infliximab, adalimumab, etanercept)	First-line treatment for RA, If patient is not responding to methotrexate	Reactivation of TB
Hydroxychloroquine	Used as a monotherapy for mild RA or combined with other DMARDs	Macular damage
Rituximab	Combined with DMARDs when they fail to control symptoms	Immune reaction, infection

Other important facts of RA:

- Atherosclerosis of coronary artery disease (CAD) is the most common cause of death in a patient with RA
- RA patient has a subluxation of C1 and C2 of the spine. It is imperative to get patient's lateral cervical spine X-ray before intubating the patient otherwise patient may develop quadriplegia.

Differential diagnosis of RA

Felty syndrome	Caplan syndrome
• Rheumatoid arthritis • Splenomegaly • Neutropenia	• Rheumatoid arthritis • Pneumoconiosis

SERONEGATIVE ARTHROPATHIES

Seronegative arthropathies are group disorders that **affect joints**, but do **not have rheumatoid factor**. Seronegative arthropathies disorders include:

- Psoriatic arthritis
- Reactive arthritis
- Ankylosing spondylitis

Common characteristics of seronegative arthropathies disorders are:

- Involve sacroiliac joint and lower back
- Negative rheumatoid factor (RF)
- Negative anti-nucleic acid (ANA)
- Associate with HLA- B27

1. ANKLOSING SPONDYLITIS

Ankylosing spondylitis is an inflammatory disease that causes some of the vertebrae in the spine to fuse together, which makes the spine less flexible. It is more common in men, in **mid 20s.**

Si/Sx: Low back **pain and stiffness after waking up,** which usually lasts more than an hour and **relieves with activity**

Diagnosis:

- **Schober's test**: this test is used to measure the flexibility of the spine. A mark is made approximately at L5, and then one mark is 5 cm below this mark and another 10 cm above this mark. The patient is asked to touch his toes without bending knees. In a normal person the distance between these dots should increase more than 5 cm, whereas a patient with ankylosing spondylitis show dots distance < 5 cm
- **Best initial test** is X-ray of spine and hip that shows " **bamboo stick spine**" which is fusion of intervertebral discs and sacroiliitis
- **MRI** is the **most accurate test**; it detects the disease even before X-ray

Treatment:

- **Encourage physical activity and NSAIDs**
- If patient has severe disease or is not responding to NSAIDs, then give **TNF inhibitors**

Complications:

- Uveitis (30%)
- Restrictive lung disease (15-3 %)
- Aortitis (3%)

2. PSORIATIC ARTHRITS

Psoriatic arthritis is a form of arthritis that affects some people who have psoriasis

Si/Sx: Nail pitting, sausage shaped digits, arthritis of distal interphalangeal (DIP) joints

Diagnosis:

- Elevated ESR
- Best initial test is plain x-ray of joints, which shows **"pencil-in-cup deformity"** at the DIP joints

Treatment:

- **Best initial** treatment is **NSAIDs**
- DMARDs such as methotrexate are used in **severe disease or when a patient is not responding to NSAIDs**. DMARDs slow or stop the joint damage and progression of psoriatic arthritis.

- Anti-TNF (etanercept, adalimumab, infliximab) is used, when **DMARDs fail** to control symptoms. These stop the inflammation by suppressing TNF.

Key to differentiate RA, OA and Psoriatic arthritis
- **Rheumatoid arthritis** affects **MCP joints** and **PIP** joints
- **Osteoarthritis** affects **DIP** joints and **PIP** joints
- **Psoriatic arthritis** affects **DIP** joints

---

3. REACTIVE ARTHRITIS

Reactive arthritis develops **in reaction to an infection in another part** of the body such as GI or genitourinary tract infection. Most common bacteria are **Chlamydia, Salmonella, Shigella, Yersinia, and Campylobacter**
Si/Sx:

- Joint pain, **uveitis, conjunctivitis, urethritis,** mouth ulcers, skin rash

Treatment: There is no specific treatment for reactive arthritis; treatment is directed towards **symptoms**

- **NSAIDs** are given to control inflammation and joint pain.
- Interarticular corticosteroids help reduce the inflammation in severe pain or acute flare-ups
- **Doxycycline** is added to NSAIDs if patient is suspected to have reactive arthritis from **chlamydia infection**

Boards tip to distinguish reactive arthritis caused by chlamydia from other bacterial infection

- Patient with reactive arthritis due to **chlamydia** shows **arthritis, uveitis, conjunctivitis, genital lesions / genital discharge**

- Patient with reactive arthritis due **other bacterial infection** shows **arthritis, uveitis, conjunctivitis**

ADULT STILL'S DISEASE

Adult still's disease is a rare type of arthritis that cause **daily spiking fever** and **salmon colored rash**

Diagnostic tests:

- **Negative RA factor** and negative ANA
- **High ferritin** level

Treatment:

- **NSAIDs**
- If NSAIDs are ineffective, then give **methotrexate**

SYSTEMIC LUPUS ERYTHEMATOUS (SLE)

SLE is an autoimmune disease and can affect any organ. It is much more common in females than males (9:1). African-American females are often affected more than other races.

Si/Sx: Non-specific symptoms fatigue, fever, anorexia weight loss, joint pain

Diagnosis: Need 4 of the following to diagnose SLE:

Mnemonic: **DOPAMINE RASH**

1. Discoid rash: raised rim with central necrosis and atrophy
2. Oral ulcers
3. Photosensitivity
4. Arthritis
5. Malar rash: butterfly pattern on cheeks
6. Immunologic criteria (discussed below)
7. Neurologic disorder (Psychosis, seizures, or personality changes)
8. Elevated ESR
9. Renal disease (nephrotic or nephritic syndrome)
10. ANA positive
11. Serositis (pericarditis, pleurisy)
12. Hematologic disease (hemolytic anemia, thrombocytopenia, leukopenia)

Diagnostic tests: immunologic are as follow:

- **Best initial test** is ANA, is found in > 98 % of cases. It is **sensitive but not specific**
- Specific test and confirmatory test is **Anti-dsDNA or Anti-smith antibodies**

Treatment:

- NSAIDs are given to a patient with **mild joint pain**
- **Topical steroids are given** for **rash**
- **Steroids and hydroxychloroquine** are given to patients with **acute SLE flare-ups**

- If the patient with **SLE has glomerulonephritis**, then first **get the renal biopsy** and **treat the patient based on biopsy findings**.
    - if biopsy shows **sclerosis , then no treatment** is needed
    - If the biopsy shows **early and non-proliferative** disease, then give **prednisone**
    - If biopsy shows **advance and proliferative disease**, then give **prednisone and mycophenolate**

Other high-yield **SLE questions**

- Malar rash (Butterfly pattern) heals **without scaring**
- **Discoid lupus** appears as raised rim with central necrosis and atrophy, it heals **with scar.** 5% patients with discoid lupus will develop SLE
- **Anti-ds DNA** increase the risk of **lupus nephritis**
- During the disease **flare up** complement level **(C3, C4) are decreased** and anti-dsDNA is increased
- **Anti-Ro (SSA)** increases the risk of **congenital heart block**
- Atherosclerosis CAD is the most common cause of death in a patients with SLE

DRUG-INDUCED LUPUS
Lupus can also be triggered by medications such as **hydralazine, procainamide, isoniazid, and quinidine**
Diagnosis: Anti-histone antibody
Treatment: Stop the offending drug and symptoms usually resolve in one to two weeks

Broads tip to distinguish drug-induces lupus from SLE

- Drug-induced lupus
  - o **Never affects renal or CNS**
  - o **Complements and anti-dsDNA are normal**

ANTIPHOSPHOLIPID SYNDROME

Antiphospholipid syndrome is an autoimmune disorder caused by antiphospholipid antibodies. It is usually seen in other autoimmune disorders such as SLE.

Complication: it is associated with pregnancy complications such as preeclampsia, thrombosis, **spontaneous abortion**

Diagnosis:

- **Antiphospholipid** antibodies or **anti-cardiolipin** antibodies

Treatment: **Aspirin and** low-molecular-weight heparin **(LMWH) throughout the pregnancy**

SCLERODERMA

Scleroderma is a group of disorders in which normal tissue is replaced with thick fibrous tissue

Type: two types of scleroderma are:

- Diffuse scleroderma, which involves almost all organs.
- Limited scleroderma is known as CREST syndrome, it affects some organs

1. DIFFUSE SCLERODERMA

Diffuse scleroderma primarily affects skin, but may also involves lungs, renal, cardiovascular system, genitourinary system (GU), and, gastrointestinal system (GI)

Si/Sx: symptoms are as follow:

- Raynaud's phenomenon is spam in small blood vessels of fingers and toes in response to cold and emotional stress; they become numb then turn white, then blue and then red.
- Skin: hardening of skin in hands, arms, face, trunk and legs
- Gastrointestinal: esophageal dysmotility, GERD
- Renal: Malignant hypertension and renal failure

- Lungs: pulmonary fibrosis and pulmonary hypertension

Diagnosis:
- ANA
- Anti-topoisomerase antibodies (anti-scl-70)

Treatment: There is no specific treatment for scleroderma. Treatment is directed towards symptoms
- Raynaud's phenomenon: Tx. **Nifedipine**
- Skin thickening: Tx. **D-Penicillamine**
- GERD and esophageal dysmotility: Tx. **Proton pump inhibitors (PPIs) for life**
- Hypertension or renal failure: Tx. **ACE-inhibitors**
- For **pulmonary hypertension,** any of the following can be given:
  - **Bosentan** a endothelin inhibitor, which prevents the growth of pulmonary vasculature
  - **Epoprostenol or treprostinil** a prostacyclin analogues, which dilates the pulmonary vasculature
  - Sildenafil

Complication: Pulmonary fibrosis and pulmonary hypertension are the leading cause of death

2. CREST syndrome

CREST represents
- Calcinosis of fingers
- Raynaud's phenomenon
- Esophageal dysmotility
- Sclerodactyly
- Telangiectasia

Diagnosis: **Anticentromere antibodies**
Treatment: D-penicillamine

Note: CREST syndrome does not involve hands, joints, kidney and lungs Mnemonic to remember that is **HiJKL.** Involvement of any of these organs excludes CREST syndrome.

EOSINOPHILIC FASCIITIS

Eosinophilic fasciitis is a rare condition that causes thickening and inflammation of skin and fascia

Si/Sx: similar to CREST syndrome, additionally **orange peel appearance of the skin**

Diagnosis: CBC shows eosinophilia

Treatment: corticosteroids

POLYMYOSITIS AND DERMATOMYOSITIS

Polymyositis and dermatomyositis are chronic inflammatory diseases of proximal muscles. In addition to muscles in dermatomyositis skin is also affected

Si/Sx: symptoms of polymyositis and dermatomyositis

Polymyositis	Dermatomyositis
• Progressive muscle weakness • Difficult swallowing (dysphagia) • Difficulty speaking • Mild joint or muscle tenderness • Fatigue • Shortness of breath	**Same as dermatomyositis plus the** following skin findings: • **Heliotrope rash** - purple discoloration of face • **Gottron's papules** - scaly lesions over knuckles • **Shawl sign**- erythematous neck and shoulder area

Diagnosis:
- ANA
- **CPK and aldolase** are the **best initial tests**
- **Muscle biopsy** is the **most accurate test**

Treatment: Prednisone

Complications: both conditions are associated with the followings:
- Patients are at increased risk of developing **cancer** especially of the cervix, lungs, pancreas, breasts, ovaries and gastrointestinal tract
- **Anti-Jo-1** is associated with inflammatory myopathies; it **increases the risk of interstitial lung disease**

POLYMYALGIA RHEUMATICA

Polymyalgia rheumatica is an inflammatory disease that causes **pain and stiffness in shoulder, neck, upper arm and hips**

Si/Sx: **pain and stiffness in proximal muscle** with difficulty getting up from seated position. Other general symptoms include fever, fatigue, unintentional weight loss, and depression

Note: Patient with PM/DM also presents with similar complaint , but has **muscle pain and tenderness,** whereas patient with polymyalgia rheumatica has **pain and stiffness**

Diagnosis:
- Increased ESR (>100)
- Other labs such as CPK, aldolase and muscle biopsy **are normal**

Treatment: Low dose prednisone

Complication: Polymyalgia rheumatica is often associated with **temporal arteritis, also as known as giant cell arteritis.** It is possible to have both of these conditions together. Symptoms of temporal arteritis are headache, temporal tenderness, jaw claudication and visual disturbance.

FIBROMYALGIA

Fibromyalgia is a disorder of unknown etiology

Si/Sx: Patient usually presents with **widespread body pain and tenderness** with **trigger points** in joints, muscles, tendons and other soft tissues. Other symptoms includes fatigue, **non-refreshing sleep,** headache, depression

Diagnosis:
- There is **no specific test** to diagnosis fibromyalgia. It is diagnosed based on physical exam. Patient must have **pain and tenderness** at **least 11 of the 18 trigger points**; neck, shoulders, chest, rib cage, elbows, lower back, buttocks, thighs, knees
- Other labs such as ESR, CPK, aldolase are **all normal**

Treatment:
- Initial treatment involves **physical therapy, exercise and relaxation** techniques.
- If these fail to control symptoms, then give antidepressant (amitriptyline, pregabalin or milnacipran) or muscle relaxant

CHRONIC FATIGUE SYNDROME

Chronic fatigue syndrome is characterized by severe, continued tiredness that is not relieved by rest and is not caused by medical condition

Si/Sx: > 6 months of non-refreshing sleep fatigue, stiffness with no tender points

Treatment:

- Initial treatment involves **physical therapy, exercise and relaxation** techniques.
- If these fail to control symptoms, then give antidepressant (amitriptyline, pregabalin or milnacipran) or muscle relaxant

---

Boards tip:

- To distinguish between fibromyalgia and chronic fatigue syndrome, look at the pain at tender points. If the patient has pain at the tender points, then the diagnosis is fibromyalgia. However, no pain at tender points suggests chronic fatigue syndrome.

VESCULITIS

1. TEMPORAL ARTERITIS

Temporal arteritis (TA) is a condition in which temporal arteries of the head become inflamed and damaged

Si/Sx: headache and tenderness in temple area, jaw claudication, fever, vision impairment

Diagnosis:

- Erythrocytes sedimentations rate (ESR) higher than 60mm/hour, but it is usually >100 mm/hour in TA
- Most accurate test is temporal artery biopsy

(High-yield)

Treatment: high dose prednisone, which should be started immediately following ESR test results, otherwise patient may develop irreversible blindness

2. TAKAYASU'S ARTERITIS

Takayasu's arteritis is **inflammation of the aorta and its branches.** It is usually seen in young Asian female between 15-30 years of age

Si/Sx: fatigue, muscle ache, **diminished pulses or blood pressure on the affected side**
Diagnosis:
- Increased ESR
- Most accurate test is Aortic arteriography or MRA

Treatment: Steroids
Complication: If carotid artery is involved, it can lead to TIA or stroke

3. BEHCET'S DISEASE

Behcet's disease is a rare condition that affects the inflammation of blood vessels throughout the body
Si/SX: painful oral and genital ulcers
Diagnosis: there is no specific test
- Diagnosed is based on symptoms and positive pathergy test, which is **formation of sterile skin abscesses** where a sterile needle is inserted by a physician

Treatment: Prednisone and colchicine

CRYSTAL INDUCED ARTHROPATHY

1. GOUT

Gout is an inflammatory arthritis, it occurs when uric acid builds up in joints.
Etiology: Levels of uric acid can be increased by some genetic defects or acquired causes such as
- Excessive alcohol ingestion
- Steroid withdrawal
- Drugs (diuretics, pyrazinamide, ethambutol)
- Hemolysis
- Neoplasia

Si/Sx: sudden onset of intense joint pain, which is most commonly seen in first metatarsophalangeal joint (MTP). Pain increases even with the slight touch of bed sheet
Diagnosis:
- Best initial test is arthrocentesis
- Most accurate test is microscopic analysis of joint fluid, which shows **needle shaped negative birefringent crystals**

Treatment:

Acute attacks treatment is given as follow:

- If the patient has **renal impairment,** then give Interarticular or oral steroids
- If the patient **does not have renal** impairment, then give **NSAIDs (Indomethacin), or Colchicine**
  - NSAIDs are the first-line treatment
  - If the patient **can not tolerate NSAIDS or is elderly, then** give colchicine
    - Colchicine **prevents the further attacks,** it is given every hour until symptoms resolve or patient GI abnormalities
- If NSAIDs or colchicine are ineffective, then give **oral steroids**

Chronic or maintenance treatment is given to prevent future attacks. It is combination of lifestyle modification and medications

- **Lifestyle modifications** such as weight loss, limit alcohol and low purine diet.
- **Medications**: depends on uric acid level, renal failure and renal stones
  - If the patient is **under secreting uric acids,** has **no renal failure** or **no history of kidney stones,** then give **Probenecid**
  - If the patient has **renal failure** or **has a history of kidney stones,** then give **Allopurinol**. It can be used in patients, who under secret or overproduce uric acid
    - Side effects of allopurinol includes allergic nephritis, hemolysis and rash

2. PSEUDOGOUT

Pseudogout is an inflammatory arthritis caused by accumulation of **calcium pyrophosphate** crystals in joints

Si/Sx: Severely painful, warm and swollen joint. **Large joints** such as knees and wrist are frequently affected

Etiology: older age, trauma, metabolic disease such as hyperparathyroidism, hemochromatosis, hypophosphatemia, and hypomagnesemia

Diagnosis:

- Best initial test is arthrocentesis
- Most accurate test is microscopic analysis of joint fluid, which shows positive **birefringent rhomboid-shaped crystal.**
- X-ray of the affected joint shows joint damage and crystal deposit in the joint cartilage

Treatment: NSAIDs are first-line therapy. Steroids are given if patient is not responding to NSAIDs

---

Boards tip for pseudogout

- If a patient with pseudogout is <50 years of age, then make sure to rule out following metabolic cause: (4 H's)
    - Hyperparathyroidism
    - Hemochromatosis
    - Hypophosphatemia
    - Hypomagnesemia
- If **hemochromatosis** is suspected, then order **transferrin saturation levels**

PAGET DISEASE OF BONES (OSTEITIS DEFORMANS)

Paget disease of bones is caused by increased activity of both osteoblast (bone formation cells) and osteoclasts (reabsorbs bone) cells that results in abnormal bone formation

Si/Sx: Bone pain, diffuse bone fractures, hearing loss, bowing of legs, enlarged head and skull deformity, **high cardiac output failure**

Diagnosis:

- Best **initial test** is alkaline phosphate
- X-ray is the most **accurate test**, it shows sclerotic lesions
- Bone scan is the most **sensitive test**

Treatment:

- 1st choice is bisphosphonates
- 2nd choice is calcitonin

FOOT PAIN DIFFERENTIAL DIAGNOSIS

Condition	Characteristics	Treatment
Plantar fasciitis	Sharp heel pain ever time foot strikes the ground. Pain is worse in the morning	Stretching
Morton neuroma	Pain and numbness between 3rd and 4th toes, which is caused by wearing pointed toe shoes	**Wear appropriate shoes** and pain relievers. Surgery is reserved for refractory cases

BONE TUMOR

Tumor	Age	Characteristics	Treatment
Ewing sarcoma	5 -15	• 2nd most common tumor • Occurs at the diaphysis of long bone • X-ray shows **" onion skinning"**	Chemotherapy
Osteogenic sarcoma (osteosarcoma)	10 - 25	• The most common tumor • Occurs around the knee (distal femur and proximal tibia) • X-ray shows **" sun-burst sign**	Excision and local irradiation
Osteochondroma	< 25	• Benign tumor • Occurs around the knee (distal femur and proximal tibia)	Excision
Giant cell	20 - 40	• Benign tumor • Occurs in the epiphysis of the long bone • X-ray shows **" hot-spot"** at the location of the tumor	Excision and local irradiation

RHEUMATOLOGY INFECTIOUS DISEASES

SEPTIC ARTHRITS

Septic arthritis also known as infectious arthritis is caused by direct invasion of joint space by bacteria.

Cause: Septic arthritis is classified as either gonococcal or non-gonococcal.

- **Gonococcal arthritis** is caused by **Neisseria gonorrhea**; it is the most common cause in **sexually active young adults.**

- **Non-gonococcal arthritis** is caused by **staphylococcus aureus (40%), streptococcus (30%), and aerobic gram-negative rods (20%).** It is most common in adults and children older than 2 years of age. Incidence of non-gonococcal arthritis increases with the degree of joint damage joints and prosthetic joints. Rheumatoid arthritis is the greatest risk factor.

Si/Sx:

- **Symptoms of non-**gonococcal arthritis include **single affected** joint that is immobile, swollen, red, warm and tender.

- **Symptoms of non-**gonococcal arthritis include **multiple affected joints, migratory arthritis, tenosynovitis**

Diagnosis:

- **Arthrocentesis** (joint fluid aspiration) to get cell count, gram stain and culture. Results are as follow:

	Non-gonococcal arthritis	Gonococcal arthritis
WBCs	>50,000 cells predominantly PMNs	30,000 – 50,000 cell
Gram stain	Positive in 40-70 %	Positive in 25 %
Culture	Positive in 90-95 %	Positive in 50 %

- Patients with gonococcal arthritis should also have a swab of all the sites of sexual contacts such as urethra, anus, cervix, and oropharynx

Treatment: Empiric treatment is given to the patient until the definitive cause and sensitivity are known. Empiric treatment is as follow:

- Empiric treatment for **non-gonococcal arthritis is vancomycin and ceftriaxone**
- Empiric treatment for **gonococcal arthritis is IV or IM ceftriaxone**

OSTEOMYELITIS

Osteomyelitis is the infection of the bone that is caused by microbial agent. Bacteria can enter the bone via hematogenous spread, nearby infections or direct contamination.

Cause: S. aureus is the most common cause; other causes may include group B. streptococcus, and Streptococcus pneumonia

Si/Sx: Fever, chills, pain, swelling, warmth, redness over infected area

Diagnosis:

- **X-ray** is the **best initial test**
- If x-ray shows no abnormality, then get MRI
- **Bone biopsy and culture** is the **most accurate test**
- **Bone scan is only done if x-ray shows** no abnormality, and patient has **contraindications for MRI**, such as cardiac pacemakers

Treatment: Empiric treatment with IV vancomycin and 3rd generation cephalosporin's, until culture and sensitivity results become available

Note: Patients with Sickle cell anemia are at increased risk of osteomyelitis from salmonella, and IV drugs abusers from pseudomonas. However, S. aureus is still the most common cause of osteomyelitis

RHEUMATOLOGY SURGERY

SHOULDER INJURIES

Injury	Characteristics	Diagnosis	Treatment
Anterior shoulder dislocation	Arm is held close to the body and **externally rotated**, as if the patient is going to shake hands Physical exam shows **numbness on deltoid area** due to stretching of axillary nerve	X-ray of shoulder with **anterior and lateral view**	Close reduction
Posterior shoulder dislocation	Arm is held close to the body and **internally rotated.** It usually occur during **uncoordinated arm movement such as** seizure, electric shocks	X-ray of shoulder with **axillary or scapular view**	Close reduction
Rotator cuff injury	Patient experiences **shoulder pain** when arm is **raised from 60° to 120°**	MRI of the shoulder	NSAIDs and physical therapy Advise the patient that complete rest may lead to frozen shoulder
Clavicular fracture	Pain over fracture site and **inability to lift arm** because of pain	X-ray	Arm sling or figure-of-eight wrap

SHOULDER PAIN

Shoulder pain is a common complaint

Treatment:

- 1st line therapy is **heat pad, physical therapy and NSAIDs**
- If it is ineffective for > 6 weeks, then give a **steroid shot**
- Refractory cases may need **surgery**

ELBOW PAIN

Injury	Cause	Diagnosis	Treatment
Tennis elbow (Lateral epicondylitis)	Painful **lateral** elbow that is caused by overuse of the elbow. It is most common in people playing tennis or racquet sports	**Wrist extension** and **supination** against the resistance **elicits pain**	Ice, rest, NSAIDs, bracing
Golfer Elbow (Medial epicondylitis)	Painful **medial** elbow that is caused by overuse of the elbow. It is most common in golfers	**Pronation** of forearm and **flexion of wrist** against the resistance **elicits pain**	Ice, rest, NSAIDs, bracing

FOREARM AND WRIST INJURIES

CARPEL TUNNEL SYNDROME

Carpel tunnel syndrome is a painful hand and arm condition caused by median nerve entrapment in the wrist.

Si/Sx: Pain and numbness in median nerve distribution (thumb, index finger, middle finger and radial half of the ring finger), which is worst at night

Diagnosis: Clinical diagnosis

- **Phalen's test:** wrist flexion at 60 ° for 1 minute reproduces the pain.
- **Tinel's sign:** tapping median nerve over along its course reproduces the pain

Treatment: Wrist splint and NSAIDs. Surgery is reserved for refractory cases

FOREARM AND WRIST INJURY CONTINUED

Injury	Characteristics	Diagnosis	Treatment
Colles fracture	**Distal radius fracture** results from the fall **onto an outstretched hand.** It is most common in **elderly** (osteoporosis makes bone very fragile	X-ray	Closed reduction and long arm case
Scaphoid fracture	Scaphoid bone is **located at the base of the thumb.** It is usually seen in **young patient, who fell on a outstretched hand** with weight on the palm	X-ray, but may be negative for first 3 weeks	If x-ray is negative - **spica cast for 3 weeks** and then repeat X-ray If x-ray shows displaced and angulated fracture - **open reduction and internal fixation**
Monteggia fracture	**Direct hit on ulna** results in fracture of the proximal third of the ulna with dislocation of the head of the radius	X-ray	Fractured joint - open reduction and internal fixation Dislocated joint - closed reduction
Galeazzi fracture	**Direct hit on radius** results in fracture of the radius with dislocation of the distal radioulnar joint	X-ray	Same are Monteggia fracture
Nightstick fracture	**Isolated fracture of ulna** associated with direct trauma to the forearm	X-ray	Splint for minor fracture Open reduction and internal fixation for significantly displaced fractures

FINGER INJURIES

Injury	Cause	Physical exam	Treatment
Trigger finger	One of the finger or thumb gets **locked in a bent position**	Clinical diagnosis: patient have flexed fingers, which are hard to **extend without using other hand**	Steroid injection
De Quervain tenosynovitis	Painful condition that occurs when the tendons around the **base of the thumb are affected**	Clinical diagnosis; have the patient **hold the thumb in closed fist then force the wrist towards ulnar side reproduces** the **pain on the radial side** of the wrist and thumb	Steroid injection
Dupuytren contracture	**Thickening of the fibrous** tissue layer underneath the skin of the palms and fingers	Physical exam shows **fingers are flexed towards the palms and tender nodules in the palms**	Surgery
Jersey finger	Injury to **flexor tendon of distal interphalangeal** joint. It is often seen in athletes when one player grabs another player's jersey with the tip of the finger(s) while that player is running away.	**Inability to flex the distal knuckle** of the injured finger	Splint
Mallet finger	Injury to the **extensor tendon of distal interphalangeal joint**. It occurs when ball or other objects strikes the tip of the finger.	**Inability to extend distal knuckle** of the injured finger	Splint

AMPUTATED DIGITS
Amputated digits are managed as follow:
- Clean the amputated digit with saline, then wrap it in a saline gauze, then place it in a sealed bag and place the bag on ice bed

HIP AND LEG INJURIES

Injury	Cause	Leg appearance	Treatment
Posterior hip dislocation	Dashboard injury to knee during motor vehicle accident is the most common cause of hip dislocation	Leg is shortened and internally rotated	Closed reduction
Hip fracture	Most common from fall or direct trauma. Some medical conditions such as osteoporosis weakens the bone and make person susceptible to break bones easily	Leg is shortened and externally rotated	Open reduction and pinning
Femoral shaft fracture	Direct trauma to the femur	Injured leg is shorter than the other leg	Intramedullary rod fixation
Tibial fracture	Direct trauma to the tibia		Casting Intramedullary nailing for open fractures, multiple bone fragments and large degree of displacement

KNEE INJURY

1. ANTERIOR CRUCIATE LIGAMENT (ACL)

ACL injury is usually caused by **hyperflexion** of knee, stopping suddenly while running, or direct trauma to the knee

Si/Sx: Pain, swelling, difficulty walking

Diagnosis:

- Positive **anterior drawer** sign
- MRI

Treatment:

- **Athletes** - Tx. Arthroscopic repair
- **For non-athletes or sedentary patients** – Tx. Immobilization and leg strengthening

2. POSTERIOR CRUCIATE LIGAMENT (PCL)

PCL injury occurs due to **hyperextension** of the knee or direct trauma to the knee

Si/Sx: Pain, swelling, difficulty walking

Diagnosis:

- Positive **posterior drawer** sign
- MRI

Treatment: Arthroscopic repair

3. MENISCAL TEAR

Meniscal tear is caused by traumatic injury to the knee

Si/Sx: Pain swelling, patient complain of catching or locking of the knee

Diagnosis:

- McMurray's test
- MRI

Treatment: Arthroscopic repair

4. TIBIAL STRESS FRACTURE

Tibial stress fracture occurs during forced marches.

Diagnosis: X-ray, it is usually normal initially

Management:

- Casting, no weight bearing, and then repeat x-ray in two weeks

5. LATERAL KNEE TRAUMA
Lateral knee trauma caused by **unhappy triad that** involves 3 structures of the knee: **anterior cruciate ligament (ACL), medial collateral ligament (MCL), and medial meniscus or lateral meniscus**

6. POSTERIOR DISLOCATION OF KNEE
Posterior dislocation of the knee occurs due to direct force on the tibia while the knee is flexed. It can cause injury to the **popliteal artery**. Make sure to check the **knee pulses**, if pulses are decreased or absent, then do **Doppler or arteriogram of the leg**

ACHILLES RUPTURE
Achilles tendon is the strongest tendon in the body. It connects calf muscles to the heel. Sudden force on the foot or ankle can rupture it.
Si/Sx: pain, inability to stand on toes on injured side, **popping or pistol-shot like noise when injury occurred**
Diagnosis: Thompson test that shows **absent plantar flexion** of the injured foot when an examiner squeezes the calf muscles
Treatment: Surgery and casting in equinus position

BACK PAIN

1. DISK HERNIATION
Disk herniation is defined as localized displacement of disk material beyond the intervertebral disk space. Most common locations are **L4-L5** and **L5-S1** part of the spine.
Si/Sx: low back pain, pain shooting down buttocks, thighs and knees which **exacerbates with coughing and sneezing**
Diagnosis:
- **Straight leg raise test**: when a patient lying is on his back on the examination table, the examiner lifts the patient's leg while knee is straight. This test is considered positive if the patient experience **pain when legs is raised between 30 - 70 degrees**
- MRI- may **confirm** the diagnosis
Treatment:
- **Bed rest and NSAIDs** are the best initial therapy. Most of the patients get better within 4 weeks
- If these are ineffective, then do **nerve block**

- Surgery is reserved for refractory cases

2. CAUDA EQUINA SYNDROME

It is an emergency medical condition in which damage to the cauda equina results in an acute loss of function of the lumbar plexus, and nerve roots of the spinal cord.

Si/Sx: Severe back pain, **sudden loss of sensation** over genitals, anus and inner thighs, sexual dysfunction, bowel and bladder incontinence

Diagnosis: MRI

Treatment: immediate corticosteroids and surgery

Boards tip for cauda equina syndrome
- If the question gives a choice between MRI and treatment, then pick treatment before MRI

---

3. METASTATIC MALIGNANCY OF SPINE

Occurs when cancer cells from primary tumor site metastasize to the bone

Si/SX: Constitutional symptoms (fever, chills, weight loss), back pain that **worst at night and is not relieved with rest**

Diagnosis:
- X-ray is the **best initial test**.
- Spine MRI is the gold standard and it is also the best initial **diagnostic test**
- Bone scan is the most sensitive test

Treatment: Steroids and radiation

4. SPINAL STENOSIS

Abnormal narrowing of the spinal canal that may occur at any part of the spine

Si/Sx: Pseudoclaudication = pain and discomfort in the buttocks, thighs, legs and feet with walking or prolonged standing; **pain is relieved by sitting or leaning forward.** Other symptoms include weakness, numbness, and sexual dysfunction

Diagnosis: MRI

Treatment:

- **Mild to moderate symptoms** is treated with **exercise and pain relievers.**
- **Laminectomy** is reserved for patient with disabling symptoms or refractory cases

COMPARTMENT SYNDROME

Compartment syndrome is a serious condition that occurs when the pressure in the muscle compartment increases and compromise the blood supply to the muscle and nerve cells. It is commonly seen in lower extremities after trauma to them.

Si/Sx: pain out of proportion, paresthesia, numbness, paralysis and pallor. Pulses may be present, but absence of pulses considered ominous

Diagnosis:

- Clinical diagnosis, but it can be confirmed by measuring the compartment pressure, which is usually > 30 mm Hg in compartment syndrome

Treatment: immediate fasciectomy to lower the compartment pressure and restore tissue perfusion. Delay in fasciectomy can lead to permanent damage

RADIAL NERVE INJURY

Radial never injury is caused by oblique fracture of distal humerus

Si/Sx: Patient **unable to extend the wrist**

Management:

- Close reduction
  - If patient **regains function after** the fractures is reduced, then manage the patient with **arm cast or sling**
  - If patient **does not regain** function after the fractures is reduced, then **surgery** may be needed

RHEUMATOLOGY CCS

CASE # 1

Case introduction
A 60-years-old Caucasian male comes to the office because of joint pain
and stiffness from last 1 month.

Initial vitals signs
Temperature: 37.2 degrees
Pulse: 68 beats/min, regular rhythm
Respiration rate: 19/ minutes

Blood pressure, systolic 134 mm Hg
Blood pressure, disystolic, 85 mm Hg

Height: 63.0 inches
Weight: 120.0 lbs.
Body mass index: 21.3 Kg/m2

History of present illness (HPI)
A 60-years-old Caucasian male comes to the office because of joint pain
and stiffness from last 1 month. He says has joint stiffness every morning,
which lasting less than 20 minutes that increases with exercise and relieves
with rest.. She says it is affecting her walking ability and preventing her to
go up or down stairs. She denies any chest pain, shortness of breath and
dizziness, weight loss. She has had hypertension from last 10 years and
taking hydrochlorothiazide.

Past medical history
Hospitalization: For C-section delivery at age 25
Other medical condition: HTN
Current medication: hydrochlorothiazide.
Allergies: none
Vaccination: up to date

Family history

Father died of MI, and mother died of lung cancer.

Social history

Marital history: married, 1 child

Occupation: retired; bank teller

Recreational: gardening, cooking, bingo

Personal habits: Does not drink smoke, or use drugs

Review of system:

General: see HPI

Skin: see HPI

HEENT: see HPI

Musculoskeletal: see HPI

Cardiology: see HPI

Abdominal: see HPI

Genitourinary: see HPI

Please see pages 1-5 for general CCS cases approach

Step 1. None (patient is stable does not require any emergency measures)

Step 2. Order the complete physical exam, and then move the clock to get
the results
- Results show:
  o Upper extremity exam shows nodules on DIP, PIP
  o Rest of the physical exam is within normal range

Step 3. Order labs, and then move the clock forward to get the results
- CBC
- UA
- BMP
- Chest X-ray
- X-ray of lower knees

- Following labs are usually ordered for all joint disease
  o ANA
  o RF factor
  o Anti-CCP
  o Joint fluid
  o Leukocytes, C&S, gram stain

- Results show:
  o Joint fluids aspiration show clear fluid, leukocytes count
    1,500/mm3
  o X-ray shows joint osteophytes
  o Rest of the labs are within normal limit

Step 4.
- Acetaminophen
- Advise weight lose and joint strengthening exercises
- Diet modification

Step 5. Make a follow-up appointment after a month and send patient
home

Step 6. None

Step 7. Move the clock forward to next appointment date.
- Patient comes to the office and usually feels better

Step 8. None

Step 9. None

Step 10. Basic counseling, age and gender specific screening
- No smoking, drinking, illegal drug use
- Weight lose
- Seat belt use,
- Drug compliance
- Advance directive
- Colonoscopy
- PAP/mammography
- Influenza shot

Diagnosis: Osteoarthritis

CASE # 2

Case introduction
A 35-years-old while male comes to the ER because of sudden pain and swelling in the joint of the first toe on his right foot

Initial vitals signs
Temperature: 38.9 degrees
Pulse: 98 beats/min, regular rhythm
Respiration rate: 19/ minutes

Blood pressure, systolic 124 mm Hg
Blood pressure, disystolic 72 mm Hg

Height: 66.0 inches
Weight: 150.0 lbs.
Body mass index: 24.2 Kg/m2

History of present illness (HPI)
A 35-years-old while male comes to the ER because of sudden pain and swelling of the joint of the first toe on his right foot. He describes his pain as sharp pain and rate 7 on a 10-point scale. He has a fever. He denies nausea, vomiting or trauma. He sexually active with multiple partners but uses condoms every time he engages in sexual activity. He is generally healthy and denies any medical condition.

Past medical history
Hospitalization: None
Other medical condition: none
Current medication: none
Allergies: none
Vaccination: up to date

Family history
Parents are healthy and alive.

Social history
Marital history: none
Occupation: physical therapist
Recreational: football, basketball, snowboarding
Personal habits: Does not smoke, or use drugs. Drink 3-5 beers a day

Review of system:
General: see HPI
Skin: see HPI
HEENT: see HPI
Musculoskeletal: see HPI
Cardiology: see HPI
Abdominal: see HPI
Genitourinary: see HPI

Please see pages 1-5 for general CCS cases approach

Step 1. None (patient is stable does not require any emergency measures)

Step 2. Oder complete physical exam, and then move the clock to get the
results
- Results show:
  - Lower extremities exam shows first toe of the right foot is
    warm and swollen. It has limited range of motion and pain
    with passive movement.
  - Rest of the physical exam is normal

Step 3. Order the following labs, and then move the clock forward to get
the results
- CBC
- UA
- Chest X-ray
- BMP
- X-ray of toe
- ESR
- Joint aspiration
- Joint fluid for cell count, protein,
- Joint fluid stain,
- Joint fluid culture
- Joint fluids culture and sensitivity (C& S)
- Serum uric acid
- PT/PTT/INR

- Results show:
  - CBC shows 12,000 WBC with 84% PMN and 11%
    lymphocytes
  - ESR- 8
  - Joint fluid analysis shows clear fluid, WBC 38,000 PMN 93%,
    needle shaped negative birefringent crystals
  - Urine acid level: 19

Step 4. Medicine
- Indomethacin

Step 5. Move the patient in the wards

Step 6. Order the followings:
- Low protein diet
- Bed rest with /bathroom privileges

Step 7. None

Step 8. None or may order rheumatologist consultation

Step 9: follow-up every 8 -12 hours, until patient feels better

Step 10. Consult and age and gender specific screening
- No smoking, drinking, illegal drugs
- Safe sex, seat belt
- Low protein diet
- Weight reduction

Diagnosis: Gout

CASE # 3

Case introduction
A 26-years-old male comes to the ER with left knee pain

Initial vitals signs
Temperature: 38.9 degrees
Pulse: 98 beats/min, regular rhythm
Respiration rate: 19/ minutes

Blood pressure, systolic 124 mm Hg
Blood pressure, disystolic, 72 mm Hg

Height: 66.0 inches
Weight: 150.0 lbs.
Body mass index: 24.2 Kg/m2

History of present illness (HPI)
A 26-years-old male comes to the ER with left knee pain. He said the pain
started yesterday and has difficulty walking without using assistance. He
knee is red, swollen, left knee that is painful to touch. He describes his pain
as sharp pain and rate 8 on a 10-point scale. He denies prior knee
condition, recent trauma, knee surgery and illegal drug use. He sexually
active with multiple partners and does not use condoms. He denies any
history of STDs or other medical conditions.

Past medical history
Hospitalization: None
Other medical condition: none
Current medication: none
Allergies: none
Vaccination: up to date

Family history
Parents are healthy and alive.

Social history

Marital history: none

Occupation: physical therapist

Recreational: football, basketball, snowboarding

Personal habits: Does not smoke, or use drugs. Drink 3-5 beers a day

Review of system:

General: see HPI

Skin: see HPI

HEENT: see HPI

Musculoskeletal: see HPI

Cardiology: see HPI

Abdominal: see HPI

Genitourinary: see HPI

Please see pages 1-5 for general CCS cases approach

Step 1. None (patient is stable does not require any emergency measures)

Step 2. Order complete physical exam, and then move the clock forward
to get the results
- Results show:
- o Extremities exam shows left knee is red, swollen and tender.
  Patient has limited range of motion and pain with passive
  movement
- o Rest of the physical exam is normal

Step 3. Order the labs, and then move clock forward to get the results
- CBC
- UA
- Chest X-ray
- BMP
- ESR
- Joint aspiration
- Joint fluid for cell count, protein,
- Joint fluid stain,
- Joint fluid culture
- Joint fluids C& S
- Serum uric acid
- PT/PTT/INR
- Throat C& S
- Urethral C& S
- Rectal C& S

- Results shows:
- o CBC shows 15,000 WBC with 83 % PMN & 12% Lymphocytes
- o Knee x-ray shows soft tissue swelling
- o Joint fluids analysis shows WBC 80,000 with PMN 93%, no
  crystals
- o Gram-negative diplococcus

Step 4. Empiric medicine Do not wait for C& S results give empiric
medicine

- **IV access**
- Empiric treatment with IV ceftriaxone and vancomycin
- Acetaminophen (for fever)

Step 5. Move the patient in ward

Step 6. Order the followings
- Bed rest with bathroom privileges
- NPO

Step 7. Labs
- Check if medicines need to be changed based on C& S

Step 8. Order orthopedics surgeon consult, and them move the clock forward to get the consult recommendations

Step 9. Follow-up every 4-6 hours
- If the patient still has pain, then order arthroscopy to drain the joint fluid, and do follow-up every 4 -6 hours

Case usually ends here

Step 10. Counsel and screening
- No smoking, drinking, illegal drugs
- Wear seat belt
- Safe sex
- Age and gender specific screening

Diagnosis: Septic arthritis

PULMONOLOGY

UPPER REPARATORY CONDITIONS

1. ACUTE PHARYNGITIS
Pharyngitis is a sore throat caused by inflammation of pharynx
Cause: it can be caused by bacterial or viral infection
- **Bacterial**: Group A beta-hemolytic streptococcus (GABHS) is the most common cause
- **Viral:** Adenovirus, EBV, HSV, measles, rhinovirus, RSV, parainfluenza virus

Si/Sx: Symptoms of sore throat vary, depending on the cause, which are as follow:
- A symptomatic criterion that is used to diagnose Group A beta-hemolytic streptococcus (**GABHS**)
  - **Sore throat**
  - **Tonsillar exudate**
  - **Cervical adenopathy**
  - **Absence of cough**
- Symptoms for **non-GABHS includes** fever, body ache, enlarged lymph node in armpits, rhinorrhea, conjunctivitis,

Diagnosis:
- Best initial test is **rapid GABHS antigen test** also known as **rapid strep test**
- Most accurate test is throat culture

Note: In adults negative rapid step test excludes the GABHS pharyngitis, no tests or treatment is required. However, if a child has a negative step test, then get a throat culture.

Management: depends on the followings
- **Viral** pharyngitis is treated with **conservative management** such as fluids, rest, gargling with warm water, or antipyretics

- If **GABHS** is suspected, then manage the patient as follow:

○ If the patient has **all 4 symptoms**, then give **penicillin; there is no need to do diagnostic tests.** If the patient is allergic to penicillin, then give azithromycin or clindamycin
○ If the patient has **2 or 3 symptoms**, then **do rapid strep test**
○ If the patient has **0 or 1 symptom**, then give **symptomatic treatment** such as acetaminophen, gargles

Complication: GABHS can lead to rheumatic fever and acute poststreptococcal glomerulonephritis (APGN)

Note: Penicillin or other antibiotics given during GABH pharyngitis reduces the risk of rheumatic fever, but not the risk of APGN

2. SINUSITIS
Sinusitis is an inflammation of the tissue lining the sinuses
Si/Sx:

- **Acute sinusitis** symptoms include fever, **headache, pain behind the eyes, facial tenderness, maxillary tooth pain, bad breath,** nasal discharge.
- **Chronic sinusitis** symptoms include high fever, darkened nasal discharge, and **respiratory illness that was getting better and then begins to get worse**

Types and causes:

- **Acute sinusitis:** when symptoms of sinusitis present for **< 4 weeks**. It is commonly associated with bacterial infection: **S. pneumonia, H. influenza non-type b, and M. catarrhalis**
- **Chronic sinusitis:** when symptoms of sinusitis lasts **> 12 weeks or 3 months**. It is associated with anaerobic bacteria or fungus. (Diabetic patients are at increased of getting sinusitis from mucormycosis).

Diagnosis:

- Transillumination test
- Best initial test is CT of the sinus
- Most accurate test is sinus culture

Treatment:
- **Acute sinusitis is treated as:**
  o Symptomatic treatment such as **fluids, humidifier, nasal saline and inhale steam 2-4 times per day**
  o Give Amoxicillin, if patient has any of the followings:
    - Fever and pain
    - Purulent nasal discharge
    - Symptoms do not resolve after 7 days of symptomatic
  o If patient continues to have symptoms after 3-5 day of amoxicillin, then give **amoxicillin-clavulanate**
- Chronic and fungal sinusitis are surgical drained and antibiotics

Complications:
- Periorbital edema (no pain with eye movement)
- Periorbital cellulitis (Pain with eye movement)
- Meningitis

3. INFLUENZA

Influenza, which is commonly known as flu

Cause: RNA virus of the family orthomyxovirus

Si/Sx: fatigue, fever, arthralgia, runny, nose cough, sore throat

Treatment: treatment depends on the onset of symptoms and time of presentation.
- If the patient presents **< 48 hours** of onset of symptoms, then treat the patient with **neuraminidase inhibitors** such as oseltamivir, or zanamivir. Neuraminidase inhibitors help by **shortening the duration of symptoms**
  o Side effects of **zanamivir** include **bronchoconstriction,** therefore it should not be given to a patient with COPD
  o Side effects of **oseltamivir** include **nausea and vomiting**
- If the patient presents **> 48 hours of onset of symptoms,** then give **symptomatic treatment** such as acetaminophen for fever and pain, fluids, and the rest.

Prevention: Influenza vaccination is given annually to protect against influenza. It is given to high-risk patient such as:

- All healthcare workers
- All nursing home patient
- All patients with chronic diseases lung, kidney
- All immunosuppressed patients
- All pregnant women, regardless of trimester
- Everyone >50 years of age

4. ALLERGIC RHINITIS

Allergic rhinitis is an allergic inflammation of the nasal cavity
Cause: pollen, dust, animal dander
Si/Sx: itching, sneezing, wheezing, boggy and **bluish turbinate**
Diagnosis:

- Patient's history
- Skin testing or IgE RAST tests may be needed to identify the allergen

Treatment:

- **Best initial management is to avoid the** known allergen
- **Intranasal corticosteroids** is the drug of choice

5. VASOMOTOR RHINITIS

Vasomotor rhinitis is a condition that causes constant runny nose, sneezing, and nasal congestion
Cause: there is no exact known cause, but risk factors may include air pollution, spicy food, strong emotions, alcohol
Diagnosis: diagnosis of exclusion
Treatment: depends on symptoms

- If the patient has **clogged nasal cavity,** then give **topical corticosteroids**
- If the patient has **postnasal drip,** then give **intranasal antihistamine (azelastine)**
- If the patient has pure **rhinorrhea, then** give Ipratropium bromide

LOWER RESPIRATORY TRACT INFECTION

OBSTRUCTIVE LUNG DIEASE

Obstructive lung disease is characterized by narrowing of lungs or damage to lungs, which results in obstruction of the airway, and difficulty with exhaling.

Cause: the most common causes of obstructive lung diseases are:

- Asthma
- Bronchiectasis
- Chronic obstructive pulmonary disease (COPD), which includes chronic bronchitis and emphysema

Diagnosis: Diagnosis depends on the specific cause. However, all obstructive lung diseases show:

- **Increased** total lung capacity (**TLC**), functional residual capacity (**FRC**), and residual volume (**RV**)
- **Decreased FEV1, FEV and FEV1/FVC ratio**

Treatment: treatment depends on specific cause (discussed below)

1. ASTHMA

Asthma is a chronic lung disease, characterized by inflammation and narrowing of airway

Cause: common triggers include pollen, pet dander, dust mites, tobacco smoking, respiratory infection, and medicines such as NSAIDs

Si/Sx: recurring episodes of expiratory wheezing, shortness of breath, chest tightness, and cough. Symptoms often are worst at night or early morning

Diagnosis:

- ABG shows **mild hypoxia and respiratory ankylosis**
- Pulmonary function test shows:
  - Increased TLC, FRC and RV
  - Decreased FEV1, FEV and FEV1/FEV ratio
- CBC may show eosinophilia
- Chest X-ray may show hyperinflation
- Diffusion Lung Capacity of Carbon monoxide (**DLCO) is increased**

Bronchodilator test

Bronchodilator test is used to diagnose asthma, when a patient experiences symptoms of asthma, but **diagnostic tests are inconclusive.** FEV1 is measured before and after administering nebulized albuterol. Asthmatic patient shows >20 % **increase** in FEV1 after receiving nebulized albuterol

Methacholine stimulation test

Methacholine stimulation test is used to diagnose asthma, when a patient complains of asthma like symptoms, but **symptoms are not clear.** Methacholine is an artificial form of acetylcholine, which provokes bronchoconstriction. FEV1 is measured before and after administering nebulized methacholine. Asthmatic patient shows >20 % **decrease** in FEV1 after receiving nebulized methacholine

Note: Everyone shows decreased FEV1 after methacholine stimulation test, but asthmatic patient shows FEV1 decreased more than 20%.

Treatment: avoid known trigger and treat as follow (see table below)

Treatment for stable asthma

Type	Daytime symptoms	Nighttime symptoms	PFTs	Treatment
Intermittent	2 times a week	2 times a month	FEV1 >80%	Inhaled albuterol, as needed
Mild persistent	>2 times a week	>2 times a month	FEV1 >80%	**Add inhaled** corticosteroids
Moderate persistent	Everyday	>2 per week	FEV1 60 – 80%	**Add** inhaled salmeterol and oral montelukast
Severe	Continuous	Frequent	FEV1 <60%	**Add oral** corticosteroids

- **Exercise induced asthma** is managed with **inhaled albuterol prior to exercise**
- Extrinsic asthma is caused **by high levels of IgE** in response to extrinsic factors and it is treated as follow
  - **1st line** treatment is **cromolyn**
  - **2nd line** treatment is **omalizumab**

2.   ASTHMA EXACERBATION

Asthma exacerbation is characterized by acute episode of progressive **worsening wheezing, shortness of breath, chest tightness**
Management: is as follow

- If the patient is **losing conscious** or has **silent lungs** (no wheezing), then **intubate the patient**

- If the patient is **not losing conscious and has airflow in lungs, then manage the patient in following steps:**
  - o Get Arterial Blood Gas (ABG) and give oxygen
  - o Nebulized albuterol, it works instantly
  - o Inhaled ipratropium
  - o IV prednisone, it usually take 4-6 weeks to be effective

Note: silent lungs signifies no airflow, and without a airflow nebulized medication may not get delivered to the lung, and render useless

---

Boards often try to confuse asthma with two following condition

I.   **ALLERGIC BRONCHOPULMONARY ASPERGILLOSIS (ABPA)**
      It as an exaggerated immune system response to Aspergillus fungus
- Look for asthmatic patient with sudden worsening of asthma symptoms and coughing up **brownish mucoid** plugs
- Diagnosis:
  - o Chest X-ray shows central bronchiectasis
  - o Specific test:
    - - **Skin-prick** Aspergillus fumigatus test
    - - Circulating precipitating antibodies
- Treatment:
  - o 1st line treatment is **corticosteroids**
  - o If corticosteroids are ineffective, then give **Itraconazole**

II. METHEMOGLOBINEMIA

In this condition hemoglobin cannot pick up oxygen because hemoglobin is locked in an oxidized state

- Look for a patient **with sudden shortness of breath after exposure of drugs such as dapsone, nitroglycerin, amyl** nitrate, nitroprusside or anesthetic
- Diagnosis:
  - Physical exam **shows clear lung sounds**
  - ABG shows **normal Po2**
  - Peripheral smear **shows brown blood**
- Treatment: Methylene blue

3. BRONCHIETASIS

Bronchiectasis is characterized by destruction of smooth muscles and elastic tissues of the bronchial tree. This damage leads to abnormal dilation of the large airway.

Cause: cystic fibrosis, Kartagener syndrome, infection (Tuberculosis, whooping cough), IBD, rheumatoid arthritis

Si/Sx: foul smelling sputum production, recurrent lung infection, and hemoptysis

Diagnosis:

- **Best initial test is chest x-ray,** which shows **"tram-tracks sign"** that is caused by thickened, dilated airway
- **Most accurate test is high resolution CT**
- Sputum culture to find the bacteria responsible for infection

Treatment: There is no specific cure for bronchiectasis. Supportive care includes:

- Postural drainage, chest physiotherapy, cupping and clapping of secretion
- Bronchodilator, expectorants and hydration
- Antibiotics based on sputum culture, but **keep rotating antibiotics** to prevent development of drug resistance
- **Surgical resection** for **localized bronchiectasis**

4. CHRONIC OBSTRUCTIVE PULMONARY DISEASE (COPD)

Chronic obstructive pulmonary disease includes **emphysema** and **chronic bronchitis**

4a. CHRONIC BRONCHITIS

Chronic bronchitis is characterized by inflammation of bronchi and bronchioles, which causes excessive secretion of mucus into the airway, leading to narrowing and obstruction of the bronchial tree.

Causes tobacco smoking is the leading cause

Si/Sx: cough and sputum occur **daily for 3 months for at least 2 consecutive years**, dyspnea, wheezing

Diagnosis:

- ABG shows **hypoxia with increased pCO2**
- Chest x-ray shows **increased pulmonary marking**
- Pulmonary function test shows
  - **Decreased** FEV1, FVC, & EFV1/FVC
  - **Increased** TLC and RV
  - Diffusion lung capacity of carbon dioxide (DLCO) is **normal**
- Diagnosis is confirmed with lung biopsy, which shows **increased Reid index** (bronchial wall thickness increased more than .04)

Boards clue to distinguish chronic bronchitis from emphysema

- Diffusion lung capacity of carbon dioxide (DLCO) is **normal in chronic bronchitis, whereas it is decreased in emphysema**

Treatment:

- **First line** therapy is **anticholinergics** such as tiotropium (once a day) or ipratropium (every 4-6 hrs.)
- If **it is ineffective**, then add **inhaled albuterol or other beta-adrenergic**
- If **treatment is still ineffective**, then **add theophylline**

4b. EMPHYSEMA

Emphysema is characterized by loss of elasticity of terminal airway, leading to permanent abnormal enlargement of terminal bronchioles, and destruction of the alveolar wall.

Cause: Tobacco smoking is the leading cause. In rare case, alpha1-antitrypsin deficiency

Types of emphysema

- **Centrilobular emphysema** is associated with **tobacco smoking**. It predominantly affects the upper half of the lungs
- **Panlobular emphysema** is associated with **alpha1-antitrypsin deficiency**. It uniformly affects the entire alveolus.

Diagnosis:

- ABG shows hypoxia with increased pCO_2
- Chest x-ray shows **flat diaphragm and increased anterior posterior diameter of lungs and bullae** (bullae are collection of alveoli that can rupture and cause pneumothorax)
- Pulmonary function test shows
  - **Decreased** FEV1, FVC, & EFV1/FVC, a
  - **Increased** TLC and RV.
  - Diffusion lung capacity of carbon dioxide (DLCO) is **decreased**

Treatment:

- Same as chronic bronchitis. However, patient with panlobular are also given alpha-1 antitrypsin infusion

Additional management for COPD patient

1. FEV1 is the best predictor of survival of a COPD patient: higher the FEV1, better the survival

2. Following measures may lower the mortality of a COPD patient
   - Smoking cessation
   - Lung volume reduction
   - Home oxygen therapy

Home oxygen lowers the mortality in COPD patients. It is given when any of the following is present:

- PO2 is < 55 mmHG or pulse oxygen saturation is <88 %
- Patient with cor pulmonale with signs of right heart failure, elevated hematocrit, PO2 < 59 mmHG or pulse oxygen saturation < 90 %

3. All COPD patients must receive the followings:
   - Yearly influenza virus
   - Pneumococcal vaccine every 5 year
   - H. Influenza vaccine once per lifetime

4c. COPD EXACERBATION

COPD exacerbation is characterized by acute onset of shortness of breath, exercise intolerance, fatigue

Management: patient is managed in a following stepwise manner

- Get Arterial Blood Gas (ABG) and give oxygen
- Nebulized albuterol and ipratropium simultaneously
- IV prednisone
- Antibiotics: ceftriaxone and macrolides such as azithromycin, clarithromycin. These lowers the mortality in a patient with COPD exacerbation, therefore these should be given to all patients regardless of X-ray findings

RESTRICTIVE LUNG DIEASE

Restrictive lung disease is a group of disorders that restrict lung expansion, which results in decreased lung volume and inadequate oxygenation.

Diagnosis: Diagnosis depends on the specific cause. However, all restrictive lung disease all shows, the following:

- Decreased total lung capacity (TLC), functional residual capacity (FRC), residual volume (RV
- Increased or normal FEV1/FVC

1. INTERSTITIAL LUNG DISEASE

Disease	Risk factors	Diagnosis
Asbestos	Mining, welding, shipyard, plumbing, boilers	• Chest x-ray shows pleural thickening, **pleural plaques and calcification in lower lungs** • Lung biopsy shows **barbell shaped asbestos fiber**
Silicosis	Pottery barns, brickyards, sandblasting	• Chest x-ray shows **eggshell calcification** in upper lungs • Lung biopsy shows **barbell shaped asbestos fiber**
Pneumoconiosis	Metal mining, dust	• Chest x-ray **shows irregular opacities**
Coal miner's lung disease	Coal mining	• Chest x-ray shows **circular densities in apical lungs**
Berylliosis	Electronics, ceramics, dental work	• Lung biopsy shows **noncaseating granuloma**

Compilation of interstitial lung disease:
- Asbestos increases the risk of adenocarcinoma
- Silicosis increases the risk of Tuberculosis (TB). Patient should have yearly PPD. PPD induration > 10 mm is considered positive TB in a patient with silicosis.

Treatment: there is no treatment for interstitial lung treatment, other than berylliosis, which is treated with steroids

2. SARCOIDOSIS
Sarcoidosis is characterized by abnormal collection of chronic inflammatory cells (granulomas). It can affect any organ, but lungs are commonly affected.
Cause: there is no known cause of sarcoidosis
Risk factors: African-American, women, and age 20-40
Symptoms: fever, **dry cough**, malaise, shortness of breath, weight loss, arthritis, raised red firm skin sore (erythema nodosum) on lower legs

Diagnosis:

- **Best initial test is chest X-ray**, which shows bilateral hilar adenopathy
- **Most accurate test** is biopsy of lungs or other involved organ, which shows noncaseating granuloma (Make sure to **start biopsy at the least invasive site,** if it is inconclusive, then move to next site, such as first do skin biopsy, then lymph nodes, then parotid, and then lungs)
- Increased Angiotensin converting enzymes (ACEs)
- Hypercalcemia, which is secondary to increase in vitamin D production by granuloma
- Increased alkaline phosphatase

Note: Erythema nodosum is not diagnostic for Sarcoidosis because it is also seen in other systemic diseases

Treatment: Steroids

3. EXTRAPULMONARY DISEASE

Extrapulmonary diseases that causes restrictive disease are Myasthenia gravis, Guillain barré, kyphosis, chest wall deformities, diaphragmatic hernia, and ascites
Treatment: supportive

PULMONARY HYPERTENSION

Pulmonary hypertension is increased blood pressure in pulmonary arteries that leads to decreased output from the right ventricle of the heart
Cause: overgrowth and obliteration of pulmonary vasculature
Si/Sx: right **ventricular heave at sternal border, loud p2,** cyanosis, fatigue
Diagnosis:

- Best initial tests is **transthoracic echocardiography**
- Most accurate test is **right heart catheterization**

Treatment:

- **Endothelin inhibitor** – Bosentan (prevents the growth of pulmonary vasculature)
- **Prostacyclin analogue** - Epoprostenol or treprostinil (pulmonary vascular dilator)
- Sildenafil

PLEURAL EFFUSION

Pleural effusion is an abnormal accumulation of fluid in pleural space (thin layer between lungs and chest cavity)

Types:

- **Transudate** is low in protein content, which is caused by **CHF, cirrhosis, pulmonary embolism**
- **Exudates** is high in protein content, which is caused **by lung infection, TB, lung cancer, rheumatic disease, pulmonary embolism**

Si/Sx: fever, chest pain, cough, shortness of breath, dullness to percussions, decreased tactile fremitus

Diagnosis:

- **Best initial test is decubitus chest x-ray**, which shows blunting of the costophrenic angle
- **Most accurate test is thoracocentesis**: pleural fluid is removed from the chest with a needle. Fluid is then analyzed to determine the followings:
  - Type of effusion by LDH, protein content
  - Cause of effusion by gram stain and cultures, acid-fast stain, pH, glucose, cell count

Light criteria

	Exudate	Transudate
LDH effusion	> 200 IU/ml	<200 IU/ml
LDH effusion/serum ratio	> 0.6	< 0.6
Protein effusion/Serum ratio	> 0.5	< 0.5

Note: Transudate effusion must have all three values (< 200 IU/ml, < 0.6, and < 0.5); otherwise it is considered as exudate

Management:

- If pH is < 7.0, then the diagnosed is **empyema**, it is treated with **chest tube drainage**
- If acid-fast stain, gram stain and culture are positive for **TB**, then next step is to confirm the diagnosis with pleural biopsy. Tx. **TB medications**
- If cytology shows malignancy, then further diagnosis and treatment is based on **malignancy**

- If any of the above mentioned are not the cause of pleural effusion, then treat the effusion as follow:
  - o For small effusions- Tx. **Diuretics**
  - o For large effusions- Tx. **Chest tube drainage**
  - o If effusion is recurrent –Tx. **Pleurodesis**
  - o If pleurodesis is ineffective- Tx. **Decortication**

ADULT RESPIRATORY DISTRESS SYNDROME (ARDS)

Adult respiratory distress syndrome is a life-threatening condition in which fluids accumulates in air sacs that prevents oxygen diffusion from the lungs to blood

Cause: trauma, aspiration, septic shock, pneumonia, inhalation of toxic fumes, and near drowning

Si/Sx: dyspnea, resistance hypoxia, tachypnea, and diffuse alveolar infiltrate

Diagnosis:

- ABG shows **hypoxemia with normal CO2**
- Chest x-ray shows complete " **white-out"** of both lungs
- Pulmonary artery catheterization shows **normal capillary wedge pressure (12 -18)**
- **PaO2 -to FIO2 ratio more than 200 is required for the diagnosis**

Note: Capillary wedge pressure is high (> 18) in cardiogenic shock

Treatment:

- Oxygen,
- Positive end-expiratory pressure (PEEP) of 6 cm to keep alveoli open
- Low tidal volume of 6 ml per kg.
- Place the patient in prone position
- Diuretics and dobutamine

Boards often ask ventilator-setting questions in the context with ARDS. Know the followings you should be able to answer most of the ventilator settings questions

- CO_2 level is controlled by respiratory rate and tidal volume
  - If the patient has high CO_2 levels, then manage it by increasing the respiratory rate or tidal volume that lowers the CO_2 levels in the patient
  - If the patient has low CO_2 levels, then manage it by lowering the respiratory rate or tidal volume that increases the CO_2 levels in the patient

- Oxygen level is controlled by PEEP and FIO2
  - If the patient has low oxygen levels, then manage it by increasing the PEEP or FIO2 that increases the oxygen levels in the patient

  - If the patient has high oxygen levels, then manage it by lowering the PEEP or FIO2 that lowers the oxygen level in the patient

---

PULMONARY EMBOLISM
Pulmonary embolism (PE) is sudden blockage in a lungs artery by fat droplet, blood clot, air bubble or tumor cells
Cause: most common cause is a blood clot in the deep veins of the proximal legs (above knees). Other less common causes may include fat droplets, amniotic fluids, air bubble
Risk factor: Virchow's triad (endothelial damage, hypercoagulable, and stasis), estrogen-containing hormonal contraception, genetic thrombophilia (factor V Leiden, protein C deficiency, protein S deficiency, antithrombin deficiency, prothrombin mutation), antiphospholipid syndrome, nephrotic syndrome, cancer
Si/Sx: chest pain, sudden dyspnea, tachypnea, tachycardia, leg pain and swelling

Diagnosis:

- ABG shows respiratory alkalosis
- EKG may show S wave in lead 1, Q wave in lead II, and T wave in lead III.
- EKG may show sinus tachycardia
- **Best initial test is chest x-ray**, it is usually normal in PE
  - If **chest x-ray is positive**, then get **CT spiral**
  - If **chest x-ray is positive**, but the patient is **allergic to dye**, then get **V/VQ scan**
  - If **chest x-ray is negative**, then get **V/VQ scan**
- If the diagnosis is **still inconclusive after V/VQ scan**, then do **venous ultrasound**

Treatment:

- If the patient is **stable patient** and has **no active** bleeding, then give **oxygen, heparin and warfarin**
- If the patient is **stable patient** and has **active bleeding**, then put a **inferior vena cava filter**
- **If the patient is unstable** and has **no active bleeding**, then give tPAs
- If the patient is **unstable** and has **active bleeding**, then perform embolectomy

SOLITARY PULMONARY NODULE

If solitary nodule is found incidentally on a chest X-ray, next best step in management is to get an old chest x-ray and compare it with current one, and manage it is as follow:

1. If an old x-ray is available then compare the size of nodule with the new x-ray:
   - **Benign** nodule doubles in **< 1 month or more than 480 days**
   - **Malignant** nodule **doubles in > 1 month or < 480 days**.
2. If an old x-ray is **not available**, then use the following to determine if nodule is cancerous or a benign:

Characteristic of benign and malignant nodule

Benign nodule	Malignant nodule
• Non-smoker • < 35 years of age, • Calcification of nodule • Nodule <2 cm • Nodule has smooth margin	• Smoker • 50 years of age, • No calcification of nodule • Nodule> 2 cm • Nodule has irregular margin

- If the patient has **benign nodule**, then **follow-up in 3-6 months.**
- If the patient has **malignant nodule,** then get a **CT scan and sputum cytology**

3. **CT scan and sputum cytology**
   - If CT scan and sputum cytology shows tumor, then do **bronchoscopy, and treat the patient according to the tumor's stage**
   - If CT scan and sputum cytology is inconclusive, then do **bronchoscopy and biopsy**
     o If the diagnosis still inconclusive, then **do needle aspiration biopsy**

Note: If the chest x-rays shows a suspicious nodule that is **close to the periphery,** then do Video-assisted thoracic surgery (VATS)

Other frequently asked lung cancer related questions

1. What is the most common lung cancer in the smokers?
   Answer: Bronchogenic carcinoma (small cell and squamous cell)

2. What is the most common lung cancer in non-smokers?
   Answer: Adenocarcinomas

Differential diagnosis of lung cancer

Cancer	Characteristic
Squamous cell carcinoma	• Centrally located tumor • Most common in smokers • Secrets PTH-like peptide that causes **hypercalcemia**
Small cell carcinoma	• Centrally located tumor • Most common in smoker • Can lead **to SIADH, Lambert-Eaton syndrome**
Large cell carcinoma	• Peripherally located tumor • Highly anaplastic, undifferentiated tumor
Adenocarcinoma	• Peripherally located tumor • Most common cause of lung cancer in non-smokers
Bronchoalveolar syndrome	• Peripherally located tumor • Subtype of adenocarcinoma

Diagnosis:
- Chest X-ray
- CT guided fine-needle aspiration
- Thoracoscopic biopsy

Treatment:
- **Surgical resection and radiation** for **localized tumor or non-small cell carcinoma**
- **Chemotherapy and radiation** for **small cell carcinoma, metastatic cancer or unresectable tumors**

SMOKING CESSATION

All patients should be screened and counseled against smoking at each visit

Treatment: Best initial step is to assess if the patient is **willing to quit** smoking, because if the patient is not willing to quit smoking, then the treatment may not be successful. However, if the patient is willing to quit, then the management is as follow:

- Nicotine **patch and gums** are controlled release nicotine thus help reduce abrupt effects of nicotine withdrawal
- **Bupropion** is the best initial treatment for patients with depressed mood and wanting to quit smoking. However, it is **contraindicated** in patients with **seizures or epilepsy** because it lowers the seizure threshold.
- **Varenicline** can be safely used in patients with seizures and epilepsy

SLEEP APNEA

Sleep apnea is characterized by infrequent breathing during sleep

Types and causes:

- **Obstructive sleep apnea**, in this condition there is a partial or complete collapse of upper airway. This type of apnea is more in overweight people
- **Central sleep apnea**, there is no known cause of central sleep apnea, but it is often caused by **poor ventilatory drive** in conditions such as CNS disease, alcohol, hypnotic medicines

Diagnosis: Sleep study (polysomnography)

Treatment:

- **Obstructive sleep apnea:** best initial treatment is weight loss, continuous positive airway pressure (CPAP)
  - If it is ineffective, then perform surgical resection of palate, uvula and pharynx
- **Central sleep apnea:** avoid alcohol, hypnotic medicines before going to sleep. Other treatment options include oxygen, acetazolamide (causes metabolic acidosis that stimulate respiration) or medroxyprogesterone (central respiratory stimulant)

PULMONOLOGY INFECTIOUS DISEASES

PNEUMONIA

Pneumonia is an infection of lungs caused by bacteria, virus or fungi.

Typical and atypical pneumonia

	Typical pneumonia	Atypical pneumonia
Symptoms	• Abrupt onset of high fever (>102 F) • Chills • Progressive cough • Thoracic pain	• Progressive onset of fever (<102 F) • No chill • Dry cough • Myalgia, • Headache
Prodrome	Short duration (<2 days)	Long duration (> 2 days)
Chest x-ray shows	Lobar or segmental involvement	Multilobar or diffuse Involvement
Cause	S. Pneumoniae, H. influenza, S. aureus	Mycoplasma pneumonia, Legionella pneumonia, chlamydia

DIFFERENTIAL DIAGNOSIS OF PNEUMONIA

1. TYPICAL PNEUMONIA

Organism	Association
	Typical bacterial pneumonia
Streptococcus pneumonia	• Most common cause of typical pneumonia
Pseudomonas	• Common in cystic fibrosis
Klebsiella	• Common in alcoholics, diabetics • Associated with **"current jelly"** sputum
Anaerobes	• Seen in patient with altered consciousness, poor dentition, dementia

2. ATYPICAL PNEUMONIA

Organism	Characteristics
Legionella	• Common in patient exposed to contaminated water source, such as air conditioner • Si/Sx: **altered mental status, hyponatremia, diarrhea, high LDH** • **Diagnosis**: charcoal extract, urine antigen test or direct fluorescent antibodies
Mycoplasma	• Common in young adults (College students) • **Diagnosis:** PCR, cold agglutinin
Chlamydia pneumonia	• Common in elderly • Si/Sx: sore throat, hoarseness, • **Diagnosis:** serology titer
Chlamydia Psittaci	• Contracted from birds
Coxiella burnetii	• Contracted from farm animals (cattle goats), ingestion of infected milk
Actinomyces	• Common in Immunocompetent patient with dental or facial trauma • **Diagnosis:** gram stain • **Treatment:** penicillin
Nocardia	• Common in Immunocompetent patients, mimic TB • **Gram-positive acid-fast aerobe** • **Treatment:** Bactrim

Diagnosis:
- Best initial test is chest x-ray
- Most accurate test is sputum gram stain and culture

Treatment: empiric treatment is started until gram stain and culture results are available. Empiric treatment can be **outpatient or inpatient** (discussed below)

Patient is treated in hospital (Inpatient) if patient has any one of the followings: Mnemonic- **CURB 65**
- Confusion
- Uremia
- Respiratory rate >30/minute
- Blood pressure: systolic <90 mmHG or diastolic <60 mmHG
- Age >65

Inpatient empiric treatment regimen
- IV ceftriaxone and azithromycin

    Or
- IV fluoroquinolone such as levofloxacin, gatifloxacin, or moxifloxacin

Note: Ciprofloxacin is ineffective in pneumonia

Outpatient empiric treatment regimen
- Oral fluoroquinolone such as levofloxacin, or gatifloxacin, or moxifloxacin

    Or
- Oral macrolides: Azithromycin, or clarithromycin

Note: Erythromycin is ineffective in pneumonia

3. **HOSPITAL ACQUIRED PNEUMONIA / HEALTHCARE ASSOCIATED PNEUMONIA**
Pneumonia that starts **within 48 hours of admission or within 90 days after hospitalization**
Risk factor: hospitalized patient that are alcoholics, have chronic lung disease, immunocompromised, or had major surgery
Treatment: combination **of 2 drugs** with IV piperacillin/tazobactam or fluoroquinolone with imipenem or meropenem

4. VENTILATOR ASSOCIATED PNEUMONIA

This is a sub-type of hospital-acquired pneumonia that develops **within 48 hours** or longer **after** receiving **mechanical ventilation**

Treatment: 3 drugs combination: Imipenem, gentamicin and vancomycin or linezolid

- Side effect of linezolid include thrombocytosis and serotoninergic syndrome

5. ASPIRATION PNEUMONIA

Aspiration pneumonia occurs when mouth anaerobes **are aspirated in the lungs usually with food, saliva, or gastric content. Right lower lung** is the most commonly affected

Risk factors: it is often seen in hospitalized stroke patients, ICU patients or elderly patients with dysphasia

Treatment: Piperacillin/ Tazobactam

High-yield boards question

- What is the best way to prevent aspiration pneumonia?

- Answer: Head end elevated at 45° or upright supine position

6. ASPIRATION PNEUMONITIS

Aspiration pneumonitis occurs when **gastric content** is aspirated in the lungs and cause **inflammation in the lungs**

Risk factors: it is usually seen in drug overdose, intoxicated, depressed level of consciousness

Treatment:

- No treatment is required
  - Clinical symptoms usually **resolves within 24 to 48 hours**
  - Chest X-ray usually **clears within 7 to 10 day**

7. FUNGAL PNEUMONIA

Organism	Characteristics
Pneumocystis carinii	• Common in AIDS patient with CD 4 cells count < 200 • **Diagnosis**: Increased LDH, sputum silver stain • **Treatment**: Bactrim (TMP/SMX)
Histoplasmosis	• Common in people living in wet areas such as Mississippi river valley, and Ohio • Associated with bat droppings • **Diagnosis**: Urine antigen is the most sensitive test • **Treatment**: Itraconazole
Blastomycosis	• Common in people living in southeast and south-central Unites States • **Diagnosis**: sputum cytology shows **broad-based budding yeast** • **Treatment**: oral itraconazole
Coccidioides immitis	• Common in people traveled to southwest desert • **Diagnosis**: sputum cytology shows **budding yeast** • **Treatment**: itraconazole
Aspergillus	• Common in neutropenic patients • **Diagnosis**: chest X-ray shows **"fungus ball"** with cavitation • **Treatment**: Amphotericin B/ itraconazole

7a PNEUMOCYSTIS CARINII PNEUMONIA (PCP)

PCP is **fungal pneumonia** that is caused fungus *pneumocystis jiroveci.* It is usually seen in HIV-positive patient with CD 4 cells count < 200

Si/Sx: **dry cough, shortness of breath** (SOB), fatigue

Diagnosis:
- Increased LDH
- Chest x-ray- shows **bilateral ground glass infiltrate**
- Most accurate test is **bronchoalveolar lavage**

- Pulmonary artery oxygen (p02)
- Alveolar–arterial gradient (A–a gradient) of oxygen

Treatment:
- 1st line of treatment is IV Trimethoprim/sulfamethoxazole (TMP/SMX)
  - If patient is **allergic to sulfa drugs**- Tx. Pentamidine or atovaquone

- 2nd line of treatment is pentamidine
  - Pentamidine causes low blood sugar, which may cause seizures

- If p02 < 70 or A–a gradient >35 mmHg, then **add prednisone** to the treatment

8. TUBERCULOSIS (TB)

Tuberculosis is an infection caused by mycobacterium tuberculosis.
Si/Sx: depends on the type
- **Latent tuberculosis** has no symptoms
- **Active tuberculosis**: cough, fever, night sweat, weight loss

8a Latent tuberculosis
Si/Sx: Patients usually are asymptomatic
Diagnosis: as follow
- **Best initial test is PPD**, it is considered positive (see table below)

Induration	Considered positive in population
≥ 5 mm induration	HIV positive, close contact with active TB, taking immunosuppressive medicine
≥ 10 mm induration	Alcoholics, homeless, prisoners, prisoners, healthcare worker, new immigrant
≥ 15mm induration	General population

- If PPD test is positive, then **get chest X-ray**. If chest X-ray also shows active TB, then get 3 acid –fast bacilli (AFB) sputum stain

Note: A **normal chest x-ray** or **an abnormal chest x-ray with 3 negative AFB** is enough to **exclude activity TB**

Treatment: as follow
- If **PPD test is positive**, but **chest x-ray is negative**, then treat the patient with Isoniazid (INH) plus Vitamin B 6 for 9 months
- If **PPD is positive** and **chest x-ray is positive, then** treat the patient as active TB (discussed below)

8b ACTIVE TB

Si/Sx: fever, night sweats, weight loss, hemoptysis

Diagnosis:
- **Best initial test** is chest X-ray
- Diagnosis is confirmed with **acid-fast sputum stains and culture**

Note: After confirming TB with acid- fast stain, get blood culture and start a patient on TB medications but do not wait for culture results because culture takes 4 to 6 weeks to grow

Treatment: see table below

Active TB treatment

Treatment	Duration	Side effects
Rifampin	6 months	Turns **bodily fluids orange,** hepatotoxic
Isoniazid	6 months	Peripheral neuropathy (prevented by co-treatment with vitamin B6), hepatotoxic
Ethambutol	First 2 months	Optic neuritis, hepatotoxic
Pyrazinamide	First 2 months	Hyperuricemia, hepatotoxic

Summary of TB medication duration
- **Latent TB - 9 months**
- **Active TB:**
    - **6 months** - general population
    - **9 months –** pregnant woman, osteomyelitis, cavitary TB
    - **12 months –** TB meningitis

Other high-yield TB related points

- Do not give pyrazinamide or streptomycin to a pregnant woman

- If a patient has TB meningitis or TB pericarditis, then **add steroids** to the treatment

- If a healthcare worker is exposed to a patient with active tuberculosis, then do PPD test and give INH + vitamin B 6. Repeat PPD test in three months, if PPD is negative then stop the treatment

- If a HIV-positive patient or a child comes in close contact with a patient with active tuberculosis, then do PPD test, and give INH and Vitamin B 6 for 9 months regardless of PPD test results

- If a patient with latent TB already has received 9 months of INH and Vitamin B6, and comes backs worried that he has active TB, but has no symptoms of active TB, then have the patient **fill active TB questioner**

PULMONOLOGY SURGERY

SECURE THE AIRWAY
- In field, preform intubation or cricothyroidotomy
- In emergency room, do induction and orotracheal intubation
- If patient has **severe maxillofacial injury, then do cricothyroidotomy**

OPEN PNEUMOTHORAX
Open pneumothorax is characterized by a defect in the chest wall that draws the air during inspiration
Si/Sx: shortness of breath, **decreased breath on the affected side,** hypotension
Diagnosis:
- Clinical diagnosis
- Chest x-ray shows **trachea is in the midline**

Treatment:
- Intubation
- Positive pressure ventilation
- Tape on three sides of the open wound, as this will allow excessive pressure to escape

Complication: tension pneumothorax

TENSION PNEUMOTHORAX
Tension pneumothorax is a life-threatening condition in which large amount of air enters in the plural space, but cannot escape
Cause: penetrating or blunt trauma to the chest
Si/Sx: shortness of breath, **decreased or absent breath sounds on the affected side,** hypertympanic breath sounds, JVD, hypotension
Diagnosis:
- Clinical diagnosis
- Chest X-ray shows **trachea shifted to the opposite side of the chest**

Treatment:
- Immediate **needle thoracentesis in the 2nd intercostal** space in the **mid-clavicular line**

- Followed by **chest tube insertion** in the **4th or 5th intercostal** space in the **mid-axillary line**

Note: Tension pneumothorax is a clinical diagnosis, if patient present with symptoms of tension pneumothorax, then do immediate **needle thoracentesis,** do not waste time in doing chest x-ray

HEMOTHORAX

Hemothorax is the collection of blood in the pleural cavity
Si/Sx: decreased breath sounds in the affected side, dullness on percussion, hypotension, **collapsed neck veins**
Diagnosis: clinical diagnosis
Treatment:

- **IV fluids and chest tube,** in most patients bleeding stops spontaneously
- **Thoracotomy** is indicated if a patient has any of the following:
  - 1,500 ml of blood on initial drainage
  - 600 ml of blood in 6 hours
  - 2, 500 ml of blood in 24 hours

PULMONOLOGY CCS

CASE # 1

Case introduction
A 23-years-old Caucasian male comes to ER because of shortness of breath cough, and wheezing.

Initial vitals signs
Temperature: 37.2 degrees
Pulse: 115 beats/min, regular rhythm
Respiration rate: 30/ minutes

Blood pressure, systolic 134 mm Hg
Blood pressure, disystolic, 85 mm Hg

Height: 63.0 inches
Weight: 120.0 lbs.
Body mass index: 21.3 Kg/m2

History of present illness (HPI)
A 23-years-old Caucasian male comes to ER because of shortness of breath, cough, and wheezing from last 1 hour. He sitting upright, breathing forcefully and rapidly. He says he was playing baseball when the symptoms started. He was diagnosed with asthma 1-year age and has been stable on albuterol. He denies history of similar symptoms. He has no other medical condition. He is sexually active with his girlfriend.

Past medical history
Hospitalization: None
Other medical conditions: none
Current medication: Albuterol
Allergies: eggs, peanuts
Vaccination: up to date

Family history
Parents are healthy and alive.

Social history
Marital history: none
Occupation: physical therapist
Recreational: football, basketball, snowboarding
Personal habits: Does not smoke, or use drugs. Drink 3-5 beers a day

Review of system:
General: see HPI
Skin: see HPI
HEENT: see HPI
Musculoskeletal: see HPI
Cardiology: see HPI
Abdominal: see HPI
Genitourinary: see HPI

Please see pages 1-5 for general CCS cases approach

Step 1. Order all the following, under " stat"
- Pulse oximetry × every hour
- Oxygen
- ABG
- IV access
- IV normal saline
- Vitals

Step 2. Order focused physical exam: heart & lungs
- Results show:
  - Patient is breathing forcefully
  - Lungs: Bilateral wheezing
  - Rest of exam is normal

Step 3. Order following labs, and then move the clock forward to get the results
- CBC
- UA
- BMP
- PEV1
- PEFR
- EKG
- Chest X-ray

- Results show:
  - Pulse oximetry shows 87% oxygen saturation
  - ABG shows pH 7.34, PaO2: 59 mm Hg, PaCO2
  - EKG shows sinus tachycardia
  - Chest x-ray shows hyperinflation of lungs

Step 4. Medicine
- Albuterol (inhaled)
- Ipratropium (Inhaled)
- Bolus Prednisone

Step 5. Do rest of the physical exam +Admit the patient in wards

Step 6. Order
- NPO

Step 7. Order following labs, and then move the clock to get the results
- FEV1
- PEFP

Results show:
- FEV1 < 2.3 1min
- PEFP < 305 1min

Step 8. Order pulmonology consultation, and then move the clock forward to get the results

Step 9. Check the oxygen every hour, and usually after **4 -6 hours patient's oxygen normalizes.** Patient feels better

Case usually ends here

Step 10. Counsel and screening
- No smoking, drinking, illegal drugs
- Safe sex, wear seal belt,
- Medicine compliance
- Age and gender specific screening

Diagnosis: Asthma Exacerbation

GASTROENTEROLOGY

ESOPHAGUS DISORDERS

1. ACHALASIA

Achalasia is a failure of the lower esophageal smooth muscles fibers relaxation that causes lower esophageal sphincter to remain closed during swallowing

Causes: loss of the nerve plexus, but there is no known cause for loss of the nerve plexus. A small percentage of cases occur secondary to other conditions such as Scleroderma, Chagas' disease

Si/Sx: chest pain, weight loss, **non-progressive dysphagia to solids and liquids simultaneously**, regurgitation of undigested food

Diagnosis:

- Chest x-ray may show dilated esophagus and no air in the stomach. However, chest x-ray is not sensitive or specific for the diagnosis of achalasia and further tests are required.
- **Barium swallow** is the **best initial test**. It shows dilated esophagus with a tapered narrowing of the lower end, referred as " bird beak."
- **Esophageal manometry** is the **most accurate test**. It shows high pressure in the lower esophageal sphincter (LES) at rest, and failure of LES to relax with swallowing.
- Endoscopy may be needed to exclude the malignancy

Treatment: There is no cure for achalasia. Treatment is given to reduce the pressure in the LES and allow the passage of food into the stomach

- **Pneumatic dilatation** is the **best initial treatment**. Complications of pneumatic dilations are chest pain, GERD, esophageal perforation.
- If it is ineffective, then perform **myotomy**. In this procedure, LES muscle fibers are cut and weakened. Complication of myotomy is GERD

- **Botulin toxin injection** is given if the patient **does not want to have pneumatic dilation and myotomy.** It relieves the obstruction by **temporarily paralyzing the nerve** that contracts the LES. Botulin toxin is **not a primary treatment** because the effect of the injection is short-lived (3 months to 1 year), and multiple re-injections are usually required.

2. ESOPHAGEAL SCLERODERMA
In esophageal scleroderma, normal esophageal tissue is replaced with fibrous tissue. LES it becomes immobile, and valves does not close
Si/Sx: non-progressive dysphagia to solids and liquids, some patients may have GERD symptoms
Diagnosis:
- **Barium swallow** is the **best initial test**
- **Esophageal manometer** is the **most accurate diagnostic test.** It shows **immobile esophagus** and **decreased LES resting pressure**

Treatment: There is no cure for scleroderma. **Proton pump inhibitors (PPIs) are given for life** to relieve GERD

3. ZENKER DIVERTICULUM
Zenker diverticulum is the **out-pouching of posterior pharyngeal constrictor, at the junction** of the pharynx and esophagus
Si/Sx: non-progressive dysphagia, bad breath, **regurgitation of previously eaten food**
Diagnosis: Best initial test is barium swallow, which shows diverticulum in proximal esophagus
Treatment: Surgical resection of diverticulum

Note: Endoscopy and nasogastric tube should be avoided in patients with Zenker diverticulum because of fear of pharynx perforation

4. ESOPHAGEAL RING AND WEBS
Esophageal rings and webs are thin folds of tissue that leads to partial or complete obstruction of the esophagus.
Types: Plummer-Vinson syndrome, Peptic stricture, and Schatzki's ring.

Differential diagnosis of esophageal ring and webs

Disease	Symptoms	Diagnosis	Treatment
Plummer-Vinson syndrome	Dysphagia, chest pain, acid reflux, **iron deficiency anemia**	Barium swallow shows **proximal esophageal** stricture	**Iron replacement**
Peptic stricture	Dysphagia, chest pain, acid reflux **(GERD)**	Barium swallow shows **distal esophageal** stricture	Pneumatic dilation
Schatzki ring	Dysphagia, chest pain, acid reflux, intermittent dysphagia to solids	Barium swallow shows ring in the **mid-esophagus**	Pneumatic dilation

5. DIFFUSE ESOPHAGEAL SPASM

Diffuse esophageal spasm is **uncoordinated contractions** of esophageal muscles. These contractions prevent forward movement of food from esophagus to stomach

Si/Sx: dysphagia, chest pain felt right **after meals or after drinking a cold beverage. (Chest pain that may mimic myocardial infarction**, but has no effect with exertion)

Diagnosis:

- **Best initial test is barium study**, which may show " corkscrew" pattern **during the time of spasm**
- **Most accurate test** is esophageal manometry, which shows **high-intensity uncoordinated contractions**

Treatment: Calcium-channel blockers or nitrates are given to relax the esophageal muscles

6. ESOPHAGITIS

Esophagitis is irritation or inflammation of esophagus

Cause: Infection (virus, yeast, fungi), medicine, GERD, surgery or chest radiation

Si/Sx: Painful swallowing, difficulty swallowing, sore throat, hoarseness, heartburn

Management is as follow:

1) Most common **drugs responsible** for esophagitis are iron sulfate, vitamin C, NSAIDs, doxycycline, bisphosphonates (alendronate, risedronate)

    Boards tip look for

    - Postmenopausal woman taking **alendronate or risedronate**
    - Anemic patient taking **iron sulfate**
    - Young patient taking **vitamin C**
    - Patient taking **NSAIDs**
    - Patient with acne taking **doxycycline**

    Treatment for drug induced esophagitis:

    - Advise the patient **to sit upright** then take medicine with **lots of water** and **stay upright for 30 minutes after taking the medicine**

2) Most common **viruses responsible** for esophagitis are candida, herpes simplex virus (HSV), and cytomegalovirus (CMV)

    Treatment for viral induced esophagitis is as follow:

    - **Candida** is the most common cause of esophagitis in an immunocompromised patient. So if a **HIV**-positive patient with **CD 4** count < 100 presents with esophagitis, then give him **fluconazole**
        - If the patient's symptoms improve, then **continue treating the patient with fluconazole.**
        - If the patient is not getting better, then **endoscopy** should be done (endoscopy findings and treatment options are discussed on the next page)
    - If the patient is **HIV-negative**, then do **endoscopy biopsy** (endoscopy findings and treatment options discussed on the next page)

Esophagitis differential diagnosis

Endoscopy findings	Most likely diagnosis	Treatment
Multiple punched-out ulcers	Herpes simplex virus (HSV)	Acyclovir
Single large ulcer or intracytoplasmic inclusions	Cytomegalovirus (CMV)	Ganciclovir plus acyclovir
Sterile ulcer	Aphthous ulcers	Steroids

7. MALLORY-WEISS SYNDROME

Mallory-Weiss syndrome is a tear in the mucus membrane at the gastroesophageal junction

Cause: retching, vomiting, binge drinking

Si/Sx: Painless bloody vomiting

Treatment:

- **IV fluid** is the **best initial treatment**, and in most cases bleeding stops spontaneously.
- If the bleeding does not stop, then **cauterization or epinephrine** injection near the bleeding site may be given to close the bleeding blood vessels.

Complication: Mallory–Weiss syndrome is associated with **hiatal hernia**

8. BOERHAAVE SYNDROME

Boerhaave syndrome is spontaneous esophageal perforation

Cause: iatrogenic, binge drinking, during medical instrumentation such as an endoscopy or paraesophageal surgery

Si/Sx: Severe retching and bloody vomiting followed by retrosternal chest pain and upper abdominal pain

Diagnosis:

- Chest x-ray shows mediastinal or free peritoneal air
- Water-soluble contrast esophagram (Gastrografin) can be used to confirm the diagnosis

Treatment: IV fluids, IV antibiotics and left thoracotomy

Note: Barium swallow is not used to diagnose Boerhaave syndrome because the spillage of barium into the mediastinal and pleural cavity can induce inflammation and may cause fibrosis. However, if Gastrografin study is negative, then barium study can be performed.

9. ESOPHAGEAL VARICES

Esophageal varices are abnormally dilated sub-mucosal veins in lower third of the esophagus. They are often caused by portal hypertension and cirrhosis (liver disease). These veins can leak or even rupture and cause life-threating bleeding.

Si/Sx: Painless bloody vomiting and signs of liver disease such as gynecomastia, splenomegaly, spider angiomata and palmar erythema.

Diagnosis: Endoscopy

Treatment:

- **IV fluids, blood** transfusion (if hematocrit is < 30 % in an older individual and < 25% in a young individual), **fresh frozen plasma** to correct PT or INR, and platelet transfusion if the platelet count is < 50,000.
- **Initial treatment is octreotide and antibiotics** (quinolone or ciprofloxacin).
    - Octreotide is given to lower the portal hypertension
    - Antibiotics are given to prevent infection from gram-negative bacteria that can cause spontaneous bacterial peritonitis.
- If the patient continues to bleed, then perform upper **endoscopy with band ligation is done.** Endoscopy is **diagnostic and therapeutic.** It obliterates the bleeding vessels.
- If the **patient is still bleeding,** then do **transjugular intrahepatic portosystemic shunt (TIPS).** In TIPS, a small tube is placed between the portal vein and hepatic vein that carries blood from the liver to the heart, which reduces the portal pressure.
    - **Complication and contraindication** of TIPS is **hepatic encephalopathy**
- Once **bleeding is under control,** then give **non-selective beta-blockers** (Propranolol) it decreases the re-bleeding frequency

Boards tip for esophageal varices

1. If the patient is **bleeding** and the question asks, which **drug will lower the mortality**? Answers: **ciprofloxacin**
2. If **bleeding has stopped,** and the question asks, which drug will lower the mortality? Answer: **Propranolol**

10. GASTROESOPHAGEAL REFLUX DISEASE (GERD)

GERD is a condition in which stomach content (food, acid) refluxes back into the esophagus

Cause: Alcohol, smoking, abnormal lower esophageal sphincter relaxation, hiatal hernia, scleroderma, pregnancy and medicines

Si/Sx:
- Metallic taste in mouth
- Nocturnal cough
- Sore throat
- Burning chest pain
- Wheezing

Diagnosis:
- GERD is diagnosed **based on signs and symptoms.**
- If the diagnosis is not clear, then do 24-hour pH monitoring

Treatment:
- **Lifestyle modification** is the best initial treatment for all the patients with GERD:
  - Weight loss
  - Elevate head of bed 6-8 inches
  - Avoid alcohol, nicotine, caffeine
  - Avoid chocolate, spicy food, fatty food and peppermint
  - Avoid eating within 3 hours of bedtime
- If lifestyle modification is ineffective, then give **PPIs**
- If PPIs are ineffective as well, then perform **Nissen fundoplication or endocinch**; it tightens the lower esophageal sphincter.

Complication: Patient with long-standing GERD is at risk of developing Barrett's esophagus. Patient should have serial monitoring with endoscopy starting 5 years after they were first diagnosed with GERD.

11. BARRETT'S ESOPHAGUS

Barrett's esophagus is caused by **long-standing GERD (> 5 years)**. In this condition **lower esophageal epithelium** (squamous cell epithelium) is replaced by **columnar epithelium**.

Barrett's esophagus is a premalignant condition. It can lead to **adenocarcinoma** of the lower esophagus.

Diagnosis: Endoscopy biopsy

Treatment: depends on endoscopy biopsy. (Discussed below)

Endoscopy biopsy findings	Treatment
Barrett's esophagus or columnar metaplasia	PPIs and repeat endoscopy every 2-3 years
Low-grade dysplasia	PPI and repeat endoscopy every 3-6 months
High-grade dysplasia	Distal esophagectomy

12. ESOPHAGEAL CANCER

Esophageal cancer is a malignancy of esophagus. Two most common esophageal cancers are squamous cell cancer and adenocarcinoma.

- Squamous cell cancer arises from the cells of the upper part of the esophagus.
- Adenocarcinoma arises from the cells of the lower part of the esophagus.

Risk factors:

- Risk factors for the **squamous cell carcinoma** are **smoking, ethanol** and **Plummer venison syndrome.**
- Risk factor for the **adenocarcinoma** is **Barrett's esophagus**

Si/Sx: Progressive dysphagia initially to solids, and later to liquids, weight loss, heartburn, coughing, hoarseness

Diagnosis:

- Best initial test is barium swallow to rule out obstruction
- Best initial diagnostic test endoscopy biopsy
- X-ray or CT of the chest is usually performed to check for **metastases** disease

Treatment: depends on the location of the tumor

- **Localized tumors** are treated with **surgical resection** and **chemotherapy (5-fluorouracil)**

- **Metastatic tumors** are treated with **radiation and chemotherapy (5-fluorouracil)**
- **Metal stent** is placed to keep esophagus open for palliation and improve dysphagia

---

Boards tip for esophageal disorders

- For any esophagus dysfunction, best initial step in management is always barium swallow. Even if you suspect that the patient has cancer, initial step is still barium swallow to rule out obstruction

- If patient is > 60 years of age, has anemia, heme-positive stool, symptoms present > 6 months and weight loss, then make sure to endoscopy biopsy to check for esophageal cancer

---

STOMACH DISEASES

1. GASTRITIS

Gastritis is a condition in which the inner lining of the stomach becomes inflamed

Cause: NSAIDs, alcohol, Helicobacter pylori, pernicious anemia

Si/Sx: Painless melena, vomiting blood, nausea, vomiting, pain in the upper part of the abdomen, loss of appetite

Management:
- If gastritis is caused by drugs –Tx. **stop offending drug**
- If gastritis is caused **H.pylori** infection -Tx. **treat H.pylori**

Any patient >45 of age with gastritis should have upper endoscopy to exclude gastric cancer

---

High-yield questions

- what is the most common cause of **gastritis**?
  Answer: **NSAIDs**

- What is the most common cause of **peptic ulcer**?
  Answer: **H.pylori**

---

2. PEPTIC ULCER DISEASE (PUD)

Peptic ulcer is a condition in which lining of the stomach or duodenum is affected.

- A peptic ulcer in the stomach is called gastric ulcer
- A peptic ulcer in the duodenum is called duodenal ulcer.

Cause: Helicobacter pylori (H. pylori) is the **most common cause** of peptic ulcer, but causes may include NSAIDs, alcohol, smoking, burns, head trauma and Zollinger-Ellison syndrome.

Si/Sx: Gastric ulcer and duodenal ulcer both cause epigastric pain, bloating, nausea, hematemesis and melena. To distinguished them read the following:

- **In gastric ulcer pain increases soon after eating and gets better 2-3 hours after eating**
- **In duodenal ulcer pain occurs 2-3 hours after eating and relieves soon after eating**

Diagnosis:

- **Endoscopy** helps determine the location of the ulcer
- **Urease breath test and stool antigen detection test** are the **best initial tests**
  - These tests are non-invasive tests, but make sure that the patient is not taking PPIs for at least two weeks prior to performing these tests otherwise tests may come out false positive.
- **IgG serology** is the **most sensitive test**
  - If IgG serology test is negative, then one can safely exclude the possibility of H. pylori infection.
  - If IgG serology test is positive for H. pylori, then this test has no value because once serology is positive, it stays positive for life. Therefore, the positive test will not differentiate old infection from new infection
- **Endoscopy biopsy** is the **most accurate test**

Treatment for H.pylori

- **Best initial treatment** is the combination of **three medicines -** PPIs, Amoxicillin and clarithromycin.
  - If a patient is **allergic to penicillin,** then replace amoxicillin with tetracycline drugs.

- H.pylori is capable of **developing resistance to antibiotics**. If a patient is not responding to initial treatment, then **perform urease breath test or stool antigen test** to see if H.pylori is present.
  - If any of the test is positive for H.pylori, then treat the patient with a **combination of 4 antibiotics – PPIs, metronidazole, tetracycline and bismuth.**
  - If urease breath test or stool antigen test is negative for H.pylori, then check gastrin levels to check if the patient has f **Zollinger-Ellison syndrome**

Complication of PUD: Perforation, gastric outlet obstruction, and hemorrhage

3. ZOLLINGER-ELLISON SYNDROME (ZES)
Zollinger-Ellison syndrome is a small tumor of pancreas or duodenum in which a **large amount of gastrin is secreted. High levels of gastrin increases the production stomach acid.**
Si/Sx: patient often presents with recurrent signs and symptoms of peptic ulcer disease
Diagnosis:
- **Gastrin level** is best **initial test**
- If **gastrin levels** are **inconclusive**, then do **secretin stimulation test**. In this test, a small amount of secretin is injected, and **gastrin hormone and gastric acid output are rechecked.**
  - In a normal person, these are suppressed after the test
  - In a patient with ZES, gastrin hormone and gastric acid output **remains high** after the test
- Once the diagnosis is known, and then it is important to localize the tumor.
  - **Endoscopy ultrasound** is performed first to **localize the tumor.**
  - If these fail to locate the tumor, then **nuclear somatostatin scan** is performed **detect metastatic ZES.**
Treatment: depends on location of the tumor
- **Localize** tumor is **surgically removed.**
- **Metastatic** ZES is treated with **lifelong PPIs**

4. NON-ULCER DYSPEPSIA

Non-ulcer dyspepsia is a diagnosis of exclusion, all the tests including endoscopy is negative

Management: There is no specific treatment; PPI's, H2 blocker, or antacids can be tried

5. GASTROPARESIS

Gastroparesis is a condition in which forward movement of food from the stomach to the small intestine is slowed or stopped.

Cause: nerve damage or loss of nerve sensitivity, in conditions such as diabetes, gastrectomy, systemic sclerosis, or anticholinergic medicines

Si/Sx: abdominal distension, **early satiety, postprandial nausea, and unintentional weight loss**

Diagnosis:

- Clinical diagnosis.
- Diagnosis can be confirmed with gastric emptying scan, but often not necessary

Treatment:

- **Initial treatment** for gastroparesis is **diet modification- high protein, low fiber and low fats.**
- If **diet modification is ineffective,** then drugs such as **erythromycin or metoclopramide** may be given, these increase the GI motility

6. DUMPING SYNDROME

Dumping syndrome is a condition in which ingested food bypass the stomach and enters small intestine undigested.

Cause: It is seen in patients who had surgery to remove all or some parts of stomach, or patients who have had stomach bypass surgery to lose weight

Si/Sx: Symptoms of dumping syndrome are seen during the meal or within **15-30 after the meal.** Symptoms include nausea, vomiting, **sweating, flushing, lightheadedness, heart palpitations, confusion, and fainting**

Diagnosis:

- Clinical diagnosis
- Gastric emptying scan can be used to confirm the diagnosis

Treatment:

- Initial treatment for gastroparesis is **diet modification- eat multiple small meals that are high in protein, high fats and low carbohydrates.**
- If diet modification is ineffective, then **somatostatin (Octreotide)** may be given; it slows down the emptying of food into the intestine.

INFLAMMATORY BOWEL DISEASE (IBD)

Inflammatory bowel disease is an inflammatory condition of all or part(s) of the digestive tract. Two types IBD are Crohn's disease (CD), and ulcerative colitis (UC)

Si/Sx of CD and UC

	Ulcerative colitis	Crohn's disease
History	<ul><li>**Bloody diarrhea**</li><li>Tenesmus</li><li>Lower abdominal pain</li></ul>	<ul><li>**Watery diarrhea**</li><li>Weight loss</li><li>Abdominal pain</li></ul>
Extraintestinal manifestation	<ul><li>Toxic megacolon</li><li>Erythema nodosum</li><li>Pyoderma nodosum</li><li>Arthralgia</li><li>Uveitis</li></ul>	<ul><li>Same as ulcerative colitis **plus** the followings:<ul><li>Kidney stone</li><li>Gallstones</li></ul>Vitamin B12 deficiency</li></ul>

Diagnosis:

- **Barium study** is the **best initial test**
- **Endoscopy biopsy** is the **most accurate test**.
- If the diagnosis is still not clear, then serology test is performed (results are discussed on the next page)

Diagnostic findings of UC and CD

	Ulcerative colitis (UC)	Crohn's disease (CD)
Barium study	Diffuse and continuous involvement, Lead-pipe colon, edema, pseudopolyps	Skip lesion, creeping fat, cobblestoning, stricture
Endoscopy biopsy	Transmural granuloma	Crypt abscess
Serology	Antineutrophil cytoplasmic antibody (ANCA)	Antisaccharomyces cerevisiae antibody (ASCA)

Treatment:

- Best **initial treatment** for UC is **sulfasalazine or 5-ASA (mesalamine)**
- Best **initial treatment** for CD is **sulfasalazine**
- **High-dose steroids** are useful in **acute exacerbation** of UC or CD.
- **Azathioprine and 6-mercaptopurine** are given if the patient develops **acute flare-up of IBD while weaning the patient off of steroids.**
- **Tumor necrosis factors** (TNF) such as infliximab is given if a patient with **CD develops fistula**
  - Patient must be tested for latent TB (PPD test) before starting infliximab because it can reactivate latent TB from granuloma. If **PPD** induration > 5mm – Tx. **INH** before giving Infliximab
- If a patient with Crohn's disease has **perianal involvement**, then give **metronidazole and ciprofloxacin**

Colon cancer surveillance in IBD

- Start colonoscopy **8 years after** the time of diagnosis, **then every year thereafter**
- If only **left side of colon is involved, then start** colonoscopy **beginning 15 year** after the time of diagnosis, **then every year thereafter**

Management: If any grade of dysplasia is found during the surveillance, then do **total colectomy**

COLON CANCER SCREENING

- Patient with no family history of colon cancer screening- start screening at the age 50
  - o Yearly FOBT
  - o Sigmoidoscopy every 3-5 years
  - o Colonoscopy every 10 year

- Colonoscopy is very sensitive for colon cancer. If it is performed, and it shows no abnormality, then there is no need to do FOBT for next 10 year

If a question asks, which test is the **best screening test for** colon cancer?
Answer: Colonoscopy

COLONOSCOPY FINDING AND MANAGEMENT

- **Hamartomas and hyperplastic** polyps are **benign polyps.** They do not increase the risk of colon cancer and require colonoscopy follow-up **every 10-year**

  - o *Easy way to remember*: Hamartomas and hyperplastic polyps are happy polyps. They **do not increase the risk of colon cancer.**

- Adenoma or villous polyps **increase the risk of developing** colon cancer. They require close monitoring (discussed in the table below)

Management for Adenomas and villous polyps

Colonoscopy findings	Follow-up
• 1 polyp, <1 cm adenoma polyp or villous polyp	• Colonoscopy after 3 years, then after 10 years
• > 3 polyps, > 1cm adenoma polyps or villous polyps	• Colonoscopy after 3 years, then after 5 years
• **Cancerous** polyp removed and **margins are clear**	• Colonoscopy 1 year after removal of cancerous polyp, then after 3 years

Colon cancer screening

Condition	Screening
No family history of colon cancer or general population	Start colonoscopy at the age 50, then every 10 years
IBD (Crohn's disease, Ulcerative colitis)	Start colonoscopy **8 years after the diagnosis of IBD**, then every year thereafter
One family member with colon cancer	Start colonoscopy at **40 years of age or 10 years prior** to the age at which the youngest family member was diagnosed with colon cancer (**Which ever come first**), then every 10 years
Colon cancer in three family members, in two generations, one death before the age of < 50	Start **colonoscopy** at age **25 or 10 years prior** to at which the youngest family member was diagnosed with colon cancer, then every **1-2 years thereafter**
Turcot's syndrome, Gardner syndrome, Familial adenomatous polyposis	Start **sigmoidoscopy 10-12 years** of age then **every year** thereafter

- Turcot's syndrome is characterized by the presence of multiple adenomatous colon polyposis with increased risk of colorectal cancer and increased risk of **medulloblastoma**
- Gardner's syndrome characterized by the presence of multiple adenomatous colon polyposis, **desmoid tumors**, and **osteomas of the skull or mandible**

DIARRHEA

1. INFECTIOUS DIARRHEA
Infectious diarrhea is characterized by **fever, bloody diarrhea and WBCs** in stool

1a. CAMPYLOBACTER
- This is the most common cause of infectious diarrhea; it is caused by ingestion of undercooked poultry.
- Erythromycin speeds the recovery
- Complication: Guillain- Barre syndrome

1b. YERSINIA
- This is caused by ingestion of undercooked pork
- Patient usually presents with **RLQ pain, joints pain and rash**

1c. SHIGELLA
- This is caused by pathogens transmitted via the fecal-oral route
- Complication -reactive arthritis, shigella secrets shiga toxin that can lead to Hemolytic uremic syndrome (HUS)

1d. SALMONELLA
- This is caused by ingesting contaminated eggs, poultry and milk
- Patients with sickle cell anemia are at increased risk of infection risk from salmonella

1e. ENTEROHEMORRHAGIC E.COLI (0517:H7)
- This is caused by consumption of undercooked beef
- Complication: **HUS**

1f. VIBRIO PARAHEMOLYTICUS
- This is caused by consumption of seafood

1g. VIBRIO VULNIFICUS
- This is caused by ingestion of raw seafood (oysters, clams)
- Patients may also have skin bullae

- Patients with hemochromatosis and liver disease are at increased risk of infection from vibrio vulnificus

- Diagnosis **of infectious diarrhea** is as follow:
  - o Best initial test is **fecal leukocytes**
  - o Most accurate test is **stool culture & Sensitivity**

- Treatment **of infectious diarrhea**:
  - o **For mild** diarrhea - Tx. **Hydration**
  - o **For severe** diarrhea – Tx. **Ciprofloxacin**

2. NON-INFLAMMATORY DIARRHEA

Non-inflammatory is characterized by **large volume watery diarrhea without blood and WBCs in the stool**

2a. ROTAVIRUS

- This is the most common cause of diarrhea **in kids**

2b. NORWALK VIRUS

- This is the most common cause of non-bloody diarrhea in **adults**
- Look for a patient, who just came back from **cruise ship**

2c. GIARDIA

- This is caused by pathogens transmitted via the fecal-oral route: **drinking contaminated water from fresh water streams**. It is also seen in **men, who have sex with men**
- Patient usually present with **steatorrhea, bloating and flatus**
- Diagnostic test: **ELISA stool antigen**
- Treatment: **Metronidazole**

2d. CRYPTOSPORIDIUM

- This is caused by pathogens transmitted via the fecal-oral route: **drinking contaminated water from fresh water streams**

- **Note:** Giardia is also acquired by drinking water from the fresh water streams, but unlike giardia, patients with cryptosporidium do not have steatorrhea, cramps and bloating

- It is commonly seen in **HIV-positive patients**
- Diagnosis: **Modified acid fast stain**, which shows **oocysts in stool**
- Treatment: depends on following:
  - If patient is **Immunocompetent** – Tx. **Supportive**
  - If patient is **HIV positive** – Tx. **Best initial therapy is HAART** to raise CD 4 count
  - Paromomycin is partially effective

2e. STAPHYLOCOCCUS AUREUS and BACILLUS CEREUS
- Both of these cause vomiting and diarrhea within few hours of ingesting of infected food
- **To distinguish in them look at the case history**
  - **Bacillus** cereus diarrhea usually occurs after ingesting **reheated rice products**
  - **Staphylococcus** aureus diarrhea usually occurs after ingesting **mayonnaise or egg products**

3. SCOMBROID POISONING
- Symptoms: **flushing, diarrhea, wheezing** and vomiting **within 10 minutes of eating food infected with scombroid**
- Causes: tuna, snapper, mackerel
- Treatment: **Diphenhydramine** (antihistamines)

4. LACTOSE INTOLERANCE
- Patients have **flatulence, gaseous distention, bloating and diarrhea after eating dairy** products **other than yogurt**
- Diagnoses: **Hydrogen breath test**
- Treatment: **diet modification**

5. CLOSTRIDIUM DIFFICILE
- Look for a patient presenting with **green diarrhea** and recent history **antibiotics uses** such as clindamycin, amoxicillin, fluoroquinolone
- Diagnosis:
  - Best **initial test: ELISA stool toxin assay**
  - Accurate test is **cytotoxicity assay**

- Management:
  - Best initial therapy is **metronidazole**
  - If patient's diarrhea was **resolved with metronidazole, and then occurs again** –Tx. **Metronidazole**
  - If patient is **not responding to metronidazole** – Tx. **Oral vancomycin** (IV Vancomycin has no effect on C-difficile)

6. OSMOTIC DIARRHEA

Osmotic diarrhea is caused by **ingestion of nonabsorbable solutes**, which remains in the bowel and draws water from the body.
Cause: Lactose intolerance, mannitol, oral magnesium
Diagnosis:

- Stool osmotic gap > 50 mOsm/kg
- Stop ingesting offending agent or **fasting usually stops diarrhea**

Treatment: Stop ingesting offending agent

Stool osmotic gap is calculated by: 290 – 2 (stool Na + stool K)

---

7. SECRETORY DIARRHEA

Secretory diarrhea is characterized as loose stool; electrolytes and water are actively secreted or are not absorbed from luminal content
Cause: Cholera toxin, enteric virus
Diagnosis:

- Stool osmotic gap is <50 mOsm/kg
- **Fasting does not stops diarrhea**

Treatment: Supportive

8. EXUDATIVE DIARRHEA

Exudative diarrhea is characterized by the presence of **blood and pus** in the stool
Cause: Crohn's disease, Ulcerative colitis
Diagnosis and treatment: see Crohn's disease and Ulcerative colitis

9. CARCINOID SYNDROME

Carcinoid syndrome is a group of symptoms associated with carcinoid tumor, which secretes high amount of serotonin.
Si/Sx: Diarrhea, heart palpitation, **wheezing, flushing**

Diagnosis: Best initial test is 5-HIAA levels
Treatment: Octreotide

10. IRRITABLE BOWEL SYNDROME (IBS)

Irritable bowel syndrome is a functional GI disorder characterized by **abdominal pain and altered bowel habits without any organic cause**. It is more common in **young females than males**
Si/Sx:
- Abdominal pain is relieved by defecation
- Pain is less at night
- Alternating bowel habits of constipation and diarrhea

Diagnosis: IBS is a diagnosis of exclusion
Treatment:
- If patient is complaining of **constipation**- Tx. **Fibers**
- If patient has **diarrhea** - Tx. **Antispasmodics** such as **dicyclomine**
- If patient is **not responding to antispasmodics** –Tx. **TCAs antidepressants**
  - Anti-depressants work by two ways: 1) anticholinergic effect, 2) relieves neuropathic pain

11. MALABSORPTION DIARRHEA

Malabsorption diarrhea is characterized inability to absorb nutrient from gastrointestinal tract
Si/Sx: Bulky stools, fatty stools, bloating, failure to thrive, weight loss, muscle wasting
Diagnosis of malabsorption diarrhea:
- Best initial test is **sudan black stain**
- Most sensitive test is **72-hour fecal fat collection**

Cause: Celiac disease, tropical sprue disease, Whipple disease, and chronic pancreatitis

11a. CELIAC SPRUE DISEASE
- Look for a patient with **symptoms of malabsorption diarrhea and iron deficiency anemia**
- Patient may also have folic acid deficiency

- Physical exam usually shows vesicular rash (**dermatitis herpetiformis**) on extensors surface of skin such as elbows, shoulders
- Diagnosis:
  - Best initial test is **anti-endomysial, antigliadin, and anti-transglutaminase antibody**
  - Most accurate test is **small bowel biopsy**, which **shows villous atrophy**
- Treatment: **Gluten free diet**. Make sure to tell patient that it may take few weeks for the symptoms to completely resolve after starting gluten free diet
- Complications: **gastrointestinal lymphomas**

11b. TROPICAL SPRUE

- Look for a patient with the **symptoms of malabsorption diarrhea** and **recent travel of tropical** island
- Diagnosis: **Small bowel biopsy**, which **shows microorganism**
- Treatment: **Oral tetracycline for 3-6 months**

11c. WHIPPLE DISEASE (Tropheryma Whippelii)

- Look for a patient with **symptoms of malabsorption diarrhea**, and **arthralgia, neurological** abnormalities **and ocular findings**
- Diagnostic test:
  - Small bowel biopsy, which shows **PAS Positive microorganism**

    Or
  - **PCR of stool** for Tropheryma Whippelii
- Treatment: **Tetracycline** for **1 year**

11d. CHRONIC PANCREATITIS

- Look for a patient with **symptoms of malabsorption diarrhea and chronic pancreatitis**
- Diagnosis:
  - Initial test is **amylase and lipase**
  - Best **initial diagnostic** test is **abdominal x-ray** or **CT without contrast**
  - Most accurate test is **secretin stimulation test**
- Treatment: **Oral pancreatic enzyme replacement**

Q. **What is the purpose of D-xylose test?**

A. D-xylose is a simple sugar that does not require enzymes for digestion prior to absorption. D-xylose test is used to **determine if malabsorption diarrhea is caused by the small intestine disease** (Celiac sprue, Tropical sprue, Whipple disease) or **chronic pancreatitis**. Oral D-xylose is given to the patient and then checked in blood or urine sample. **D-xylose is not absorbed** if the patient has any of the **small intestine disease** that affects its ability to absorb nutrients. In contrast, **D-xylose absorption is normal in chronic pancreatitis**.

Q. **What is the purpose secretin stimulation test?**

A. Secretin stimulation test measures the ability of the pancreas to release pancreatic enzyme in response to secretin in the small intestine (duodenum). In this test nasogastric tube is inserted through the nose into the duodenum. Secretin is given intravenously. Duodenum content is collected in NG tube over next 1-2 hours. **Normal person** shows **increased pancreatic enzyme in NG tube**. In contrast, person with **chronic pancreatitis** shows **no or low pancreatic enzyme** in NG tube.

GI BLEEDING

Differential diagnosis for GI bleeding

	Upper GI bleeding	Lower GI bleeding
Location	Proximal to ligament of treitz	Distal to the ligament of treitz and superior to the anus.
Cause	Esophageal varices, esophagitis, Mallory-Weiss tear, Gastric ulcer, Gastritis, duodenal ulcer,	Anal fissure, IBD, hemorrhoids, diverticulosis, colonic polyps, colon cancer
Stool	Black, "**tarry** " feces (melena)	**Bright red blood** in stool (Hematochezia)

Management of GI Bleeding

- Before doing any test, make sure to check if the patient needs **fluid resuscitation**
- Start with **Nasogastric (NG) tube** because **most common cause** of GI bleeding is **upper GI bleeding**. (See figure on the next page)

GI bleeding workup:

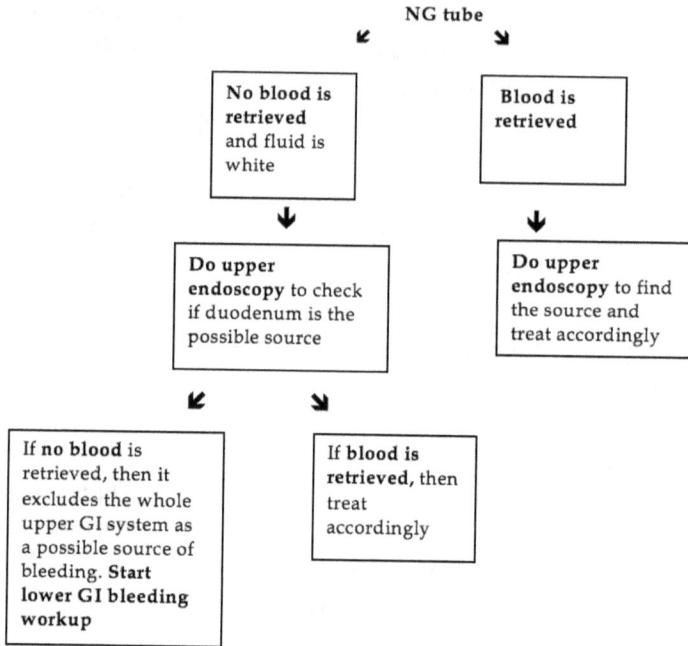

NG tube

| No blood is retrieved and fluid is white | Blood is retrieved |

| Do upper endoscopy to check if duodenum is the possible source | Do upper endoscopy to find the source and treat accordingly |

| If **no blood** is retrieved, then it excludes the whole upper GI system as a possible source of bleeding. **Start lower GI bleeding workup** | If **blood is retrieved,** then treat accordingly |

- Lower GI work up:
  - Start with **anoscopy** to exclude hemorrhoids
  - If anoscopy is negative, then further diagnostic testing depends on the quantity of the bleeding:
    - Do **colonoscopy,** if bleeding is **< .05 ml/min**
    - Do **angiography,** if bleeding is **> 2ml/min**
    - Do **tagged red cell scan,** if bleeding is **between .05 - 2 ml/min**

HEMORRHOIDS

Hemorrhoids are swollen and inflamed veins in the lower rectum and anus that can cause pain and or bleeding

Cause: Straining during bowel movement, increased pressure in veins

Si/Sx:

- Internal hemorrhoids are usually painless, but these tend to bleed easily
- External hemorrhoids are painful

Treatment:
- **Internal** hemorrhoids are treated with **rubber band ligation**
- **External** hemorrhoids are treated with **high fiber diet, sitz bath and stool softener. If this is ineffective,** then **surgical hemorrhoidectomy.**

CONSTIPATION
Most common causes are **lack of dietary fibers and insufficient fluid intake,** but other causes may include hypothyroidism, calcium channel blocker, ferrous sulfate, anticholinergic medications
Treatment: **hydration** and **increased fiber diet (psyllium & methylcellulose).** Treat the underlying cause, if applicable

LIVER DISEASES

CIRRHOSIS
Cirrhosis is advanced liver disease, in which fibrosis and nodules replace the normal liver tissue
Cause: Most common causes of cirrhosis are **alcohol, hepatitis B and hepatitis C,** other less common causes include primary biliary cirrhosis, primary sclerosis cholangitis, hemochromatosis, Wilson disease, autoimmune hepatitis, and nonalcoholic steatohepatitis.
Si/Sx: all forms of cirrhosis have following characteristics:
- Low albumin levels
- Portal hypertension
- Gynecomastia
- Spider angiomata
- Thrombocytopenia (increased PT time)
- Jaundice
- **Ascites**
- Palmar erythema
- Asterixis
- Hepatic encephalopathy
- Esophageal varices

Ascites is the accumulation of **fluid in the peritoneal cavity**. It results from high pressure in the portal system and low albumin. Most common causes of ascites are cirrhosis and severe live disease, but other causes may include CHF, cancer, pancreatitis, and portal vein thrombosis.

Diagnosis:
- Ultrasound
- Paracentesis (needle aspiration of peritoneal fluid)– it is performed **if the patient develops new ascites, abdominal pain and tenderness or fever.** Fluid is checked for its **gross appearance, protein level, albumin, and cell count.**
- SAAG (Serum ascites albumin gradient) is the difference between serum albumin and ascites albumin. See below

Differential diagnosis of ascites

SAAG = Serum albumin – ascites albumin	
<1.1 g/dL	>1.1g/dL
• Infection (TB, bacterial fungal, parasitic) • Malignancy (Pancreatic cancer, ovarian cancer) • Hypoalbuminemia (Nephrotic syndrome, protein losing enteropathy, malnutrition)	• Budd-Chiari syndrome • Portal hypertension • CHF • Constrictive pericarditis

Treatment:
There is no specific treatment for cirrhosis. Treatment is directed towards managing the complications and treating the underlying cause. (Discussed below)

Cirrhosis complications	Treatment
Ascites and edema	Spironolactone and other diuretic
Hepatic encephalopathy	Neomycin, lactulose
Portal hypertension	Propranolol(it prevents esophageal varices)
If ascites fluid shows **WBC > 500 or neutrophils > 250**	IV Cefotaxime

Prognosis: Mortality of a patient with cirrhosis can be predicted with **Model for End-Stage Liver Disease** also known as MELD score, which uses the value of the followings to predict the survival:

- Bilirubin
- INR
- Creatinine

SPONTANEOUS BACTERIAL PERITONITIS
Spontaneous bacterial peritonitis is a **life-threating complication of ascites**
Cause: E coli
Si/Sx: Fever, abdominal pain and bloating, abdominal tenderness
Diagnosis:

- Abdominal ultrasound or CT
- **Best initial test is WBCs** count, from the sample of peritoneal fluid
- **Most accurate test is peritoneal fluid culture**

Note: WBCs > 500 or neutrophil >250 confirm the infections and antibiotics should be started immediately without waiting for culture results to avoid complications

Treatment: IV cefotaxime or ceftriaxone. Additionally, IV albumin is added to the treatment to maintain renal perfusion pressure

SPECIFIC CAUSES AND MANAGEMENT OF CIRRHOSIS

1. PRIMARY BILIARY CIRRHOSIS
Primary biliary cirrhosis is an **autoimmune disease** of the bile duct of the liver. Bile builds up in the liver and leads to slow progressive liver damage, and ultimately causing scarring, fibrosis and cirrhosis. It is much more in females than male; 9:1(females to male)
Si/Sx: Fatigue, **pruritus**, jaundice, **xanthoma** (cholesterol deposit in the skin), and **xanthelasma** (cholesterol deposits around eyes)
Diagnosis:

- Best initial test: normal bilirubin, increased alkaline phosphatase and increased IgM-antibodies
- Most **accurate test: Anti-mitochondrial antibody and liver biopsy**

Treatment: Ursodeoxycholic acid

2. PRIMARY SCLEROSIS CHOLANGITIS

Primary sclerosis cholangitis is a chronic bile duct disease that causes inflammation and obstruction of bile duct, inside and outside the liver. Bile builds up in the liver and leads to slow progressive liver damage, and ultimately leads to scarring, fibrosis and cirrhosis

Cause: Autoimmune diseases, but it is **more common in patients with Ulcerative colitis (UC)**

Si/Sx: Fatigue, **pruritus,** jaundice

Diagnosis:

- Best initial test: **increased bilirubin, increased alkaline phosphate and increased Gamma-glutamyl transferase or gamma-glutamyl transpeptidase (GGTP)**

- Most **accurate test** is endoscopic retrograde cholangiopancreatography **(ERCP)**, which shows **" beads on a string"** appearance, which is narrowing and dilation of biliary tract, **anti-smooth muscle antibody or ANCA**

Treatment: Ursodeoxycholic acid or cholestyramine

3. HEMOCHROMATOSIS

Hemochromatosis is an abnormal accumulation of iron in the body

Cause:

- **Primary hemochromatosis is autosomal recessive** disease that is caused by mutation in HFE gene.

- **Secondary hemochromatosis** is found in patients with thalassemia, excess iron intake, **receiving multiple blood transfusions**

Si/Sx: Excessive iron deposited in the body leads to **darkening of skin, diabetes, pseudogout, restrictive cardiomyopathy,** and **infertility**

Diagnosis:

- Iron studies shows **increased iron, increased ferritin level, increased transferrin** and **low total iron binding capacity (TIBG)**

- **Most accurate test is liver biopsy**

Treatment:

- **Best initial treatment is phlebotomy.**

- Deferoxamine is useful in patients, who are refusing phlebotomy or cannot undergo phlebotomy.

Complication: most common cause of **death** in a patient with hemochromatosis is **cirrhosis**

4. WILSON DISEASE

Wilson disease is an autosomal recessive disorder in which copper accumulates in the body tissues. It affects liver, kidney, nervous system and blood cells

Si/Sx: **Tremors, psychosis**, seizure, cirrhosis, **hemolytic anemia**, renal tubular acidosis

Diagnosis:

- **Best initial tests** are **slit-lamp examination of eyes** for Kayser-Fleischer ring (dark circle around the eye that may be visible to the naked eye) and **low ceruloplasmin level.**
- **Most accurate test** is liver biopsy

Treatment:

- **Best initial treatment is penicillamine**; it binds to the copper and increases its urinary excretion.
- Other treatment options include **zinc acetate** that blocks the copper absorption in the intestine; **Trientine** that binds to copper and increased urinary excretion of copper

5. AUTOIMMUNE HEPATITIS

Autoimmune hepatitis is an inflammation of the liver that occurs when body's own immune system attacks liver

Type: two main types of autoimmune hepatitis are:

- **Type I autoimmune hepatitis**: this is the most common type. It can occur at any age. Most of the patients have other autoimmune disorders.
  o Diagnosis:
    - Best initial test is **ANA and anti-smooth muscle antibodies**
    - **Most accurate test is liver biopsy**

- **Type II autoimmune hepatitis**: this is most common in **young girls**.
  o Diagnosis:
    - Best initial test is **anti-liver-kidney-muscle antibody**
    - **Most accurate test is liver biopsy**

Treatment: prednisone and or azathioprine for both types

6. ALCOHOL HEPATITIS

This is the most common cause of liver disease in US

Diagnosis:
- Clinical diagnosis
- AST: ALT = 2:1 is highly suggestive of alcohol liver disease

Treatment: Abstain from alcohol can reverse the disease

7. NONALCOHOLIC STEATOHEPATITIS (NASH)

Nonalcoholic steatohepatitis (NASH) is liver inflammation caused by accumulation of fat in the liver. It resembles alcoholic liver disease, but it affects people who drinks little alcohol or do not drink at all. It is seen in obese, diabetics or patient with hyperlipidemia

Diagnosis: liver biopsy is the **most accurate test**, which shows microscope fat deposits.

Treatment: Treat the underlying cause such as lose weight, treat diabetes or hyperlipidemia.

HEPATITIS

Hepatitis is swelling and inflammation of the liver
Cause: Virus, drugs, alcohol, autoimmune

AST and ALT in hepatitis
- **Viral** hepatitis - **ALT > AST**
- **Drug** hepatitis - **AST > ALT**
- **Alcohol** hepatitis – **AST>ALT= 2:1**

1. HEPATITIS A

Hepatitis A is the most **common cause of hepatitis**. It is usually transmitted by fecal oral route

Diagnosis -IgM anti-hepatitis A virus

Treatment: Self-limited

2. HEPATITIS B

Hepatitis B is transmitted by exposure of blood or body fluids contaminated with hepatitis B infection such as blood transfusion, sexual contact or re-use of contaminated needle

Diagnosis: hepatitis B is diagnosed based on serology (discussed below)

Stage	Surface antigen (HBsAg)	e-antigen (HBeAg)	Core-antibody (HBcAb)	Surface antibody (HBsAb)
Acute disease	Present	Present	Present	Absent
Window phase	Absent	Absent	Present	Absent
Recovered	Absent	Absent	Present	Present
Vaccinated	Absent	Absent	Absent	Present
Chronic disease	Present	Present	Present	Absent

Note: Acute and chronic hepatitis B has same serology. Only way to differentiate them is to look at the duration of HBsAg. If **HBsAg** is present for < 6 months, then it is diagnosed as acute hepatitis. If HBsAg is present for > 6 months, then it is diagnosed as chronic hepatitis

Treatment:
- **Acute hepatitis** B is self-limited
- **Chronic hepatitis B** is treated with lamivudine.
  - If lamivudine is ineffective, then entecavir, telbivudine, adefovir or **interferon** may be used

Side effects of interferon include **depression**, thrombocytopenia, flu-like symptoms

---

High-yield hepatitis B related questions

1. A nurse accidently stuck herself with a needle that is contaminated with blood from a patient with hepatitis B. She received all 3 hepatitis B series shots 5 years ago. What is the next step in management?

   Answer: **check Hepatitis B surface antibody**

2. Hepatitis B surface antibody is checked and it is present in her. What is the next step in management?

   Answer: Assurance

3. If her hepatitis B surface antibody were negative, then what would have been the next step in management?

Answer: Give hepatitis B vaccine and hepatitis B immunoglobulin

4. HEPATITIS C

Hepatitis C is transmitted by blood transfusion, or re-use of contaminated needle

Diagnosis

- Best initial test is **hepatitis C antibody,** but it may be negative for 4-10 weeks after the infection
- Most accurate test is hepatitis C **PCR-RNA,** and it can be found within 1-2 weeks after the infection
- **Liver biopsy** is usually done after confirming the hepatitis C because a patient may have hepatitis C infection for years, but have little or no damage to the liver

Treatment: Interferon plus ribavirin

Q. What is the most common side effect of ribavirin?
Answer: Hemolytic anemia

Boards tip:

- If a patient, who is suspected to have hepatitis C has negative hepatitis C antibody, then order hepatitis C PCR-RNA because it is detectable earlier than hepatitis C antibody.

ACUTE PANCREATITIS

Acute pancreatitis is sudden inflammation of pancreas

Cause:

- **Alcohol** (most common cause)
- **Gallstones** (2nd most common cause)
- Medications such as hydrochlorothiazide, didanosine, stavudine
- Trauma
- ERCP
- Hypertriglyceridemia

Si/Sx:

- **Epigastric pain radiation to the back**, nausea, vomiting, fever, shock,
- Physical exam may show **Grey turner sign, Cullen sign**

Diagnosis:

- Best initial test is **amylase and lipase.** Lipase is more specific than amylase because amylase is also increased in parotid gland and perforations.
- Most accurate test is **CT abdomen**

Treatment:

- If CT scan shows < 30% necrosis, then:
  - NPO
  - Pain medications

- If **CT scans shows >30%** of necrosis, then:
  - NG suction
  - NPO
  - IV antibiotics (Imipenem, meropenem or meperidine)

- If this is ineffective then do **biopsy**
  - If biopsy **shows necrosis** - Tx. **Surgical debridement + antibiotic**
  - If biopsy **does not show necrosis** - Tx. **Elective debridement**

Note: Imipenem should not be given to a patient with a history of seizure.

PANCREATIC ABSCESS AND PANCREATIC PSEUDOCYST

	Pancreatic abscess	Pancreatic pseudocyst
Time line	Within 10 days of the episode of acute pancreatitis	5 weeks after the episode of acute pancreatitis
Si/Sx	Fever and shock	Fever and shock
Diagnosis	CT abdomen	CT abdomen
Treatment	CT-guided percutaneous drainage plus antibiotics	If the cyst is present from < 6 weeks and is < 6cm in size, then just observe. If the cyst is present for > 6weeks or is > 6cm in size, then do percutaneous drainage

PANCREATIC CANCER

Adenocarcinoma of the head of pancreas is the most common type of pancreatic cancer

Risk factors: cigarette smoking, chronic pancreatitis, first-degree relative with pancreatic cancer, high fat diet and diabetes mellitus.

Si/Sx: painless progressive jaundice, loss of appetite, weight loss, diarrhea, Trousseau's sign, and Courvoisier's sign

Diagnosis:

- Increased bilirubin and liver function test
- Best initial test is ultrasound
- **Then do CT scan**, and further diagnostic tests depend on CT findings:
  - If a **CT scan shows a mass** on pancreas, then perform **percutaneous biopsy**
  - If a CT scan shows **no mass** on pancreas, then perform Endoscopic retrograde cholangiopancreatography **(ERCP)**

Treatment: Pancreaticoduodenectomy (Whipple procedure)

GASTROENTEROLOGY SURGERY

RIGHT UPPER QUADRANT (RUQ) PAIN

1. BILIARY COLIC

Biliary colic is a transient pain that is felt when something blocks the outflow of bile from the gallbladder

Cause: Gallstones is the most common cause, other less common causes are strictures and tumor

Si/Sx: Sharp colicky RUQ pain felt within 30-60 minutes after meals, particularly **after eating food high in fats**. Pain usually lasts for 1-6 hours.

Diagnosis: Abdominal ultrasound

Treatment: Cholecystectomy

2. CHOLECYSTITIS

Cholecystitis is inflammation of the gallbladder

Cause: Obstruction of the cystic duct with gallstones leads to bile buildup in the gallbladder, which causes inflammation

Si/Sx: sharp RUQ pain **radiating to the right shoulder or back**, positive **Murphy sign** (RUQ palpitation during inspiration causes sharp pain and respiratory arrest)

Diagnosis:

- **Initial test is abdominal Ultrasound** that shows gallstones, pericholecystic fluid and thickened gallbladder wall.
- If the ultrasound is inconclusive, then get **HIDA scan.** It is a nuclear scan test, after the dye is injected you will see dye uptake in the liver and common bile duct, but not in the gallbladder because stone in cystic duct is preventing dye to get in the gallbladder.

Management:

- If the patient presents **<72 hours** after the onset symptoms, then do **emergency cholecystectomy**
- If the patient presents **>72 hours** after the onset symptoms, then the treatment includes **NPO, NG Suction, IV fluids** and **IV Piperacillin/Tazobactam**

       ○ Elective Cholecystectomy is usually performed after 4-6 weeks.
- If patient is **not responding to** IV fluids and IV Piperacillin/Tazobactam, then do **emergency cholecystectomy**

3. ASCENDING CHOLANGITIS

Ascending cholangitis is a bacterial infection of the biliary tract
Si/Sx: RUQ pain, high fever (104°-105°), jaundice, change in mental status and shock
Diagnosis:
- Labs show **high alkaline phosphatase**
- Abdominal **ultrasound shows dilation of common bile duct**

Treatment:
- Best initial treatment is **NPO, NG Suction, IV fluids, IV Piperacillin/Tazobactam and metronidazole**
- Then **Endoscopic retrograde cholangiopancreatography (ERCP)** is performed to decompress the biliary tree and remove the stone
- If ERCP is ineffective, then do **percutaneous transhepatic cholangiography (PTC)**

4. CHOLEDOCHOLITHIASIS

Choledocholithiasis is the presence of gallstone in the common bile duct
Si/Sx: RUQ pain, jaundice, increased conjugated bilirubin, increased alkaline phosphate
Diagnosis: Ultrasound
Treatment: Laparoscopy cholecystectomy

5. HEPATIC ADENOMA

Hepatic adenoma is a benign liver tumor
Risk factors: OCPs with high estrogen or anabolic steroids
Si/Sx: most of the hepatic adenomas are asymptomatic, but some patients may have RUQ pain
Diagnosis: CT of URQ
Treatment:
- Stop OCPs or anabolic steroids
- Symptomatic tumor is surgical resected

6. PYOGENIC LIVER ABSCESS

Pyogenic liver abscess is the pus-filled area in the liver

Cause: Bacteria, abdominal infection, trauma

Si/Sx: RUQ pain, fever, enlarged liver

Diagnosis: CT or Ultrasound

Treatment: Percutaneous drainage

7. AMOEBIC LIVER ABSCESS

Amoebic liver abscess is liver abscess caused by amebiasis

Si/Sx: RUQ pain, fever, weight loss, liver tenderness

Diagnosis: CT or ultrasound

Treatment:

- Metronidazole.
- If metronidazole is ineffective, then do percutaneous drainage

LEFT UPPER QUADRANT (LUQ) PAIN

1. ACUTE MESENTERIC ISCHEMIA

Acute mesenteric ischemia is a condition in which reduced blood flow in mesenteric blood vessels lead to ischemia and eventually necrosis of the bowel wall

Cause: Strangulation, arterial thrombosis, arterial embolism, surgery

Si/Sx: Weight loss, **postprandial pain, abdominal pain**

Boards clue: Look for an old patient who does not eat anymore because he/she experiences **extreme pain with food**

Diagnosis:

- Labs show **metabolic acidosis and increased amylase**
- Most accurate test is **angiography**

Treatment: Embolectomy or surgical resection of affected bowel

2. SPLENIC RUPTURE

Cause: Blunt abdominal trauma, enlarged spleen

Si/Sx: LUQ pain, LUQ tenderness, confusion, **Kehr's sign** (LUQ pain referred to the left shoulder pain)

Diagnosis:
- Physical exam
- Abdominal CT

Treatment:
- **Surgical repair**
- If surgical repair is not possible - Tx. **Splenectomy**

Important: Do not forget to give Haemophilus influenza B, pneumococcal and Meningococcus vaccines after splenectomy

RIGHT LOWER QUADRANT (RLQ) PAIN

1. APPENDICITIS

Appendicitis is inflammation of appendix
Cause: occurs when appendix is obstructed by feces, foreign object or in the rare case tumor
Si/Sx:
- Fever, nausea, vomiting, periumbilical pain, rebound tenderness
- Rovsing's sign: when one palpates left lower quadrant and then suddenly release hand, patient experiences pain at McBurney's point

Diagnosis:
- Appendicitis is a clinical diagnosis; fever and leukocytosis (10,000-15, 000 WBC predominantly neutrophils)
- If **diagnosis is not clear, then** get abdominal **ultrasound or CT**

Treatment:
- If appendix is **not perforated** – Tx. NPO, **IV fluids, IV antibiotics,** and then **laparotomy**
- If appendix is **perforated** - Tx. **NPO, IV fluids, IV** antibiotics, **until** fever and WBCs normalizes, and then perform laparotomy

Important: In **pregnant** woman **appendicitis may be pushed to the right upper quadrant**. If a pregnant woman presents with pain on the right upper quadrant, then keep appendicitis in the differential diagnosis.

LEFT LOWER QUADRANT (LLQ) PAIN

1. SIGMOID VOLVULUS

Sigmoid volvulus is twisting of sigmoid colon around its mesenteric attachment. It is the most common form of volvulus of the GI tract.

Si/Sx: Crampy LLQ pain, abdominal distention, constipation

Diagnosis: Abdominal X-ray shows " **parrot beak**" appearance

Treatment: Rigid proctosigmoidoscopy and rectal tube in usually left in place to prevent recurrence of volvulus

2. DIVERTICULOSIS AND DIVETRICULITIS

Condition	DIVERTICULOSIS	DIVERTICULITIS
Cause	Is a condition in which **pouches form** in the wall of the colon	Is a condition in which pouches form in the wall of the **colon and become inflamed** or infected
Si/SX	LLQ abdominal pain, **lower GI bleeding** (bright red blood per rectum)	**Nausea, vomiting, fever** **LLQ abdominal tenderness**
Diagnosis	Colonoscopy	**Abdominal CT**
Treatment	High- fiber diet	Ciprofloxacin and metronidazole

Note: Colonoscopy is not done in diverticulitis because of fear of colon rupture

ABDOMINAL TRAUMA AND MANAGEMENT

1. Patient with **gunshot wounds** should be taken directly for **exploratory laparotomy**
2. Management of a patient with **blunt abdominal trauma** depends on the patient's condition:
   - If a patient is **hemodynamic unstable**, then proceed directly for **laparotomy**
   - If a patient is **hemodynamically stable**, then do Diagnostic Peritoneal Lavage (DPL) or Focused Assessment with Sonography for Trauma (FAST).

3. Stab wounds: if a patient is stable then does digital exploration

WOUND INFECTION MANAGEMENT
It is common after abdominal surgery
- If physical exam shows **erythema,** and CT contrast shows **no abscess.** Tx. **Antibiotics**
- If physical exam shows **fluctuating mass,** and CT contrast shows **abscess.** Tx. **IV antibiotics and CT guided abscess drainage**

OBSTRUCTIVE JAUNDICE CAUSED BY STONES
Look for an obese, fecund woman in her 40s with recurrent abdominal pain
Diagnosis:
- Labs: high alkaline phosphate
- Best initial test is **ultrasound**
- Diagnosis is confirmed with **endoscopic retrograde cholangiopancreatography** (ERCP)

Management:
- **Sphincterotomy**, and remove the common duct stone
- Then do **cholecystectomy**

OBSTRUCTIVE JAUNDICE CASUED BY TUMOR
Patient usually present with progressive symptoms and weight loss within weeks
Cause:
- Adenocarcinoma of the ampulla of Vater
- Adenocarcinoma of the head of pancreas
- Cholangiocarcinoma arising in the common duct itself

Diagnosis:
- Best initial test is ultrasound
- Then do CT
  - If CT **shows pancreatic lesions,** then do **percutaneous biopsy**
  - If CT **does not show** pancreatic lesions then do **ERCP, to check ampullary cancer and cholangiocarcinoma**

Treatment: surgical resection

ISCHIORECTAL ABSCESS

This is a very common condition. Look for a patient with **abscess lateral to
anus** between the **rectum** and the **ischial tuberosity**
Management: Incision and drainage
Complication: **Fistula of anal**

Small bowel and large bowel obstruction

	Small bowel obstruction	Large bowel obstruction
Si/ Sx	**Intermittent crampy abdominal pain**, vomiting, abdominal distension, constipation, focal tenderness, **hyperactive bowel sounds**	Constipation, abdominal distension, cramping, **feculent vomiting**
Cause	Adhesion from prior surgery, hernia, IBD, volvulus, stricture	Diverticulitis, colon cancer, volvulus
Diagnosis	Abdominal x-ray show **multiple air-fluid** level	Abdominal X-ray show **dilated bowel with gas**, haustra, may have a cut-off point
Treatment	NPO, IV fluids & electrolyte replacement, nasogastric decompression and surgical resection	NPO, nasogastric decompression and treat the underlying cause. Surgery is reserved for refractory cases

GROIN HERNIA

Differential diagnosis for groin hernias

Types	Description	Treatment
Direct inguinal hernia	The indirect hernia protrudes **medial** to the inferior epigastric vessels. It is more common in males than females	Surgical repair for symptomatic patient
Indirect inguinal hernia	The indirect hernia passes **lateral to inferior epigastric artery into the spermatic cord**. It is the most common type of hernia	Surgical repair for symptomatic patient
Femoral hernia	Femoral hernia protrudes **below the inguinal ligament.** It is more common in females than males	Surgical repair for symptomatic patient

GASTROENTEROLOGY CCS

CASE # 1

Case introduction
An 18-years old Caucasian male come to ER because of sudden onset of abdominal pain and vomiting

Initial vitals signs
Temperature: 38.6 degrees
Pulse: 98 beats/min, regular rhythm
Respiration rate: 30/ minutes

Blood pressure, systolic 110 mm Hg
Blood pressure, disystolic 70 mm Hg

Height: 63.0 inches
Weight: 120.0 lbs.
Body mass index: 21.3 Kg/m2

History of present illness (HPI)
An 18-years old Caucasian male come to ER because of sudden onset of abdominal pain and vomiting. He said 2 hours ago he felt nauseated and vomited twice and developed pain around the umbilicus. He rates his pain 7 on a 10-point scale. He denies diarrhea, constipation and abdominal trauma. He says he does not have any appetite and has not eaten anything since last night.

Past medical history
Hospitalization: None
Other medical conditions: none
Current medication: Albuterol
Allergies: eggs, peanuts
Vaccination: up to date

Family history
Parents are healthy and alive.

Social history
Marital history: none
Occupation: cashier at fast-food restaurant
Recreational: football, basketball
Personal habits: Does not smoke drink alcohol, or use drugs.

Review of systems:
General: see HPI
Skin: see HPI
HEENT: see HPI
Musculoskeletal: see HPI
Cardiology: see HPI
Abdominal: see HPI
Genitourinary: see HPI

Please see pages 1-5 for general CCS cases approach

Step 1. Order the followings
- Pulse oximetry
- Oxygen
- IV access
- IV normal saline
- BP monitor
- NPO
- IV Morphine

Step 2. Order complete physical exam, and the move the clock forward to get the results
- Results show:
  - Patient is in pain
  - Abdominal exam shows pain at McBurney's point

Step 3. Order the labs, and then move the clock forward to get the result
- CBC
- UA
- BMP
- Chest x-ray
- Abdominal X-ray & CT
- Lipase
- Amylase

- Result shows
  - CBC shows 15,000 WBC with 79% PMN,
  - Chest X-ray is normal
  - Abdomen X-ray is normal
  - Abdomen CT is positive for acute appendicitis

Step 4. Medicine
- IV Promethazine, metronidazole and Cefazolin

Step 5. Keep the patient in ER

Step 6. Order
- NPO

Step 7. None

Step 8. Gastroenterology surgery consult

Step 9. Order pre-surgical labs, appendectomy, and the move the clock forward to get the lab results and appendectomy results
- PT/INR
- PTT
- Blood type and cross match

- Lab results show:
  o PTT/PT/INR is WNL
  o Blood type: O negative

- Surgery consult shows that surgery has been scheduled

Step 10. Consult and age and gender specific screening
- No smoking, alcohol, smoking
- Wear seat belt, safe sex
- Age and gender specific screening is usually ordered for later dates

Diagnosis: **Appendicitis**

Case # 2

Case introduction
A 56-years-old African-American man come to ER with for nausea, vomiting and severe left lower quadrant from last 6 hours.

Initial vitals signs
Temperature: 38.6 degrees
Pulse: 88 beats/min, regular rhythm
Respiration rate: 20/ minutes

Blood pressure, systolic 140 mm Hg
Blood pressure, disystolic 87 mm Hg

Height: 68.0 inches
Weight: 180.0 lbs.
Body mass index: 27.4 Kg/m2

History of present illness (HPI)
A 56-years-old African-American man come to ER with for nausea, vomiting and severe left lower quadrant from last 6 hours. He describes his pain a colicky abdominal pain and rates it 8 on a 10-point scale. He says his last stool was 2 days ago. He denies melena, diarrhea, constipation or weight loss. He has past medical history of hypertension and type 2 diabetes for which he takes lisinopril and glyburide.

Past medical history
Hospitalization: none
Other medical conditions: Hypertension, Diabetes type 2
Current medication: Lisinopril, glyburide
Allergies: Penicillin
Vaccination: up to date

Family history
Father died of MI and mother is alive and healthy

Social history
Marital history: married; 3 children
Occupation: postal delivery
Recreational: travel, football
Personal habits: smokes 1 pack a day, drink 1-2 beers a day, denies the use of drugs.

Review of systems:
General: see HPI
Skin: see HPI
HEENT: see HPI
Musculoskeletal: see HPI
Cardiology: see HPI
Abdominal: see HPI
Genitourinary: see HPI

CASE # 2

Step 1. Order the followings:
- IV access
- IV normal saline
- BP monitor
- Telemetry

Step 2. Order complete physical exam, and then move the clock forward to get the results
- Physical exam shows:
  - Abdominal exam shows distention and tenderness on LLQ
  - Rest of the physical exam is normal

Step 3. Order the following labs, and then move the clock forward to get the results
- CBC
- UA
- BMP
- Chest x-ray
- Abdominal X-ray

- Results show:
  - WBC 12,000 with 78 % PMN, 15% Lymphocytes
  - Abdominal x-ray shows Parrot's beak sign – suggesting sigmoid volvulus

Step 4. Medicine
- Get IV access and give IV morphine

Step 5. Admit the patient in wards

Step 6. Order the followings:
- NPO
- Bed rest

Step 7. None

Step 8. Order rigid sigmoidoscopy, rectal tube and GI consult. Then, move the clock forward to get consult result then move to get sigmoidoscopy & rectal tube

Step 9. Discharge patient after 24-48 hour of inpatient monitoring

Case usually ends here

Step 10. Consult and age and gender specific screening
- Advance directive
- Living will
- No smoking, drinking, illegal drugs
- High fiber diet
- FOBT, Colonoscopy, and prostate exam should be scheduled for later dates
- Influenza and pneumococcal vaccine

Diagnosis: Sigmoid volvulus

CASE # 3

Case introduction
A 21-years-old African-American man comes to the office because of abdominal pain

Initial vitals signs
Temperature: 38.6 degrees
Pulse: 78 beats/min, regular rhythm
Respiration rate: 16/ minutes

Blood pressure, systolic 126 mm Hg
Blood pressure, disystolic 74 mm Hg

Height: 68.0 inches
Weight: 170.0 lbs.
Body mass index: 25.8 Kg/m2

History of present illness (HPI)
A 21-years-old African-American man comes to the office because of abdominal pain. He says that he has been experiencing the abdominal pain from last 2 weeks. He describes the pain as a vague pain in the mid-epigastric area that the pain occurs 2-3 hours after eating and relieves soon after eating. He rates his pain as 7 on the 10-point scale. He denies melena, diarrhea, constipation or weight loss. He has no other medical condition.

Past medical history
Hospitalization: none
Other medical conditions: none
Current medication: none
Allergies: none
Vaccination: up to date

Family history
Father has DM II and mother is healthy

Social history

Marital history: single

Occupation: cahier at local grocery store

Recreational: football, hiking

Personal habits: smokes 1 pack a day, drink 1-2 beers a day, denies the use of drugs.

Review of systems:

General: see HPI

Skin: see HPI

HEENT: see HPI

Musculoskeletal: see HPI

Cardiology: see HPI

Abdominal: see HPI

Genitourinary: see HPI

Please see pages 1-5 for general CCS cases approach

Step 1. None (patient is stable and is not suicidal)

Step 2. Order complete physical exam, and then move the clock forward to get the results
- Results shows
  - Patient is in distress
  - Abdominal exam shows epigastric tenderness
  - Rest of the physical exam is normal

Step 3. Order the labs, and then move the clock forward to get the results
- CBC
- UA
- BMP
- Chest x-ray
- FOBT
- Amylase
- Lipase
- H. Pylori antibody

- Results shows:
  - CBC shows 8000 WBC with 77% PMN
  - FOBT is positive
  - H.pylori is positive
  - Rest of the labs are within normal limit

Step 4. Medicine
- Omeprazole, amoxicillin and clarithromycin

Step 5. Make a follow-up appointment after 2-6 weeks and send patient home

Step 6. None

Step 7. Move the clock forward to next appointment date.
- Patient usually feel better

Step 8. None

Step 9. Make a follow-up appointment after 2-6 weeks and send patient home

Step 10. Consult and age and gender specific screening
- No smoking, alcohol, smoking
- Wear seat belt, safe sex
- Age and gender specific screening

Diagnosis: Peptic ulcer

PSYCHIATRY

PSYCHOTIC DISORDERS

Psychotic disorders are mental disorders that cause abnormal thinking and perception. Two main characteristics of psychotic disorders are delusions and hallucinations

Types: there are many psychotic disorders, but the most common psychotic disorders are **schizophrenia, schizophreniform, brief psychotic disorder, and schizoaffective disorder**

SCHIZOPHRENIA

Schizophrenia is a psychotic disorder. Approximately 1% of the world has schizophrenia. Common age of onset in males is 18-25 and female 25-35, but male to female ratio is 1:1.

Si/Sx: Most common symptoms include delusion, hallucination, disorganized speech, behavior disturbance and impaired social function. However, it is often described in terms of positive symptoms and negative symptoms

- **Positive symptoms** include delusion, hallucination (more auditory than visual), agitation, and disorganized speech or behavior
- **Negative symptoms** include flat affect, apathy, anhedonia, poor attention, and apathy

Subtypes of schizophrenia:

1. **Paranoid type** is characterized by **hallucination and delusion,** but normal cognitive function
2. **Disorganized type** is characterized by disorganized speech and behavior, and flat affects. It is associated with worst prognosis
3. **Residual type** is characterized by lack of positive symptoms
4. **Catatonic type** is characterized by extreme distribution, which may include stupor, rigidity, negativity, mania
5. **Undifferentiated type** is characterized by presence of symptoms that are seen in all of above subtype, but not enough to have pin-point to one particular subtype

Treatment:

- Acutely psychotic patients may require hospitalization
- Antipsychotic and psychotherapy is the best treatment for schizophrenia. **Antipsychotics are given based on side effects, not the efficacy**
- When **compliance is an issue** or the patient **does not want to take oral medicine, then give IM haloperidol**
- Patients with negative symptoms respond better to atypical antipsychotics

Antipsychotics Medicines

	High potency conventional antipsychotic	Low potency conventional antipsychotic	Atypical antipsychotics
Medicine	• Haloperidol • Fluphenazine	• Chlorpromazine	• Clozapine • Olanzapine • Risperidone • Ziprasidone • Aripiprazole
EPS* side effects	• **More** EPS side effects	• **Less** EPS side effects	• **Less** EPS side effects
ANS * side effects	• **Low** incidence of ANS side effects	• **High** incidence of ANS side effects	• **Medium** incidence of ANS side effects

*EPS = Extrapyramidal side effects, *ANS= Anticholinergic side effects

*ANS side effects include dry mouth, urinary retention, blurry vision, orthostatic hypotension, and sedation

Side effects of atypical antipsychotic

Medicine	Side effects
Aripiprazole	**Minimal weight gain, No cardiac side effects**
Clozapine	**Agranulocytosis, decreases seizure threshold**
Olanzapine	**Increases weight gain, glucose intolerance**
Ziprasidone	**Increases QT interval, minimal weight gain**
Risperidone	**Increases prolactin,**
Quetiapine	**Very sedating**

EPS side effects of Antipsychotics

Condition	Time of onset	Symptoms	Treatment
Acute dystonia	• **Within hour or first week** of treatment	• **Muscle spasms** • Difficulty swallowing • Tongue protrusion • Twisting of head	• **Lower the dose of antipsychotic and give antihistamines** (diphenhydramine) or **anticholinergics** (benztropine or trihexyphenidyl)
Akathisia	• With **first few days of** treatment	• Feeling of restlessness • **Pacing constantly** • Alternating sitting and standing • Unable to sit or stand still	• **Lower the antipsychotic dose, and add beta-blockers or benzodiazepine**
Parkinsonism	• Within a first **few months of** treatment	• **Parkinson's like symptoms** (resting tremor, rigidity, akathisia, postural instability)	• **Lower the dose of antipsychotic and give antihistamines** (diphenhydramine) or **anticholinergics** (benztropine or trihexyphenidyl)
Tardive dyskinesia	• **Occurs months to years of** treatment	• **Choreoathetosis movement** of head limbs and trunk • Frog like tongue movement	• **Stop the antipsychotics and start atypical antipsychotics**
Neuroleptic malignant syndrome	• Can occur at anytime during the treatment	• High fever • **Altered metal status** • **Rigidity** • Bradykinesia • Tachycardia • Rhabdomyolysis	• **Stop offending drugs, and give IV fluids bromocriptine, and lastly dantrolene**

Prognosis: prognosis depends on the following
- **Good prognosis:** presence of positive symptoms, late onset, known precipitating factor, married, good premorbid symptoms and family history of mood disorders
- **Poor prognosis:** presence of negative symptoms, early onset, no known precipitating factor, single, poor premorbid symptoms and family history of schizophrenia

Suicide rate: 10 % of the patients with schizophrenia commit suicide

PSYCHOTIC DISORDERS AND TIME FRAME

It is necessary to pay attention to the duration of the symptoms because **symptoms** of brief psychotic disorder, schizophreniform or schizophrenia **are the same,** but the **diagnosis is given based** on the duration of **symptoms**

- **Brief psychotic disorder** is characterized by symptoms present for **more than 1 day,** but **less than 1 month.** Treatment is same as schizophrenia
- **Schizophreniform disorder** is characterized by symptoms present for **more than a month but less than 6 months.** It is treated same as schizophrenia
- **Schizophrenia** is characterized by the symptoms present for **more than 6 months** (treatment disused on pages 358 and 359)
- **Schizoaffective disorder** is characterized by combination of symptoms of **schizophrenia and depression or mania.** It is treated with antipsychotics and or mood stabilizers. Generally **worst symptoms are treated first**

MOOD DISORDERS

MAJOR DEPRESSION DISORDER

Major depression disorder is a mood disorder characterized by persistence-depressed mood that is accompanied by **low self-esteem** and **loss of interest or pleasure**

Diagnosis: diagnosis require depressed mood or loss of interest or pleasure and presence of 5 or more symptoms from mnemonic SIG E CAPS for almost every day for at least 2-week period

- Change in **Sleep** pattern   Mnemonic: **SIGECAPS**
- Loss of **Interest** or pleasure
- Feeling of worthless or **Guilt**
- Loss of **Energy**
- Difficulty in **Concentration**
- Change in **Appetite** &/or weight
- Change in **Psychomotor** activity
- Thoughts of **Suicide** or death

Treatment:
- Before initiating treatment it is important to inquire about the **suicidal thoughts**. If a patient is at increased risk of suicide, then hospitalized the patient, even if it is against patient's will.
- **Psychotherapy** (Cognitive, behavioral therapy) with **pharmacotherapy** is the most the effective treatment. Psychotherapy teaches patient to identify the concern and or problems and develop a solution to bring satisfactory results.

Important: Patients are at high risk of committing suicide when antidepressants being to work because the patient gets little more energy to carry out a suicide plan

Indications and side effects of antidepressant treatment

Medication	Indications	Side effects
Serotonin selective reuptake inhibitor (SSRIs) (Fluoxetine, sertraline, paroxetine, citalopram, escitalopram)	• First-line medicine for depression	• Weight gain • GI disturbance • Sexual dysfunction
Serotonin selective reuptake inhibitor (Venlafaxine, duloxetine, desvenlafaxine)	• Preferred in chronic pain	• Hypertension • Blurry vision • Sexual dysfunction
Bupropion	• When **sexual dysfunction or weight gain is a concern**. (It causes modest weight loss)	• Lowers seizure threshold
Mirtazapine	• Preferred in **anorexic patients** with depression because one of its side effect is weight gain	• Agranulocytosis • Weight gain
Trazodone	• Preferred in patient with **insomnia** because one of its effect is sedation	• Priapism • Sedation
Tricyclic anti-depressant (TCAs) Nortriptyline, amitriptyline, imipramine)	• Are **not given to elderly** due to their side effects	• Dry mouth, urinary retention, constipation, blurry vision, and confusion
Monoamine oxidase inhibitors (MAIOs) (Phenelzine, tranylcypromine)	• No special indications	• Sexual side effects • Hypertensive crisis if taken with food high in tyramine (cheese, red wine)
Electroconvulsive therapy (ECT)	• Acutely suicidal • Other medicines are ineffective	• Headaches • Anterograde and retrograde amnesia

HERBAL MEDICINE
St. John's wort
- Used for mild to moderate depression
- Side effects include **Serotonin syndrome, photosensitivity**

Other high-yield points of anti-depressants

- Patients are at increased of committing suicide after starting antidepressants because they get little more energy to execute their plan
- Patients are usually treated for 6 months, but patient with multiple episodes of depression are treated > 6 months
- Advise the patient that after starting anti-depressants, it takes 1 week to see symptomatic relief, and 4-6 week to see the full effect of medication
- If one medicine is not working after 4 to 6 weeks of therapy, then switch a patient to a different medication
- When switching SSRIs to MAOIs, makes sure that the patient have 4-5 weeks of washout period to prevent serotonin syndrome
- SSRIs other than paroxetine, and all TCA can be safely used in **pregnant woman**
- If the patient on TCAs develops cholinergic side effects, then the best initial step is to get EKG; if EKG shows prolong QT interval, then treat it with **sodium bicarbonate**

SEROTONIN SYNDROME
Serotonin syndrome is a potentially life-threatening reaction that may occur when there are high levels of serotonin in the body
Cause: SSRIs, SNRIs, MAOIs, lithium, St. John's wort
Si/Sx: fever, altered mental status, muscle spasms (myoclonus), hyperreflexia
Diagnosis: Clinical diagnosis, but rule out others conditions with blood test, urine test
Treatment: stop offending drug, give benzodiazepine and cyproheptadine

Boards tip
- Know how to distinguish and treat serotonin syndrome and neuroleptic malignant syndrome. See below

Condition	Neuroleptic malignant syndrome	Serotonin syndrome
Physical findings	Rigidity & bradykinesia	Clonus & hyperkinesia
Management	• Stop offending drug • IV fluids and bromocriptine • Then, give dantrolene	• Stop offending drug • IV fluids, benzodiazepine and cyproheptadine

DIFFERENTIAL DIAGNOSIS OF DEPRESSION

1. DYSTHYMIA
Dysthymia is characterized by **mild form of depression** that lasts most of the days for **more than 2 years**
Treatment: **insight-oriented psychotherapy**; SSRIs is the second choice therapy

2. SEASONAL DEPRESSIVE DISORDER
Seasonal depressive disorder is a depression that occurs at the same time every year. It is more common in **fall and winter seasons**
Treatment: **light therapy** (phototherapy, sunlight)

3. BEREAVEMENT
Normal bereavement (grief) usually begins **after the death of loved ones** and **resolves in 1 year**. Patients experience similar symptoms of depression. However, lack of self-esteem, feeling worthlessness, suicidal ideation, and psychomotor retardation are symptoms of depression, not of bereavement.
Treatment: **supportive treatment**, but make sure to inquire about suicidal thoughts

4. ATYPICAL DEPRESSION

Atypical depression is a depression in which patient experiences **increased appetite, increased sleep**, and trouble maintaining a long-term relationship due to the sensitivity to the rejection. **Depression temporarily goes away** in response to good news or positive events, but returns later. Patients also complain of heavy feeling in extremities

Treatment: SSRIs (first choice) or MAOIs

5. HYPOTHYROIDISM

Look for patient with **depression** and symptoms of **hypothyroidism**

Diagnosis: TSH

Treatment: Levothyroxine

6. PARKINSON'S DISEASE

Look for a patient with **depression** and **Parkinson's diseases**

Treatment:

- As per Parkinson's disease
- Anti-depressant, as needed

7. MEDICATION

Certain medication can also cause depression, such as

- Beta-blockers aggravates depression
- Corticosteroids cause psychosis and depression
- Interferons
- Reserpine
- Antipsychotics

Treatment: switch the medicine with different medicine

8. SUBSTANCE ABUSE

Certain substance abuse can also cause depression, such as

- Alcohol dependence or abuse
- Amphetamines withdrawals
- Cocaine **withdrawal**

Treatment: Anti-depressant and detoxification

9. PREMENSTRUAL DEPRESSION DISORDER

Premenstrual depression disorder usually starts **1 week** before the beginning of menstrual cycle

Treatment: SSRIs

10. PSEUDODEMENTIA
Pseudodementia is a condition in which patient have symptoms **similar to dementia**, but actually **suffering from depression**

Key to distinguish Pseudodementia from dementia
- In Pseudodementia, patient **looks withdrawn and usually makes no eye contact**
- In Pseudodementia patient often complain about memory loss, but careful testing shows **intact memory**
- Patient with Pseudodementia **make no effort to answer hard question**, whereas patient with dementia do not give up easily

Management:
- Best step in management is to inquire about suicidal thoughts
- SSRIs

BIPOLAR DISORDER
Bipolar disorder is a mood disorder characterized by episodes of **mania** that alternates with episodes of **depression**. It is seen in 1% of the population and male to female ratio is 1:1.

Symptoms of mania: Mnemonic: **DIG FAST**
- Distractibility
- Insomnia
- Grandiosity (increased self-esteem)
- Flight of ideas
- Increased activities
- Hypersexuality
- Talkativeness

Mania is characterized by presence of above listed symptoms for at least 1 week that affects the quality of life or symptoms severe enough to require hospitalization. **Hypomania** is **lower state of mania**, in which symptoms of mania are present, but not severe enough to affect quality of life or require hospitalization

Subtypes of bipolar disorder
- **Bipolar disorder type I is an episode of mania and depression**
- **Bipolar disorder type II is depression episodes with hypomania**
- **Rapid cycling bipolar disorder is 4 or more episodes** (depression, mania or mixed) in 12 months

- **Cyclothymia** is alternating episodes of **hypomania and depression** for $\geq$ **2 years**

Treatment of bipolar disorder is as follow:

Medicine	Indications	Adverse affects
Lithium	• First line treatment for bipolar disorder	Tremors, weight gain, nephrotoxicity, diabetes insipidus, confusion, teratogenic **(Ebstein anomaly)**
Carbamazepine	• 2nd line treatment	**Agranulocytosis**, respiratory depression, Stevens-Johnson syndrome
Valproic acid	• No special indications	GI disturbance, alopecia, teratogenic, weight gain, **liver dysfunction**
Lamotrigine	• Refractory patients • Pregnant woman in 2nd or 3rd trimester	Stevens-Johnson syndrome

High-yield
- Pregnant woman with bipolar disorders is treated as follow:
  - ECT in the 1st trimester
  - Lamotrigine in 2nd or 3rd trimester

DELUSIONAL DISORDER
Delusional disorder is characterized by presence of non-bizarre delusions for more than 1 month in the absence of mood disorders or schizophrenia. Level of function is intact.
Treatment: antipsychotics

ANXIETY DISORDERS

1. ACUTE STRESS DISORDER

Acute stress disorder is a psychological condition that **occurs within 1 month of the traumatic event, symptoms last for ≥ 2 days and maximum of 1 month**

Si/Sx: common symptoms include numbness, detachment, hypervigilance, nightmare (re-experience event), flashbacks

Diagnosis: Clinical diagnosis

Treatment: Relaxation therapy with cognitive therapy is proven to be helpful.

2. POST-TRAUMATIC STRESS DISORDER (PTSD)

Symptoms of PTSD are same as **acute stress disorder, but** when symptoms are **present for more than 1 month**, then it is diagnosed a PTSD

Depression and substance must be ruled out.

Treatment:

- SSRIs are the first-line of treatment. Short treatment (up to 4 weeks) with benzodiazepine may be given for anxiety
- Relaxation therapy with cognitive therapy is also been proven to be helpful

3. PANIC DISORDER

Panic disorder is **recurrent** attacks of intense fear along with feeling of impending doom. It is accompanied by 4 of the **autonomic symptoms** often peaks within 10 -20 minutes: chest discomfort, palpitation, shortness of breath, sweating, trembling, fear of dying, numbing or tingling in the hands or feet, nausea, fear of choking, fear of dying, dizziness

Note: panic attack is a **single attack** with the similar symptoms of panic disorder. Panic attack is often mistaken for heart attack

Diagnosis: clinical diagnosis, but it is important to rule out organic causes such as MI, drug abuse

Treatment:

- Cognitive behavioral therapy
- SSRIs are **first line-treatment**; moreover, SSRIs are also used as a long-term treatment to prevent the future attacks

- Benzodiazepines may be used to relieve immediate symptoms, but are not used as long-term treatment because of high risk of abuse

4.   PHOBIA
Phobia is defined as the fear of an object or situation, and person goes to great length to avoid it
Types: common types of phobias include:
- Specific phobia is a fear of a specific object, animal, or heights
- Social phobia is a fear of social situation such as public speaking, public restroom, or public speaking

Treatment:
- Exposure desensitization
- Beta-blockers and benzodiazepine may be given prior to the exposure
- Relaxation technique

5.   GENERALIZED ANXIETY DISORDER
Generalized anxiety disorder is a condition in which a person is **worried and anxious about many things, for > 6 months** and finds it hard to control anxiety. Patient may experience fatigue, irritability, trouble sleeping or falling asleep, muscle tension, and restless while awake
Association: it often coexists with depression, panic disorder and phobia

Treatment:
- **Cognitive behavioral therapy**
- SSRIs are the first-line of treatment. SNRIs or benzodiazepines may also be used

6.   OBSESSIVE-COMPLUSIVE DISORDER (OCD)
Obsessive-compulsive disorder is characterized by **unreasonable thought** (obsession) that produces uneasiness, fear or anxiety, which leads a person to **do repetitive act** (compulsion), and that relieves the anxiety. Patient is **aware that this behavior is irrational.**
Associated conditions: depression and substance abuse often co-exists with OCD
Treatment:
- Behavioral psychotherapy therapy and SSRIs or TCAs (particularly clomipramine)

Note: patients with **obsessive-compulsive personality disorder (OCPD)** are not aware that their behavior is irrational.

ADJUSTMENT DISORDER

Adjustment disorder is a **group of symptoms that include anxious, hopeless, feeling sad and stressed.** It usually starts within 3 months of stressful event and alleviates within 6 months of the event such as divorce or breakup. Symptoms are usually severe enough to cause functional impairment.

Treatment: Psychotherapy. SSRI or SNRIs may be used

SOMATOFORM DISORDERS

Somatoform disorders are characterized **by symptoms that indicate physical injury** or illness **but no physical cause** can be found. Symptoms are **unintentionally** created

Types of somatoform disorders:
- **Somatization disorder** is defined as distressing physical symptoms, which must include **1 sexual, 2 GI and 1 neurological symptom**
- **Conversion disorder** usually occurs **after an identifiable stress** such as divorce or breakup. Patient suffers from **neurological symptoms,** such as blindness, numbness or paralysis **that are psychological.**
- **Hypochondriasis,** in which a person worries excessively that he has a **specific disease despite constant reassurance** or extensive normal medical work-up
- **Body dysmorphic disorder,** in which a patient **worries excessively that he has a flaw in his appearance**, a flaw that is imagined
- **Pain disorder** refers to pain that is severe enough to **affect person's daily** life, but **no physical cause is found**. It may be associated with depression

Treatment:
- Best therapy is maintain a **single doctor–patient relationships**
- **Schedule brief monthly visits and psychotherapy**
- Avoid diagnostic testing

- Depression may co-exist in a patient with somatoform disorder, if it does, then SSRIs may help

FACTITIOUS DISORDER

Factious disorder is a condition in which a person **fakes an illness,** in order to get a **reward or secondary gain** such as hospital admission, attention or sympathy. For example, a nurse is injecting herself insulin to induce hypoglycemia and get medical attention.

Diagnosis: clinical diagnosis, but it is important to rule out medical conditions with similar symptoms such as causes of hypoglycemia

Treatment: Psychotherapy

FACTITIOUS DISORDER BY PROXY

Factitious disorder by proxy is a condition in which a **person fakes an illness in another person** (usually a child) who is under their care, in order to **assume the caretaker role**

Diagnosis: clinical diagnosis

Treatment:

Psychotherapy. However, if a child is involved, then child protective service may needed to be involved

Note: Factitious disorders are not produced to gain money, if patient is faking symptoms for **financial gain, then it is diagnosed as malingering disorder**

MALINGERING DISORDER

Malingering disorder is a condition in which a person fakes an illness for secondary gain such as **money or housing**. Patients are usually not co-operative

Treatment:

- Psychotherapy
- Provide minimal amount of workup and treatment

IMPULSE-CONTROL DISORDERS

Impulse-control disorder is characterized by difficulty controlling owns emotions and behavior, which may be harmful to one-self or others. Individual feel **anxiety before the act and gratification afterwards.**

Common impulse-control disorders are:

- **Intermittent explosive disorder** is an extreme expression of anger to a stressor that leads to an assault or property damage
- **Pyromania** is intentionally setting fire, on ≥ 2 occasions
- **Kleptomania** is an urge to steal items that are not needed for personal use. Person usually feels guilt after stealing and **often returns stolen item**
- **Pathologic gambling** is recurrent urge to gamble that may be harmful to patient and family
- **Trichotillomania** is an urge to pull hair that results in **irregular patchy hair loss**

Treatment of impulse-control disorder is **psychotherapy**

Boards tip:

- Questions usually try to confuse trichotillomania with tenia capitis or alopecia areata. To distinguish in them know the following:
  - Tinea capitis causes **itchy, scaly and round hairless patches** on the scalp
  - Alopecia areata causes **smooth and round hairless patches** on the scalp

---

PERSONALITY DISORDERS

Personality disorder (PD) is characterized by lifelong unhealthy pattern of behavior, emotions and thoughts, which affects person's ability to interact with others.

Common personality disorders are:

- **Paranoid PD**: Patient is **suspicious and distrusts** everything. He or she think everyone is a threat to them
- **Schizotypal** PD: Patient has **odd and eccentric** beliefs, they often feels **discomfort in social relationships**
- **Schizoid PD**: Patient has no interest in social relationship, emotionally restricted and **do not want** any friends
- **Avoidant PD**: Patient **wants friend**, but **do not have friends** because they avoids other out of **fear of criticism**
- **Dependent PD**: Patients are **very submissive and clingy**. They always need someone to meet their emotional and physical needs. They cannot do anything alone because they do not trust their ability to make decisions
- **Obsessive-compulsive PD**: Patients are very **inflexible and stubborn**. They are **preoccupied** with **orderliness, perfectionism and control**. They do not think that their behavior is irrational
- **Narcissistic PD**: Patients are **egocentric**, have a **sense of entitlement**. They lack empathy and get angry when criticized
- **Borderline PD**: Patients (mostly females) have **unstable mood, behavior and relationships**; they have fear of abandonment, and usually have a history of **multiple suicidal attempts**. They view others as either all good or all bad **(Splitting)**
- **Antisocial PD**: persistence **violation of social rules**. They lack remorse; torture animals or set fires. There is a strong association of alcoholism, drug abuse and somatization disorder.

Treatment: all personality disorders are treated with psychotherapy and mood stabilizers, as needed

EATING DISORDERS

1. ANOREXIA
Anorexia is an eating disorder in which the patient has an irrational fear of weight gain even though the **patient is 85 % below their ideal weight**. They lose weight by excessive exercise, purging, fasting, laxatives or diuretics abuse
Diagnosis: measure height and weight, CBC, electrolyte, endocrine and ECG. Psychiatry evaluation to check for comorbid conditions
Treatment:
- Hospitalize patient for IV nutrients, fluid and electrolyte replacement
- Psychotherapy, SSRIs may be used to promote weight
- Treat any comorbid condition

Note: IV nutrient therapy should be started at 40 Kcal/kg/day, and then progress to 70 Kcal/kg/day, otherwise patient may develop **refeeding syndrome. Electrolytes such as p**otassium, phosphorus, and **magnesium** should be checked every 5th day

2. BULIMIA
Bulimia is characterized by binge eating followed by purging. Patients have **normal body weight**. They usually have **abrasion on dorsal hands** surface, **parotid swelling, and dental enamel erosion.**
Diagnosis: clinical diagnosis
Treatment:
- Patient usually do not require hospitalization unless there is electrolytes imbalance
- Behavioral psychotherapy
- SSRIs (fluoxetine or imipramine) may be needed to prevent bulimia relapse

SUBSTANCE ABUSE

Substance	Intoxication symptoms & treatment	Withdrawal symptoms & treatment
Amphetamine & cocaine	• Agitation, decreased appetite, arrhythmia, MI, HTN, stroke, seizure, nosebleed, dilated pupil • Treatment: Antipsychotics	• Increased appetite, depressed, suicidal, anxiety, tremor • Treatment: Antidepressants
Opiates	• Constricted pupils, constipations, slurred speech, impaired memory, coma, death • Treatment: Naloxone	• Yawning, lacrimation, runny nose, abdominal cramps, muscle spams • Treatment: Clonidine or methadone. Clonidine, if patient has hypertension
Benzodiazepine & barbiturates	• Respiratory and cardiac depression • Treatment: Flumazenil	• Anxiety, seizure, tremors, cardiovascular collapse • Treatment: Long-acting benzodiazepines
LSD & hallucinogens	• Hallucination, dilated pupils, impaired judgment, incoordination • Treatment: Supportive, antipsychotics and benzodiazepines as needed	None
PCP	• Hallucination, horizontal/vertical nystagmus, assaultive, HTN, seizure, coma • Treatment: Supportive, benzodiazepines and antipsychotics	None
Inhalants	• Impaired judgment, blurred vision, assaultive, respiratory depression • Treatment: Antipsychotics	None
Marijuana	• Mostly teenager with red conjunctiva, dry mouth, socially withdrawn, amotivational, impaired time perception • Treatment: None	None

ALCOHOL

ALCOHOL SCREENING
CAGE questionnaire is used to screen a person for alcohol abuse, which stands for:
- C: ever felt the need to **cut** down
- A: feel **annoyed** when asked about drinking
- G: feel **guilty** after drinking
- E: need drink in the morning (**eye**-opener)

ALCOHOL INTOXICATION
Alcohol intoxication symptoms include emotional lability, slurred speech, ataxia, aggression, hypoglycemia
Treatment: usually no treatment is required. Mechanical ventilation if needed

ALCOHOL WITHDRAWLS
Alcohol withdrawal symptoms are as follow:
- **Tremor** begins within **5-10 hours** after the last drink. Symptoms include **tremors, irritability, insomnia, increase**d blood pressure
- **Alcohol hallucinosis** begins within **12 – 24 hours** after the last drink. Symptoms include **visual, auditory** and **tactile hallucination.**
- **Alcohol withdrawal seizure** are **tonic-clonic seizure**, which usually begins within **6-48 hours** after the last drink
- **Delirium tremens** begins within **2 -3 days** after the last drink. Symptoms includes hallucinations, confusion, **disorientation,** autonomic lability

Management of alcohol withdrawals is as follow:
- Benzodiazepines can lessen alcohol withdrawal symptoms.
  - Long- acting benzodiazepine such **chlordiazepoxide** (Librium) or **diazepam is the first-line of treatment.**
  - Short-acting benzodiazepine such as Lorazepam or oxazepam, are preferred in a patient with liver disease
- Give Vitamin B 12, folate, thiamine, magnesium, phosphate, glucose

Note: always give thiamine before glucose to prevent Wernicke-Korsakoff

GENDER IDENTITY

- **Sexual identity** is based on person's secondary sexual characteristics
- **Sexual orientation** is defined by whom he or she is sexually attracted to
- **Gender identity** is person's own sense of male or female
- **Gender role** is a public image of a person, a male or female

GENDER IDENTITY DISORDER

Gender identity disorder is a person's inner conflict between his or her physical gender and the gender person identifies himself or herself as. Person is not happy with the gender he or she was born.

Treatment

- Psychotherapy
- Gender reassignment, if surgery is approved

SEXUAL PARAPHILIA

Sexual paraphilia is characterized by sexual fantasies or activities that involve nonhuman objects, a non-consenting partner or in certain situations. Some of the paraphilias are mentioned below:

Paraphilia	Manifestations
Exhibitionism	Sexual arousal from showing one's genital to strangers
Fetishism	Sexual arousal from non-living objects
Pedophilia	Sexual urges towards children
Frotteurism	Rubbing against non-consenting partner for sexual gratification
Masochism	Sexual arousal from being humiliated, hurt
Sadism	Sexual arousal from inflicting pain one someone

SUICIDE

Risk factors for suicide are: Mnemonic: **SAD PERSONS**

- Male **S**ex (more females attempt, but more males succeed)
- **A**ge < 20 or > 40
- **D**epression
- **P**revious suicide attempt
- **E**thanol abuse
- **R**ational thinking loss
- **S**ocial support lacking
- **O**rganized plan
- **N**o spouse (divorced, separated or single)
- **S**ickness (chronic, severe)

Treatment: Hospitalization. ECT for acutely suicidal patient

SLEEP DISORDERS

- **Night terrors** are common in children between 3- 7 years of age, they occur during **stage 3 & 4 of sleep.** In night terrors, child wakes up from sleep terrified and often go back to sleep. Children often have **no memory about the event** when they wake up next day.
- **Nightmares** usually begin before 10 years of age and are a normal part of childhood. They usually occur during **REM sleep.** In nightmares, child wakes up from sleep terrified and can often recall dream when they wake up next day.
- **Sleepwalking** is a disorder in which people walk or do other activities during sleep. It usually occurs during **3 and 4th stage of** sleep. It is usually **treated with benzodiazepines.**
- **Narcolepsy** is characterized by excessive daytime sleep patterns, even after adequate nighttime sleep. Patient **goes to REM sleep** within 5 minutes of sleep. Other symptoms may include
  - **Cataplexy: sudden** loss of muscles tone
  - **Hypnagogic: hallucinations** while falling asleep
  - **Hypnopompic: hallucination** while awakening from sleep
  - **Sleep paralysis** temporary inability to talk or move when waking, it usually lasts few seconds to minutes

  Treatment of narcolepsy: methylphenidate or pemoline

PSYCHIATRY CCS

CASE # 1

Case introduction
A 52- year-old woman comes to the clinic because she has been experiencing difficulty concentrating, problem sleeping and feeling of hopelessness.

Initial vitals signs
Temperature: 37.1 degrees
Pulse: 78 beats/min, regular rhythm
Respiration rate: 16/ minutes

Blood pressure, systolic 126 mm Hg
Blood pressure, disystolic 74 mm Hg

Height: 60.0 inches
Weight: 120.0 lbs.
Body mass index: 23.4 Kg/m2

History of present illness (HPI)
A 52- year-old woman comes to the clinic because she has been experiencing difficulty concentrating, problem sleeping and feeling of hopelessness. She reports feeling worthless. From last 2 months she no appetite, has lost 18 lbs. and has trouble falling sleep. She says her symptoms are interfering with her ability to perform her work. She denies any suicidal thoughts. She says that her mother passed away last year of breast cancer.

Past medical history
Hospitalization: None
Other medical condition: None
Current medication: None
Allergies: latex, penicillin
Vaccination: up to date

Family history
Father has DM, and mother died of breast cancer. Sister has
hypothyroidism

Social history
Marital history: Married; 2 children
Occupation: Cashier
Recreational: Cooking, travel
Personal habits: Does not drink smoke, or use drugs

Review of system:
General: see HPI
Skin: see HPI
HEENT: see HPI
Musculoskeletal: see HPI
Cardiology: see HPI
Abdominal: see HPI
Genitourinary: see HPI

Please see pages 1 -5 for general CCS cases approach

Step 1. None (patient is stable and is not suicidal)

Step 2. Order complete physical exam, and then move the clock forward to get the results
- Results show:
  - Patient looks withdrawn and makes poor eye contact
  - Rest of the physical exam normal

Step 3. Order the labs, and then move the clock forward to get the results
- CBC
- UA
- BMP
- Chest x-ray
- TSH
- Vitamin B 12
- AST, ALT

- Results show:
  - All of the labs are with in normal limit

Step 4. Sertraline and have patient sign suicide contract

Step 5. Office

Step 6. None

Step 7. None

Step 8. Order Psychiatry consultation, and the move clock forward to get the results

Step 9. Make a follow-up appointment after 6-8 weeks and send the patient home
- Move the clock to next follow-up visit. Patient usually feels better

Case usually ends here

Step 10. Counsel, and age and gender specific screening
- Medication compliance
- No smoking, drinking, illegal drugs
- Age and gender specific screening

Diagnosis: Depression

CASE # 2

Case introduction
A 24-year-old female comes to the office with difficulty breathing, rapid pounding heart, sweating and fear of dying.

Initial vitals signs
Temperature: 37.1 degrees
Pulse: 78 beats/min, regular rhythm
Respiration rate: 16/ minutes

Blood pressure, systolic 126 mm Hg
Blood pressure, disystolic 74 mm Hg

Height: 60.0 inches
Weight: 120.0 lbs.
Body mass index: 23.4 Kg/m2

History of present illness (HPI)
A 24-year-old female comes to the office with difficulty breathing, rapid pounding heart, sweating and fear of dying. She says her symptoms started last year during a staff meeting that led her to leave work that day. Since that time the frequency of attack has increased and has experienced significant interference in her life. The symptoms usually lasts 5-10 minutes, begin and stop spontaneously. She avoids a number of activities due to fear of another panic attack.

Past medical history
Hospitalization: None
Other medical condition: None
Current medication: None
Allergies: latex, penicillin
Vaccination: up to date

Family history
Father and mother are alive and healthy

Social history
Marital history: single
Occupation: Real estate agent
Recreational: Cooking, travel
Personal habits: Does not drink smoke, or use drugs

Review of system:
General: see HPI
Skin: see HPI
HEENT: see HPI
Musculoskeletal: see HPI
Cardiology: see HPI
Abdominal: see HPI
Genitourinary: see HPI

Please see pages 1-5 for general CCS cases approach

Step 1. None

Step 2. Order complete physical exam, and then move the clock forward
to get the results
- Results show:
o Patient appears anxious.
o Rest of the physical exam is WNL

Step 3. Order the labs, and then move the clock forward to get the results
- CBC
- UA
- BMP
- Chest X-ray
- TSH
- EKG
- Urine drug test

- Results show:
o EKG shows normal sinus rata
o Rest of the labs WNL

Step 4. Lorazepam, Fluoxetine

Step 5. Make a follow-up appointment after 4 weeks and send the patient
home

Step 6. None

Step 7. Move the clock forward to next appointment date
- Patient shows up in the clinic and feeling better than
before

Step 8. None

Step 9. Make a follow-up appointment after 4 weeks and send the patient
home

Cause usually ends here

Step 10. Counseling and screening
- NO smoking, drinking, illegal drugs
- Medicine compliance
- Seat belt
- And, age and gender specific counseling

Diagnosis: Panic attack

PEDIATRIC PSYCHIATRY

PERVASIVE DEVELOPMENT DISORDERS

Pervasive development disorders are a group of disorders characterized by development delay in social interaction, behavior and language, before the age of 3.

Type: four common types of pervasive development disorders are

1. **Autism** is characterized by **impaired social interaction; impaired non-verbal communication, impaired verbal (speech) communications and purposeless repetitive movements**. It has a higher incidence in males than females

2. **Asperger syndrome** is characterized by impaired social interaction; impaired non-verbal communication, purposeless repetitive movements, but **verbal (speech) communication is preserved**. It has a higher incidence in males than females

3. **Childhood disintegrative disorder** is a condition in which all of the development milestones are normal till 2 years of age, **but between 2 -10 years of age all the skill are lost;** social skills and self care skills, motor skills, play skills, bowel and bladder control, and language. It has a higher incidence in males than females.

4. **Rett syndrome:** is a neurodevelopment disorder of the gray matter of the brain with **progressive impairment** such as verbal, and motor. Clinical features include small hands, feet and deceleration of head growth. It has a higher incidence in females than males

Treatment: family support, counseling, behavior modification, and antipsychotic, if the patient is aggressive.

ATTENTION DEFICIT HYPERACTIVITY DISORDER (ADHD)

ADHD is characterized by easy distractibility, fidgety, inability to focus, inability to complete tasks, declining school performance

Diagnosis: based on the followings:

- Patient must be < 7 years old
- Symptoms must last > 6 months
- Symptoms must be present in two or more settings (school, home)
- Symptoms must interfere with daily function

Management:
- **Behavioral modification and medication** (methylphenidate or dextroamphetamine)
- **Atomoxetine is a SNRIs that may be used if a patient is > 6 years of age and** is at high **risk of methylphenidate abuse**

Co-existing conditions with ADHD
Other conditions that usually co-exist with ADHD are
- Oppositional defiant disorder (most common)
- Conduct disorder
- Anxiety disorder
- Depression

DISRUPTIVE BEHAVIOR
Two main disruptive behaviors in children are:
1. **Conduct disorder;** in which a child **bully others, start fights, cruel to animals,** and steals. It may **progress to antisocial personality disorder**
2. **Oppositional defiant disorder,** in which a child displays **disrespect and opposition to adults or authority position.** They tend to be angry and resentful of others, blame others for their mistakes.

Treatment: individual and family therapy

TOURETTE'S SYNDROME
Tourette's syndrome is characterized by **multiple repetitive tics, which start before the age of 18 and last more than 1 year.** Vocal tics (grunting, coprolalia, throat clearing) and motor tics involve the muscles of head and neck (blinking, head shaking). It is associated with **ADHD, OCD and learning disorders.**
Treatment: no treatment needed for mild symptoms, but **severe** symptoms can be treated with **haloperidol, pimozide or clonidine.**

MENTAL RETARDATION

Mental retardation is characterized by impaired intellectual and social function. It is more common in males than females. It is associated with chromosomal abnormalities, inborn error of metabolism, congenital infective, malnutrition and exposure to certain types of toxin or infection

Types and effect on life of mental retardation is as follow:

- Person with **mild mental retardation** (IQ range 50- 70) can live independently, but will need assistant in stressful situation
- Person with **moderate mental retardation** (IQ range 35-49) may work under supervision
- Person with **severe mental retardation** (IQ range 20-34) has limited abilities to take care of him or herself
- Person with **profound mental retardation** (IQ range below 20) needs constant care

Treatment: family counseling, speech and language therapy, behavior therapy, and special education

ENURESIS

Enuresis is common condition in children that occurs usually during nighttime enuresis

Diagnosis:

- Clinical diagnosis
- Urinalysis is usually done to rule out UTI
- If signs of infection are present, then do **urine culture and ultrasound**

Treatment:

- If patient is **< 7 years old** –Tx. **Reassurance**
- If patient is **> 7 years of age** –Tx. **Behavior modification**
  - ○ If this is ineffective, **then use an enuresis alarm**
  - ○ Last resort is medication such as **imipramine, TCAs or vasopressin**

Boards tip:

- If enuresis present only during **daytime and school days**, then it is most likely a **separation anxiety**
- If enuresis is presents at **night, and as well as, daytime, then** there is probably an underlining **organic cause**

PEDIATRICS

NEWBORN SCREENING

All newborns should be screened for:

- Hypothyroidism
- Phenylketonuria (PKU)
- Galactosemia

APGAR SCORE

APGAR score is a simple method to quickly access the health of a newborn immediately after birth. The scores range from 0 to 10; score 7 and above is normal, 4 to 6 is fairly low, and 3 to 0 is critical.

If 1 minute APGAR score is < 7 then do 5 minutes APGAR score

	Score 0	Score 1	Score 2
Appearance	Whole body blue or pale	Pink body and blue extremities	Whole body is pink
Pulse rate	Absent	<100	> 100
Reflex *	No response	Grimace or feeble cry	Strong cry, pull away with stimulated
Activity	None	Some flexion	Active motion
Respiratory	None	Weak, irregular gasping	Good, Strong cry

* Reflex is measured in response to stimulation of the sole of the foot or when a catheter is inserted into the nose of a baby

EYES

- 1% silver nitrate drops or 0.5% erythromycin eye ointment is given to all neonates after birth

NEWBORN EYE DISCHARGE

Cause	Characteristics	Treatment
Chemical conjunctivitis	• **Serous eye** discharge presents within first 24 hours of life	Supportive
Gonococcal conjunctivitis	• **Purulent eye** discharge presents **within 1st week** of birth	**Saline irrigation** and **IV or IM ceftriaxone**
Chlamydia conjunctivitis	• **Purulent eye** discharge presents **after 1st week** of birth	**Saline irrigation** and **oral erythromycin**

Complications
- Untreated gonococcal conjunctivitis may cause **corneal ulceration**
- Untreated chlamydia conjunctivitis may cause **blindness, corneal ulceration**

NEWBORN SKIN CONDITIONS

1. PORT-WINE STAIN
Port–wine stain is a pink, dark red or purple color mark. It often occurs on face but may occur anywhere on the body
Cause: capillary malformation of the skin
Treatment: Pulse laser
Complication: it is associated with Sturge-weber syndrome, glaucoma

2. HEMANGIOMA
Hemangioma is an abnormal buildup of blood vessels in the skin or internal organs. When it occurs in the upper layer of the skin it is called capillary hemangioma and when it occurs in the deeper layer of the skin it is called cavernous hemangioma
Si/Sx: Bright red lesion that usually **appears around 2 months** of age and **regresses by 9 years of age**
Treatment: Pulse laser, and steroids if needed

3. Differential diagnosis of newborn skin conditions

Condition	Characteristics	Treatment
Erythema toxicum	• **Yellow-white papules and pustules** (with erythematous base	No treatment
Neonate acne	• **Acneiform rash on nose** and cheeks, which occurs due to maternal androgen	No treatment
Mongolian spots	• **Blue/gray macules** on the presacral area *(don't this confuse with child abuse)*	No treatment
Milia	• White papules	No treatment
Cutis marmorata	• **Lacy reticular** pattern	No treatment

4. DIAPER RASH

Diaper rash is a common term refers to any skin irritation that occurs in the diaper-covered area.

Types and causes:

4a. IRRITANT DIAPER DERMATITIS

Irritant diaper dermatitis is caused by **prolong exposure of urine or feces** that irritates the skin. It causes **erythema and papules in the area of contact** and usually **spares intergluteal folds**

Treatment: Topical petrolatum or topical zinc oxide and diaper holidays

4b. CANDIDA DIAPER DERMATITIS

Candida diaper dermatitis that causes **erythema and papules in the area of contact** and **intergluteal skin folds**

Treatment: topical nystatin or clotrimazole

DEVELOPMENT MILESTONES

Age	Social/cognition	Language	Fine motor	Gross motor
2 months	Social Smile	Coos	Swipe at objects, eyes follow object past midline	Holds head up
4 months	Laughs	Orient to voice	Grasp objects	Rolls over supine to prone
6 months	Stranger anxiety	Babbles	Transfer objects hand to hands	Rolls over prone to supine, sits unsupported
9 months	Waves bye-bye, plays peek-a-boo	Says mama, dada (nonspecific), says bye-bye	Pincer grasp	Pulls to stand, crawls
12 months	**Separation anxiety**	Says mama dada (specific)	Mature grasp	**Stands**, plays with ball
15 months	**Temper tantrum**	Knows 4-6 words	Uses cup, Stacks 3 cube	**Walks** alone
18 months	Imitate parents at task	Knows 10 words, name common objects	Use spoon for solid food, Stacks 4 cubes	Walks downstairs
2 years	Follows 2 step command	Says 2-3 words sentence	Use spoon for semisolid food, Stacks 6 cubes **Copies a line**	Walks up and down stairs
3 years	Knows first and last name	Use 3 word sentence	Use utensils to eat, Stacks 9 cubes **Copies a circle**	Walks down stairs with alternating feet
4 years	**Participates in group play**	Counts to 10	Grooms self, **Copies a cross**	Rides tricycle

- Moro reflex disappears by 3-4 months of age
- Rooting and grasp reflex disappear by 4-6 months of age
- Parachute reflex disappears by 6-8 months of age

CARDIOLOGY

CONGENITAL HEART DISEASE

Exam tip: Most of the pediatrics cardiology questions will describe the murmur and ask, what is the most likely diagnosis?

Remember: Innocent murmurs as systolic murmurs, and <2/6 in intensity

MOST COMMOMON CONGENITAL HEART DISEASES

1. TRANSPOSITION OF THE GREAT VESSELS
In this condition aortic and pulmonary veins and arteries have switched their positions
Risk factors: it is associated with infant of diabetic mother
Si/Sx: neonates present with severe **cyanosis** immediately **after delivery**
Diagnosis:
- Murmur: may or may not have single loud S2 murmur
- **Chest X-ray** shows "**egg on string**" appearance

Treatment:
- Initial step is to give **prostaglandin** E1 (PGE1) to keep ductus arteriosus patent (PDA). PDA may prolong neonate's life until surgical correction is possible.
- Surgery correction is the definitive treatment

- TGA is the most common cyanotic condition of infancy
- TOF is most common cyanotic condition in children
---

2. TETRALOGY OF FALLOT
Tetralogy of Fallot is the most common cyanotic heart disease that presents **later in life**. It is a combination of four different defects: pulmonary stenosis, right ventricle hypertrophy, overriding aorta, and VSD.
Si/Sx: patient usually present with irritability, cyanosis that occurs during exertion and **relives with squatting**
Diagnosis:
- Systolic thrill heard along the left sternal border
- Chest x-ray shows decreased pulmonary marking and" **boot-shaped heart**" appearance of the heart

Treatment:

- Place the patient in **knee- to–chest,** give **oxygen, beta blocker, PGE1**
- Surgical repair at 4- 12 months

3.   VENTRICULAR SEPTAL DEFECT (VSD)

Ventricular septal defect is the most common congenital heart defect. It is defined as one or more hole in the ventricle septum that separates right and left ventricle

Risk factor: it is associated with fetal alcohol syndrome, TORCH syndrome, and trisomy 13, 18, and 21

Si/Sx: some babies may not have any symptoms, but symptoms may include shortness of breath, failure to thrive, cyanosis, edema

Diagnosis:

- Physical exam **shows harsh holosystolic murmur over left lower sternal border,** loud pulmonic S2 murmur
- Chest x-ray shows increased vascular marking
- Echocardiogram shows normal heart with small VSD defects and RVH or large VSD defects with LVH

Treatment:

- Small VSD **closes spontaneously** within 6 months of age. However, if patient develops pulmonary HTN, shut is >2:1, or failure to thrive, then it is surgical repaired
- Large VSDs require surgical repair
- Preexisting CHF is treated with diuretics and digoxin

Complication: CHF, infective endocarditis, pulmonary hypertension, failure to thrive

4.   ATRIAL SEPTAL DEFECT (ASD)

ASD is defined as one or more hole in the atrial septum that separates right and left atria

Types:

- Ostium primary
- Ostium secundum (most common)

Si/Sx: patient with small defects may not have any symptoms, or symptoms may not occur until middle age or later. Symptoms includes shortness of breath, fatigue, edema, heart palpitations, cyanosis

Diagnosis:
- Physical exam shows loud S1, wide **fixed-split S2 with systolic murmur**
- Chest x-ray shows increased pulmonary marking and cardiomegaly
- Echocardiograph with color Doppler shows blood flow between atria

Treatment:
- Majority of **Ostium secundum** ASD **closes spontaneously** by age 4
- **Ostium primary** ASD or symptomatic ASD are **surgical repaired**

Complications: Pulmonary HTN, MVP, dysrhythmia

5. COARCTATION OF THE AORTA

Coarctation of the aorta is narrowing of the aorta. **Almost in all cases it occurs at the origin of left subclavian artery**

Risk factors: Turner syndrome, bicuspid aortic valve, patent ductus arteriosus

Si/SX: depends on the severity of the condition. Babies with the severe condition usually are symptomatic soon after birth. Symptoms may include irritability, heavy sweating, difficulty breathing

Diagnosis:
- Physical exam shows
  - **Pink upper body and blue lower body**
  - **Blood pressure that is higher in arms than legs**
- Chest X-ray shows rib notching and narrowing of aorta at the site of the coarctation giving number **"3" appearance**
- Cardiac catheterization is the definitive diagnosis

Treatment
- Initial step is to give **prostaglandin** E1 (PGE1) to keep ductus arteriosus patent (PDA).
- Surgery correction is the definitive treatment

6. PATENT DUCTUS ARTERIOSUS (PDA)

Ductus arteriosus is a blood vessel that connects the left pulmonary artery to aorta, which allows blood to bypass the fetus' lungs. Soon after birth ductus closes, but when the ductus fails to close, then this condition is called patent ductus arteriosus.

Risk factor: female gender, **congenital rubella**, prematurity

Si/Sx: Patient with small PDA may not have any symptoms, but symptoms may include poor feeding habits, shortness of breath, poor growth, rapid pulse

Diagnosis:

- Physical exam shows " **Machinery" like, to-and-fro murmur,** wide pulse pressure and bounding arterial pulses
- Diagnosis is confirmed with echocardiography or cardiac catheterization

Treatment:

- **Best initial treatment is Indomethacin,** it blocks the prostaglandin production and close the patent ductus
- If indomethacin **is ineffective** or if the **patient is > 6-8** months old, then do **surgery** to close PDA.

7.   ENDOCARDIAL CUSHION DEFECT

Endocardial cushion defect is characterized by involvement of the ventricular septal defect, atrial septum and one or both the AV valves
Cause: it is usually associated with **Down syndrome**
Symptoms: patient presents with combination of symptoms: **VSD, ASD and AV valve insufficiency**
Diagnosis:

- Murmur: ASD **and VSD type murmur**
- Chest X- ray: shows cardiomegaly

Treatment:

- Surgical correction before pulmonary HTN develops

CHILDHOOD HYPERTENSION (HTN)

Diagnosis:

- **BP> 95%** on **two separate occasion**

Cause:

- Common cause of HTN in **children** includes **renal disease, coarctation of aorta, endocrine disorder**
- Common cause of HTN in **adolescent** is **essential HTN**

Management:

- If the patient has a renal disease, then the best initial treatment is ACEIs
- Initial management for **obese** children is weight loss, exercise and diet modification
- Best initial treatment **for children** is beta-blockers or diuretics
  - If it is ineffective, then **add** calcium channel blocker
- Initial treatment for **adolescents** is ACEIs and calcium channel blocker

GASTROENTEROLOGY

1. NEWBORN ABDOMINAL MALFORMATION

Diagnosis	Characteristic	Treatment
Omphalocele	• Intestine and abdominal organs **protrudes through the umbilicus** (belly buttons), • Intestine is covered with a thin layer of tissue • Associated with trisomy 13, 18 and 21	Surgical repair
Gastroschisis	• Intestine and abdominal organs **protrudes from lateral to midline,** • Intestine is not covered with a layer of tissue	Surgical repair
Umbilical hernia	• Outward **bulging of abdominal** organs through trough the area **around the belly button** • Associated with congenital hypothyroidism.	None, most closes spontaneously

2. NECROTIZING ENTERCOLITIS

Necrotizing enterocolitis is a medical condition seen mostly in **premature infants**, in which portion of bowel undergoes inflammation and necrosis. If it is not treated promptly, then it can be life-threatening

Si/Sx: symptoms usually develop within **first 2 weeks of life, and may include apnea, abdominal distention, bloody stool, fever, lethargy**

Boards tip: look for a **premature** infant with apnea, abdominal distention and bloody stool with first feeding

Diagnosis:
- Based on symptoms and abdominal X-ray, which shows **pneumatosis intestinalis** (air bubbles in the bowel)

Treatment:
- Stop feeding, decompress the gut by inserting small tube in the stomach, IV antibiotics
- Then, surgical removal of necrotic bowel

Boards tip:
- If boards gives you a choice between diagnostic testing and stop all the feeding and ask which one would you do first? Answer: stop all the feedings before diagnostic testing

3. MECONIUM ILIUM

Meconium is the first stool that a newborn has that is usually very thick and stick. When meconium gets even thicker and stickier than the normal meconium, it blocks the small intestine (ileum), and it is called meconium ilium.

Cause: it is associated with **cystic fibrosis**

Si/Sx: abdominal distention, **bilious vomit**, and **no passage of the first stool (meconium)**

Diagnosis: best initial test is abdominal x-ray, which shows bowel distention

Treatment: Gastrografin enema

4. MECONIUM PLUGS

Meconium plug refers to functional colonic obstruction in a newborn

Cause: it is associated with

- Hirschsprung disease
- Cystic fibrosis
- Maternal opioid use
- Small left colon in infant of diabetic mother

Si/Sx: abdominal distention, **bilious vomit**, and **no passage of the first stool (meconium)**

Diagnosis: best initial test is abdominal x-ray, which shows bowel distention

Treatment: Gastrografin enema

5. HIRSCHSPRUNG DISEASE

Hirschsprung disease is a congenital defect in never fibers of distal bowel that results in improper peristalsis and obstruction in the bowel.

Si/Sx: failure to pass meconium shortly after birth, failure to pass stool is first 48 hours of life

Diagnosis:

- Rectal exam shows **patent anus**
- Abdominal X-ray shows distended bowel loop with no air in rectum
- **Barium enema** shows **megacolon** proximal to the obstruction
- Most accurate test is **rectal suction biopsy**

Treatment: Surgical resection of **aganglionic colon** (proximal colon)

6. IMPERFORATE ANUS

Imperforate anus is congenital defect in which opening of anus is blocked or missing

Si/Sx: failure to pass meconium shortly after birth, failure to pass stool in first 48 hours of life

Diagnosis: Rectal exam shows **imperforate anus**

Treatment: surgery

Boards tip:

- If a patient presents with failure to pass meconium shortly after birth or failure to pass stool in first 48 hours of life, then the best initial test is do a rectal exam because both Hirschsprung disease and imperforated anus have these symptoms.

7. DUODENAL ATRESIA

Duodenal atresia is a congenital condition in which first part of small intestine (duodenum) is partially or completely blocked

Si/Sx: bilious (greenish) vomiting, upper abdominal swelling, absent of bowel movement after few meconium stool

Diagnosis:

- Abdominal **X-ray** shows air in the stomach and in the first part of the duodenum, which is known as **double bubble sign**

Treatment:

- **Initial treatment - place a** nasogastric tube to decompress the stomach, IV fluid and electrolytes replacement to correct the fluids and electrolyte imbalance.
- Then, perform **surgical correction, which is the definitive treatment for duodenal atresia**

8. INTUSSUSCEPTION

Intussusception is a medical condition in which one part of the small intestine slides into another and leads to bowel obstruction

Si/Sx: crying and **drawing knees up to the chest**, "Currant jelly stool" in diaper, lethargy, fever

Risk factors: previous infection with rotavirus, Meckle's diverticulum, intestinal lymphoma, Henoch-Schonlein purpura,

Diagnosis:

- Physical exam shows **sausage shaped mass in RLQ**
- Ultrasound may be helpful
- **Air enema** is diagnostic and therapeutic

Treatment:

- IV fluids and electrolytes to correct the fluids and electrolytes imbalance.
- **Air enema** is diagnostic and therapeutic

9. INTESTINAL MALROTATION

Intestinal malrotation is a congenital anomaly in which intestine is incompletely rotated around the superior mesentery artery

Si/Sx: bilious vomiting, bloody diarrhea, poor appetite, fever, lethargy

Diagnosis:

- Abdominal X-ray may show intestinal obstruction
- Ultrasound is the best initial diagnostic test

Treatment:
- IV **fluids and electrolytes** to correct the fluids and electrolytes imbalance.
- **Surgery is the definitive** treatment and it should be done immediately after fluid and electrolytes replacement.

10. PYLORUS STENOSIS

Pylorus stenosis is narrowing of the pylorus, the opening of the stomach into the small intestine. This prevents the stomach from emptying into the small intestine

Cause: hypertrophy of pylorus sphincter

Si/Sx: **non-bilious projectile vomiting** after feeding that usually presents 2 weeks to 4 months after birth, persistent hunger, dehydration

Diagnosis:
- Physical exam shows **olive -shaped epigastric mass**
- Labs may show hypochloremic hypokalemic metabolic acidosis due to persistent vomiting
- Ultrasound of abdomen shows **"target- like"** cross-section

Management:
- Patients often have hypochloremic **metabolic alkalosis, make sure to** check hydration and electrolytes **and give IV hydration and electrolyte replacement,** if needed
- **Pyloromyotomy** is the definitive care

Important: Oral erythromycin increases the risk of developing pylorus stenosis

Boards tip:
- Bilious vomiting only: Dx. Duodenal atresia
- Bilious vomiting and bloody diarrhea: Dx. Malrotation/ Volvulus
- Non-bilious vomiting: Dx. Pylorus stenosis

11. MECKEL'S DIVERTICULUM

Meckel's diverticulum is the only true congenital diverticulum in the small intestine and is remnant of the omphalomesenteric duct (also known as vitelline duct or yolk stalk).

Rule of 2s of Meckel's diverticulum is:
- It seen in 2% of the population
- Normally found 2 feet proximal to ileocecal valve
- 2 inches in length
- Contains 2 types of ectopic tissue (gastric and pancreatic)
- Commonly seen in less than 2 years of age
- Male to female ratio is 2:1

Si/Sx: most of the patients are asymptomatic, but the most common presenting symptom is **painless rectal bleeding** (melena, hematochezia)
Diagnosis: Tc-99 pertechnetate scan (also known as radionucleotide scan)
Treatment: Surgical resection of diverticulum

12. GASTROESOPHAGEAL REFLUX DISEASE (GERD)

GERD may also occur in infants
Si/Sx: most common symptoms - infant **spit ups after feeding**; other symptoms may include **coughing, wheezing and episodes of apnea after feeding**
Diagnosis:
- Clinical diagnosis is sufficient in most cases
- Best initial test: Esophageal pH monitoring

Management:
- **Initial treatment - give small and frequent thick feeds**
- If this is ineffective, then give **H2 blockers**
- If even H2 blockers are ineffective, then give **proton pump inhibitors (PPIs)**
- Last resort is **fundoplication**

13. CONSTIPATION

It is most commonly seen in school-aged children due to voluntary withholding
Diagnosis:
- Physical exam shows large volume of stool palpated cecum/suprapubic area
- Rectal exam shows rectal vault filled with stool

Treatment:
- Initial step **is manual stool disimpaction, and then diet modification and mild laxatives**

14. DIARRHEA
- Rotavirus is the most common cause of viral diarrhea in children

Treatment: fluid and electrolyte replacement

15. CHRONIC DIARRHEA
- Look for patient with **chronic diarrhea, but normal height, weight and normal stool. It is usually caused by drinking excessive fluids**

PULMONOLOGY

1. RESPIRATORY DISTRESS SYNDROME (RSD)
Respiratory distress syndrome is seen in infants **born before 32 weeks of gestation. It is due to insufficient surfactant**

Si/Sx: tachypnea, nasal grunting, intercostal retractions

Diagnosis:
- **Best initial test:**
  - o **Chest X-ray**, which shows ground-glass lung appearance
  - o **Atelectasis**
  - o **Air bronchogram**
- **Most accurate test is lecithin-sphingomyelin ratio** (<2:1 in RSD)

Treatment: oxygen and inhaled exogenous surfactant

Prevention: give IM betamethasone to the mother going under labor before 32 weeks of gestation

2. TRANSIENT TACHYPNEA OF NEWBORN
Transient tachypnea of newborn is a respiratory disorder seen shortly after birth in **full-term or near-term babies,** who are **delivered by C-section or had 2nd stage of labor**

Cause: decreased absorption of fluids in lungs

Si/Sx: labored breathing, cyanosis, tachypnea intercostal retractions

Diagnosis: Chest X-ray shows fluids in fissure, air trapping, perihilar streaking

Treatment:
- **No treatment is required,** it usually resolves within 24-48 hours after delivery
- **Oxygen, if needed**

3.   MECONIUM ASPIRATION SYNDROME

Meconium aspiration syndrome **occurs when neonates aspirates meconium with first breath**. It is usually seen in term infants

Si/Sx: cyanosis, labored breathing, tachypnea intercostal retractions

Diagnosis:

- Chest X-ray shows patchy infiltrate, increased AP diameter and diaphragmatic flattening

Management:

- Initial treatment is **oxygen**
  - If still hypoxic, then give **positive pressure ventilation**
  - If patient is still unresponsive, then give **high frequency ventilation**
  - Last resort is **extracorporeal membrane oxygen**

4.   TRACHEOESOPHAGEAL FISTULA (TEF)

Tracheoesophageal fistula is a condition in which there is an abnormal connection between esophagus and trachea

Type: there are 4 types of TEF, but the most common type is proximal esophageal atresia and distal tracheoesophageal fistula

Si/Sx: coughing, choking, **gagging and cyanosis that coincide with feeding**

Diagnosis:

- Chest x-ray with nasogastric tube shows **nasogastric tube coils in the chest, rather than going to the stomach**
- Abdominal x-ray shows air in the stomach

Treatment: Surgery

Complications: Tracheoesophageal fistula is associated with other anomalies, most commonly described as **VACTERL** syndrome. It is important to rule out these disorders, as well.

- Vertebral defect
- Anal atresia
- Cardiac abnormality
- TEF
- Renal and radial anomaly
- Limb syndrome

5. CHOANAL ATRESIA

Choanal atresia is a congenital condition in which there is an abnormal blockage of nasal passage (choana)

Si/Sx: classic symptom is that a newborn turns **blue** when **trying to breathe through nose** and **pink when crying,** inability to feed and breath at the same time

Diagnoses: Inability to pass nasogastric tube through nasopharynx

Treatment: establish the airway, and then surgical resection of obstruction

Complications: Choanal atresia is associated with other anomalies, most commonly described as **CHARGE syndrome.** It is important to rule out these disorders, as well.

- Coloboma
- Heart defects
- Atresia of nasal choana
- Growth Retardation
- Genitourinary abnormalities
- Ear abnormality

6. PERTUSSIS

Pertussis (also known as whooping cough) is highly contagious respiratory disease caused by *Bordetella pertussis*

Stages: Pertussis presents in three stages:

- **Catarrhal stage,** which usually lasts from 1-2 weeks. It begins as "cold-like" symptoms such as rhinorrhea, sneezing, but later in phase, cough develops and symptoms become worse
- **Paroxysmal stage,** which lasts 2-4 weeks. It usually begins as harsh and dry cough, but later in phase, it becomes "whooping" cough
- **Convalescent stage,** which lasts for 1-2 weeks, and patient usually recovers in this period, frequency of cough decreases

Diagnosis:

- Clinical diagnosis, patient often have history of **incomplete immunization**
- Initial test is **PCR of nasopharyngeal** aspiration
- Accurate test: **Culture**

Treatment: Oral **erythromycin** to **the patient** and all **close contacts**

Important:

- Erythromycin increases the risk of developing pylorus stenosis in infants

7. CROUP

Croup also known as laryngotracheobronchitis is an **acute inflammatory condition around the larynx (vocal cord)**, mostly in the subglottic space. It is usually seen in fall and winter seasons, in 3 months to 3 years of age children

Cause: most common cause is **parainfluenza virus type 1 and 2**; other causes include influenza A and B, RSV, adenovirus, measles and mycoplasma pneumonia

Si/Sx: barking cough, inspiratory stridor, hoarseness and difficulty breathing which is **worse at night**

Diagnosis:

- Clinical diagnosis
- **Anterior-posterior neck x-ray** shows **steeple sign (rarely done)**

Treatment: treatment depends on the symptoms

- Patients with **mild** symptoms are managed **outpatient with cool mist therapy**
- Patient with **moderate or severe** symptoms may need **corticosteroids and racemic epinephrine** to reduce airway inflammation
- **Unstable patient** or patients with **severe symptoms** may need **intubation**

8. EPIGLOTTITIS

Epiglottitis is a life-threatening condition characterized by inflammation of epiglottis

Cause: Strep. Pyogenes, S. Pneumonia, S. aureus, Mycoplasma and H. Influenza type B

Si/Sx: sudden onset of **dysphagia, drooling in tripod-sitting position**, high fever, stridor, **"hot potato"** voice

Diagnosis:

- Clinical diagnosis
- **Lateral neck** x-ray shows the **thumbprint sign,** but is rarely needed and negative X-ray does not rule out epiglottitis

Treatment:

- Epiglottitis is a **medical emergency**; do not waste time in doing neck X-ray, immediately **transfer the patient to OR and do the following:**
  - **Then get ENT consult**
  - **Give patient anesthesia and perform** intubation or tracheostomy
  - Give antibiotic (ceftriaxone or 3rd generation cephalosporin's) and steroids

Complication: H. Influenza type B is the rare cause of epiglottitis, but it is very contagious. If it is the known cause of epiglottitis, then give **rifampin prophylaxis to all close contacts**

Boards tip:

- Following two conditions are caused by build of pus in the back of the throat, but these are commonly mistaken for epiglottitis.

I. **RETROPHARYNGEAL ABSCESS**

Patient present with **dysphagia, drooling,** fever, **torticollis, refuse to turn head/ neck, "hot potato" muffled voice**

Physical exam shows:

- **Mid line** tonsil and uvula, posterior or lateral wall bulging

Management:

- IV ampicillin/sulbactam or clindamycin
- If the patient has respiratory distress or initial antibiotics fails –Tx. **Surgical drainage**

II. **PERITONSILLAR ABSCESS**

Patient present with **dysphagia, drooling,** fever, **torticollis, refuse to turn head/ neck "hot potato" muffled voice**

Physical exam shows:

- Uvula **deviated** to the affected side

Management:

- IV ampicillin/sulbactam or clindamycin and needle aspiration or incision and drainage

---

9. BACTERIAL TRACHEITIS

Bacterial tracheitis is a secondary bacterial infection of trachea and it can cause airway obstruction

Cause: S. aureus is the most common cause

Si/Sx: brassy cough, high fever, toxic appearance, respiratory distress, stridor

Diagnosis:

- Clinical diagnosis
- Labs show leukocytosis
- Neck X-ray shows **ragged tracheal air column and subglottic narrowing**

Management:

- If the patient is in severe condition, then intubate the patient
- Nafcillin or ceftriaxone is given to treat S.Aureus

10. DIPHTHERIA CROUP

Diphtheria croup is caused by *Corynebacterium diphtheria*

Si/Sx. Chills, fatigue, sore throat, cyanosis, **gray-white pharyngeal membrane on soft palate, which bleeds easily**

Diagnosis: throat culture

Treatment: symptomatic treatment

11. FOREIGN BODY ASPIRATION

Foreign body aspiration is a life-threatening condition caused by aspiration of an object that may lodge in the larynx or trachea.

Si/Sx: sudden onset of **respiratory distress, choking coughing** and **wheezing**

Diagnosis:

- Chest X-ray, but it may not show some objects because radiolucent objects do not appear on X-ray
- Bronchoscopy is diagnostic

Treatment: rigid bronchoscopy

12. BRONCHIOLITIS

Bronchiolitis is characterized by inflammation and mucus plugs in the smallest airway (bronchioles)

Si/Sx: mild upper respiratory tract infection symptoms (fever, rhinorrhea, cough fever), that soon progress to dyspnea, tachypnea, apnea, intercostal retractions

Cause: RSV (most common cause), parainfluenza, adenovirus

Diagnosis:
- **Chest X-rays** shows intestinal infiltrate, atelectasis, **hyperinflation** of lungs
- Most specific test is **ELISA** of nasopharyngeal swab

Treatment:
- Patient with mild symptoms is managed outpatient with fluids, nebulized beta-2 agonist and oxygen, if needed
- Patient with respiratory distress is hospitalized and may require IV fluids, oxygen and nebulized beta-2 agonist

Prevention: high-risk patients should receive RSV IVIG or RSV monoclonal antibodies to prevent bronchiolitis

13. PNEUMONIA

Differential diagnosis of pneumonia

Age group	Most common cause of pneumonia
Newborn	Streptococcus agalactia, Gram negative rod Chlamydia trachomatis
Infants	Streptococcus agalactia, Gram negative rod Chlamydia
Preschool	RSV, Mycoplasma
Adolescent	Mycoplasma, Chlamydia S. Pneumonia

14. CHLAMYDIA TRACHOMATIS

Chlamydia trachomatis is the common cause of pneumonia in infants of **1-3 months of age.** Patient may have history of chlamydia conjunctivitis

Si/Sx: staccato cough, no fever and no wheezing

Diagnosis:
- CBC with peripheral smear shows **eosinophilia**
- Chest X-ray shows mild interstitial disease

Treatment: erythromycin or other macrolides

15. VIRAL PNEUMONIA

Viral pneumonia is a common in children **less than 5 years of age**. RSV is the most common cause

Si/Sx: low-grade fever, tachypnea and symptoms is upper respiratory tract infection

Diagnosis

- Labs show WBCs < 20,000 **predominantly lymphocytes**
- Chest x-ray shows **hyperinflammation with bilateral interstitial infiltrate and peribronchial cuffing**

Treatment:

- Patient with mild pneumonia or no respiratory symptoms usually requires **no treatment.**
- If patient's symptoms are worsening, then give antibiotics

16. BACTERIAL PNEUMONIA

Bacterial pneumonia is common in children **more than 5 years of age**. Streptococcus pneumonia is the most common cause of bacterial pneumonia

Si/Sx: high fevers, chills, cough

Diagnosis

- Chest exam shows rhonchi, diminished breath sounds and dullness to percussion
- Labs show WBCs between 15,000 to 40,000 **predominantly granulocytes**
- Chest X-ray shows **lobar consolidation**

Treatment:

- Patient with **mild symptoms** can be managed **outpatient** with **amoxicillin** (1st choice) **or cefuroxime** (2nd choice)
- Patient with **severe pneumonia** may require **inpatient** treatment with **cefuroxime**

17. MYCOPLASMA PNEUMONIA

Mycoplasma pneumonia is most common in adolescents **more than 15 years of age**

Si/Sx: mild symptoms appear over the period of 1-3 weeks. Symptoms may include fever, chest pain, dry cough, sore throat, rash

Diagnosis:
- CBC may show anemia
- Sputum culture
- IgM viral titer
- Chest x-ray shows lower lobe interstitial pneumonia

Treatment: Erythromycin or other macrolides

18. CYSTIC FIBROSIS

Cystic fibrosis is a genetic disorder characterized by formations of cyst and fibrosis of exocrine glands

Cause: autosomal recessive defect in CFTR gene on chromosome 7

Si/Sx:
- **Multiple** respiratory tract infections, failure to thrive, greasy stools, salty sweat
- Most common symptom in newborn is meconium ileus

Diagnosis:
- Best initial test is sweat chloride concentration of > 60 mEq/L, simultaneously taken from **two different body sites**, on **two separate days**
- If sweat chloride test is not diagnostic, **then test potential difference across nasal epithelium**

Treatment:
- Encourage adequate fluid intake
- Oral replacement of pancreatic enzymes and fat-soluble vitamins (A, D, E, and K)
- Nutritional counseling
- **Chest physiotherapy, nebulized albuterol or saline**
- **Long-term ibuprofen to slow the disease progression**
- Pneumococcal and influenza vaccine
- Lung transplant for advance disease

- Antibiotics:
  - **Mild** disease –Tx. **Macrolides** or **ciprofloxacin**
  - **Severe** disease –Tx. Inpatient treatment with **IV piperacillin and tobramycin** or **ceftazidime**
  - For **resistance cases** – Tx. **Aerosolized tobramycin**

19. EPISTAXIS

Epistaxis or nosebleed is usually caused by **nose picking**

Management:

- Most resolve spontaneously; have the patient lean **head forward and compress the nares**
- If it is ineffective, then use **local vasoconstrictors** such as phenylephrine
- If patient continues to bleed, then use **nasal packing**

Prevention: use air humidifiers

MUSCULOSKELETAL DISORDER

1. NEWBORN BRACHIAL NERVES INJURIES

Disorder	Characteristics	Management
Erb-Duchenne palsy	• Injury to C5-C6 • Unable to abduct the shoulder, external rotation and supination of forearm, • **"Waiters tip"** appearance of the arm	Most cases resolve spontaneously but if it does not resolve in first 6 months of life, then patient may have permanent damage
Klumpke paralysis	• Injury to C7-T1 • Hand paralysis with Horner syndrome • **"Claw hand"** appearance of the hand	Same as above

2. CLAVICULAR FRACTURE

Clavicular fracture in a newborn is common during vaginal delivery. X-ray is the best diagnostic test. Clavicular fracture often self-resolves and requires no treatment other than **immobilization of the arm**

3. CLEFT LIP

Cleft lip is a birth defect caused by **failure of fusion of the maxillary and medial nasal processes.**

Treatment: surgical correction at 3 months of age

4. CLEFT PALATE

Cleft palate is a birth defect caused by **failure of fusion of the lateral palatine processes, nasal septum, and median palatine processes.**
Treatment: surgery between 9- 18 months of age.

5. BRANCHIAL CLEFT CYST

Brachial cleft cyst is a congenital epithelial cyst that is remnant of the second branchial cleft.
Symptoms: small neck mass present **lateral to midline**
Treatment: Surgical removal

6. THYROGLOSSAL DUCT CYST

Thyroglossal duct cyst is a congenital epithelial cyst that is remnant of the thyroglossal tract
Symptoms: **Midline** neck mass that moves with swallowing
Treatment: Surgical removal

7. MUSCULAR TORTICOLLIS

Muscular torticollis is caused by **mass on sternocleidomastoid** muscle
Diagnosis: **Cervical spine x-ray**, it is usually done to check the cervical spine
Treatment: Tx. **Passive stretching exercises**

8. KLIPPEL-FEIL SYNDROME

Klippel-Feil Syndrome is caused by **fusion of cervical vertebrae**
Diagnosis: **Cervical spine x-ray**
Treatment: **Surgery and physical therapy**

9. CONGENITAL HIP DYSPLASIA

Congenital hip dysplasia is dislocation of the hip in infants
Diagnosis
- Physical exam shows positive **Barlow maneuver and Ortolani maneuver. Barlow maneuver;** mild adduction of the hip while applying pressure on the knee causes hip dislocation. Ortolani maneuver moves the dislocated hip back into the socket. In **Ortolani maneuver,** index and middle finger are placed along the greater trochanter of femur and thumb along the inner thigh. Place the infant with hip and leg at 90 degrees and gently abduct the hip while lifting forward on the femur.
- Ultrasound of the hip is the diagnostic test

Treatment: Pavlik harness

10. CLUB FOOT

Clubfoot is a common foot abnormality in neonates

Symptoms: neonate is unable get **heel flat on the exam surface**

Management:

- Serial **casting, splints, orthesis and corrective shoes**
- If no complete resolution occurs in 3 months, then do **surgery**

11. NURSEMAID ELBOW

Nursemaid elbow also known as **radial head subluxation** that is caused by sudden traction or pulling the arm

Symptoms: physical exam shows affected arm is **pronated, adducted and flexed**

Treatment: combination of **extension, supination and abduction at 90°**

12. LEGG-CAVLÉ-PERTHES (AVASCULAR NECROSIS OF FEMORAL HEAD)

Legg-cavlé-perthes is childhood hip disorder caused by the disruption of blood flow to the head of the femur. Lack of blood supply leads to bone death (avascular necrosis). It is common in children between 2 to 8 years of age

Si/Sx: hip, knee or groin **pain that may exacerbate** with hip or leg movement, painful limp

Diagnosis

- Labs show **normal WBS and ESR**
- X-ray shows femoral **head sclerosis and femoral head widening**

Treatment: goal of management is to reduce pain and prevent permanent damage; casting, **rest, NSAIDs and get surgical consult**

13. SLIPPED CAPITAL FEMORAL EPIPHYSIS

Slipped capital femoral epiphysis refers to the separation of the ball of the hip joint from the femur. It is often seen in obese adolescence males

Si/Sx: knee pain, hip pain, **painful limp, externally rotated leg**

Diagnosis:

- X-ray of anterior posterior and frog lateral leg **view**
  - Early x-ray shows **widening of physis** without any slippage

- o **Later** x-ray shows **slippage** of acetabulum of femoral neck that gives " **ice-cream cone sign"**

- Management:
  - Immediate intervention with **surgical pinning** otherwise, the patient may develop **avascular necrosis**

14. TRANSIENT SYNOVITIS

Transient synovitis of the hip is a **self-limited inflammatory condition**. It is common in children between 5-10 years of age. It occurs following **viral infection** (most commonly an URI) or **trauma**

Si/Sx: low-grade fever, insidious onset of hip pain, pain in **groin, thigh and knee**

Diagnosis:
- Transient synovitis is a **diagnosis of exclusion**
- WBCs, ESR and x-ray are all normal

Treatment: Bed rest and NSAIDs

15. OSGOOD -SCHLATTER DISEASE

Osgood-Schlatter disease refers to **overuse knee injury**

Symptoms: Physical exam shows **tenderness and swelling** at **tibial tuberosity**

Treatment:
- Rest, knee immobilization and isometric exercise; complete resolution usually occurs in 1 -2 year

COLLAGEN VASCULAR DISEASE

1. JUVENILE RHEUMATOID ARTHRITIS (JRA)

Juvenile rheumatoid arthritis is the most common type of arthritis in children between 6 months to 16 years of age

Cause: Autoimmune

Types: three most common are of JRA are:
- **Systemic still's disease,** which causes joint pain, **daily spiking fever that returns to normal daily,** salmon colored rash, generalized lymphadenopathy, hepatosplenomegaly
- **Polyarticular arthritis,** which involves > 5 joints, causes low-onset fever and lethargy. It may progress to rheumatoid arthritis

- **Pauciarticular arthritis**, which involves < 4 joints, primarily knee, ankle and elbows

Diagnosis:
- Rheumatoid factor (RF)
- ESR
- ANA
- X-ray of joints

Treatment:
- NSAIDs are best initial therapy.
- If NSAIDs are ineffective, then give methotrexate

Follow-up: Routine slit-lamp ophthalmic examination to check for the development of uveitis

Prognosis: positive RF signifies poor prognosis, whereas positive ANA signifies good prognosis

2. KAWASAKI DISEASE

Kawasaki disease is an autoimmune disorder that affects the mucus membrane, lymph nodes, large and medium size blood vessels and heart. It is common in children < 5years of age, mainly Japanese children

Diagnosis: fever> 104°F for > 5 days, not responding to any antibiotics, plus 4 out of 5 criteria: (mnemonic CRASH)

1. Conjunctivitis
2. Nonvascular Rash
3. Coronary Artery aneurysm
4. Strawberry tongue, oropharyngeal erythema, dry & cracked lips
5. Hand and feet swelling, desquamation of fingertips

Treatment:
- Immediate **IVIG and high dose aspirin**
- If patient has platelet count > 1 million, then **add warfarin** to prevent hypercoagulable state
- Get baseline **2D echocardiogram;** follow **up 2D echo in 2-3 weeks** and **again at 6-8 weeks**

Complications of Kawasaki diseases are coronary artery aneurysm, myocarditis MI, CHF

Note: Kawasaki disease is the only exception in which aspirin is given to the children.

Boards tip:
Patient with scarlet fever may present with similar symptoms as Kawasaki disease. To distinguish them look at the rash; rash in scarlet fever is characterized as" Sand paper"

3. HENOCH-SCHÖNLEIN PURPURA (HSP)
Henoch-Schönlein purpura is an immunoglobulin (IgA) mediated vascular damage that causes the inflammation and bleeding in the small blood vessels in skin, joints, intestines and kidney
Si/Sx: abdominal pain, **petechiae and purpura on legs and buttocks,** hematuria
Diagnosis:
- Urinalysis may show RBC casts
- Blood test shows **increased platelet**
- **Increased WBCs and ESR**
- **Increased IgA and IgM immunoglobulins**

Treatment:
- Symptomatic treatment for mild disease
- Patient with severe disease may require steroids

Boards tip:

Patients with ITP also present with similar symptoms. To distinguish them look at the platelet count; which are increased in HSP, and decreased in ITP

NEUROLOGY

1. NEWBORN HEAD CONDITIONS

Condition	Characteristics	Treatment
Caput Succedaneum	• **Diffuse swelling** of the scalp that crosses **the midline suture**	No treatment, resolves itself in days
Cephalohematoma	• **Subperiosteal hematoma** that **does not cross** the midline suture • May need do CT head to rule out fracture	No treatment, resolve itself in weeks to months

Anterior fontanelle usually closes by 18 months of age. Delayed closure or abnormally large fontanelle usually suggests IUGR, rickets, hydrocephalus or hypothyroidism

2.   SPINA BIFIDA
Spina bifida is a congenital disorder of the spinal cord. It is caused by incomplete closure of the embryonic neural tube. Three types of spina bifida are:

2a. **Spina bifida occulta** (occulta means hidden) is often **hidden by newborn's skin.** In some patients, it is found incidentally during x-ray or other imaging. However, in some cases classic clues may be helpful such as **abnormal tufts of hair on the back, dimple on the skin, collection of fat or skin discoloration on the skin** above spinal defect.

2b. **Meningocele** is a rare form, in this condition **meninges** (membrane of the spinal cord) **comes out of the vertebral opening**

2c. **Myelomeningocele** is a severe form, in this **condition meninges** and **spinal cord** comes out of the vertebral defect.

Prevention: neural tube defects can be prevented
- Pregnant woman **without risk factors** should take **1mg folic acid** per day
- Pregnant woman **with risk factors** should take **4 mg folic** acid per day

3.   NEUROFIBROMATOSIS
Neurofibromatosis is a genetic disorder of the nervous system. Two main types of neurofibromatosis are:

3a. **Type 1 neurofibromatosis** is an autosomal dominant defect in chromosome 7. Patients usually present with **café-au-lait spot, axillary freckles, pigmented Lisch nodules**

3b. **Type 2 neurofibromatosis** is an autosomal dominant defect in chromosome 22. Patient usually present with bilateral acoustic neuroma (**bilateral hearing loss**), gait disturbance

Management for both types of neurofibromatosis:
- Supportive treatment
- **Annual ophthalmologic exam**

4. FEBRILE SEIZURE

Febrile seizure is characterized by seizure lasting < 15 minutes, which is triggered by a fever (> 102° F). It is common in otherwise healthy children between 9 months to 5 years of age

Diagnosis:
- Physical exam is usually normal
- No imaging is needed
- Rule out meningitis and other causes of fever

Treatment: Acetaminophen is given to control fever

Other important points about febrile seizure
- Patients with **simple febrile seizure** are **not at risk of** developing epilepsy
- **Risk of epilepsy is increased** if patient has:
  - Atypical seizure lasting >15 minutes and focal findings
  - First seizure before < 9 months of age
  - Pre-existing neurological disorder or abnormal development
  - Family history of epilepsy

5. SEIZURE

Type	Presenting features	EEG	Treatment
Absence Seizure	Complete loss of facial expression, motor and speech with eyes and facial fluttering	3 sec spike & wave	Ethosuximide
Juvenile myoclonic Epilepsy	**Jerky movements in the morning**	Irregular spike & wave	Valproic acid
West syndrome (Infantile spams)	**Flexor and extensor** Spams **of trunk and extremities**	Irregular interspersed spikes and waves	**ACTH,** If ACTH is ineffective, then give **Prednisone**

6.   TUBEROUS SCLEROSIS

Tuberous sclerosis is a multi-system genetic disorder that affects the skin, nervous system, kidneys, heart

Si/Sx: **acneform facial** nodule, **orange-peel skin** lesion on lumbosacral region, **hypopigmented skin lesions**

Diagnosis:

- **CT head shows** calcified ventricle, which can lead to obstructive hydrocephalus
- Ultrasound of the kidney
- Slit lamp examination of skin shows **hypopigmented skin lesions** that darkens with slit lamp examination

Treatment: there is no specific treatment; treatment depends on the symptoms

HEMATOLOGY

1.   LEAD POISONING

Lead poisoning screening is usually done in children at 12 months of age, but it is done at 6 months of age in children with high risk factors

High risk factors: living in building built before 1960's or painted before 1978, eating paint, live near battery recycling plant

Si/Sx: **change in behavior, stomach pain, constipation, lead lines on gums**

Diagnosis:

- Labs: MCV< 90, hypochromic anemia, basophilic stippling, increased free erythrocyte porphyrin
- Best initial test is **blood lead level**
- Confirmatory test is **venous blood level**
- **X-ray** of the long bone shows dense lead lines

Treatment: usually depends on blood lead level (discussed on the next page)

Blood lead level and management

Blood lead level (BLL) g/dl	Management
10 – 14	Educate patient and family, repeat BLL **in 3 months**
15 - 19	Educate patient and family, repeat BLL **in 2 months**
20 - 44	Educate patient and family, repeat BLL **in 1 month**
45 - 70	Remove patient from source, and give **EDTA*** or **DMSA***
≥ 70	Hospitalization + 2 medicines • If a patient has **encephalop**athy, then give **EDTA*+ BAL*** • If a patient has **no encephal**opathy, then give **EDTA*+ BAL* or DMSA***

*EDTA = Ethylenediaminetetraacetic acid
*BAL = Dimercaprol or British anti-lewisite
*DMSA= Succimer or 2,3-dimercaptosuccinic acid

2. ANEMIA

Anemia in infants usually seen around 9-24 months of age
Cause: most common in infant is **feeding cow's milk before 6 months of age**
Diagnosis:
- Best initial test is CBC, which shows **decreased ferritin**
- Most accurate test is **bone marrow biopsy**

Treatment:
- Oral sulfate
- Limit intake of cow's milk and increase dietary iron

Follow-ups:
- Reticulocytes should increase in 72-96 hours after the initiation of therapy and hemoglobin increases over 4-30 days
- Once the iron store is replenished continue iron therapy for the next 8 weeks

3. SICKLE CELL ANEMIA

Sickle cell is an autosomal recessive trait, caused by point mutation, which results in glutamic acid being substituted for valine at position 6 of the beta chain or change in base pair thiamine for adenosine

Diagnosis:

- Best initial test: peripheral smear –shows sickling of RBC
- Confirmatory test: **Hemoglobin electrophoresis**

Management:

- Regular immunization
- **Influenza given** at age 6 months and annually
- Give **pneumococcal** at age 2 months, **meningococcal** at 2 years of age
- **Penicillin prophylaxis** starting at age of 2 months, then continue it until 5 years of age
- **Daily folate** replacement
- Hydroxyurea is usually give to prevent painful crisis
- Transfusion as needed
- **Definitive therapy**: Bone marrow transplant

Complication:

- Patients are at increased for auto-splenectomy around 6 months of age. After auto-splenectomy patient are at increased risk of infection from encapsulated bacteria such as S. Pneumococcus, H. influenza, N.meningitidis
- Most common cause of mortality is acute chest syndrome
- Patient should have yearly ophthalmology exam and transcranial Doppler

4. VON WILLEBRAND DISEASE (VWD)

Von Willebrand disease is the most common heredity bleeding disorder. It is an autosomal dominant disorder caused by a deficiency of von Willebrand factor (vWF). vWF is required for platelet adhesion

Si/Sx: Platelet type bleeding: petechia, purpura, epistaxis, bleeding form gums, and heavy menstrual flow in women

Diagnosis:

- CBC shows normal platelet count
- Bleeding time shows **increased aPTT**
- Factor VIII level

- **Most accurate is VWF level and ristocetin cofactor test** (detects VWF function)

Treatment:
- **Best initial treatment is desmopressin (DDAVP)**, which releases the vWF from endothelial cells.
- If it is ineffective, then give factor **VIII replacement.**
- VIII replacement is best treatment during emergency or for major surgery

5.   IDIOPATHIC THROMBOCYTOPENIC PURPURA (ITP)

Idiopathic thrombocytopenic purpura is characterized by isolated low platelet count (thrombocytopenia)

Cause: there is no specific known cause. Some known causes include viral illness (such as mumps, measles or flu), leukemia, lymphoma, anti-platelet antibody

Si/Sx: petechiae, purpura, prolong bleeding from cuts, epistaxis, bleeding gums, heavy menstrual flow in women and **normal size spleen**

Note: enlarged spleen size suggests possible other causes of thrombocytopenia

Diagnosis:
- Idiopathic thrombocytopenic purpura is a diagnosis of exclusion. It is important to rule out other cause of thrombocytopenia
- CBC shows **low platelet count**, and normal RBCs and WBCs
- **Normal clotting factors with prolong bleeding time**

Treatment:
- Initial treatment is **prednisone**
- If prednisone is ineffective, then give **IVIG**

6. HEMOPHILIA

Hemophilia is a rare **x-linked recessive disorder**, in which blood does not clot properly. It is more common in males, and female are asymptomatic carriers

Types: Hemophilia A (Factor VIII deficiency), Hemophilia B (Factor IX deficiency)

Si/Sx: signs and symptoms depend on the level of the deficient factor. Patient with very low level of factor may experience spontaneous bleeding, whereas, patients with slight deficiency may only bleed after trauma or surgery.

Diagnosis:
- Normal bleeding time and PT, **increased PTT**
- **Mixing study:**
  - If mixing study corrects the PTT time, then it means that the patient has factor deficiency.
  - If mixing study does not fix corrects the PTT, then that patient may other condition (discussed in mixing studies evaluation below)
- **Most accurate** test is **specific factor assay,** this test is performed if mixing study corrects the PTT

Treatment: discussed below

Hemophilia treatment

Condition	Treatment
Hemophilia A	• Vasopressin for mild bleeding • Factor VIII replacement for severe bleeding
Hemophilia B	• Factor IX replacement

MIXING STUDIES EVALUATION

- If prolongation is **corrected** - Dx. Clotting **factor deficiency**
- If prolongation is **not corrected** or **partially corrected-** Dx. Coagulation factor **inhibitor**
- If prolongation is **increased -** Dx. **Antibody** is present
- If prolongation is **increased,** as well as **PTT-** Dx. **Lupus anticoagulant**

RENAL AND URINARY TRACT MALFORMATION

1. HYPOSPADIAS
Hypospadias is a congenital defect in which there is an **abnormal opening on the ventral (underside) side of the penis.** In this condition parents of the patients are advised to **not to have circumcision in newborn** because the foreskin of the penis is used to close the hypospadias

2. EPISPADIAS
Epispadias is a congenital defect in which urethra ends in an abnormal opening on the **dorsal (upper) side of the penis.** This condition is often associated with exstrophy of the bladder. Therefore, it is essential to get an urologist consult before repairing the epispadias

3. CRYPTORCHIDISM
Cryptorchidism or undescended testes is a condition in which **one or both testes fail to descend** in the scrotum. Normally testes are fully descended in the scrotum by 1year of life. Patient is **observed until 1 year of age** and if tests **do not descend by that time, then surgery is performed.** Cryptorchidism is associated with **testicular cancer; higher the testes are found higher the risk.** Moreover, risk of testicular cancer **does not decrease after the surgery.**

4. HYDROCELE
Hydrocele is fluid-filled sac in the scrotum. It is common is newborn infants. However, in some cases it may occur with an inguinal hernia.
Diagnosis:
- Physical exam: **scrotum** may **light up** with transillumination test (shine a light through scrotum)
- Ultrasound can confirm the diagnosis

Treatment: Hydroceles usually resolves within 6 months. However, if hydrocele is caused by inguinal hernia, then it should be surgically corrected

5. VARICOCELE
Varicocele is an abnormal **dilation of the pampiniform venous plexus** in the scrotum
Si/Sx: aching pain in the scrotum, feeling of heaviness in the testicles

Diagnosis:
- Scrotum exam shows visibly enlarged veins " **bag of worms**"
- Most accurate test is ultrasound

Treatment: treatment may not be necessary, but it is surgically repaired if it is causing severe pain, testicular atrophy or infertility

6. OBSTRUCTIVE UROPATHY

It a structural abnormality that affect the flow of urine

Symptom: look for a newborn, who is unable to **urinate first day of life** or has weak urinary stream

Physical exam: walnut-shaped mass above pubic symphysis

Diagnostic test: voiding cystourethrogram

Management:
- Best initial step is to empty the bladder with **foley catheter**
- Treatment of obstructive uropathy is **transurethral ablation**

7. URINARY TRACT INFECTION (UTI)

Urinary tract infection is the infection of urinary tract (kidney, ureters, bladder or urethra). Infection of the bladder is called **cystitis,** infection of the kidney is called **pyelonephritis**

Symptoms:
- Cystitis: urgency, frequency, suprapubic pain, no fever
- Pyelonephritis: fever, CVA tenderness, nausea and vomiting

Cause
- Most common cause in males and female is **E.coli**
- In males it is usually due to **uncircumcision**
- In females it is usually caused by **wiping from back to front,** sexual activity, pregnancy

Diagnosis: **Urine culture**
- If child is toilet trained, then get **midstream collection**
- If child is not toilet trained, then get **suprapubic tap or catheterization**

Management:
- Cystitis – Tx. Outpatient treatment with oral amoxicillin, or nitrofurantoin or TMP-SMX
- Pyelonephritis – Tx. Inpatient treatment with **IV gentamicin and ceftriaxone or ampicillin**

Further management:

- **Renal ultrasound** is performed is patient has **febrile UTI**
- **Voiding cystourethrogram is performed if any of the following is present:**
  - Male patient
  - Females < 5 years of age
  - Febrile UTI
- **Urine culture** is usually preformed **1weeks** after **stopping antibiotics**

8. VESICOURETERAL REFLUX (VUR)

Vesicoureteral reflux is retrograde flow of urine

- During urination urine goes from **bladder to ureteral and kidney,** which may leads to **hydronephrosis and renal fibrosis,** and leads to **ESRD**

Symptom: **burning or painful urination**

Diagnosis:

- **Initial test** is Fluoroscopic voiding cystourethrogram (VCUG) **to check the grade of VUR**
- **Then, perform renal scan** to check for renal **scarring**
  - If scarring is found, then check creatinine periodically

Management:

- Most VUR resolve spontaneously
- **Prophylactic** medicine (TMP-SMX, Nitrofurantoin or trimethoprim) is given **for a year** to **prevent kidney damage**
- **Surgery is performed** if any of the following is present:
  - VCUG shows bilateral grade IV or V reflux
  - Patient develop UTI while taking antibiotic
  - Renal scan shows severe scarring

9. WILMS' TUMOR

Wilms' tumor is a rare tumor that may affect one or both kidneys. Usually seen in children between 2-4 years of age

Risk factors: Wilms tumor is associated with aniridia, hemihypertrophy, hypospadias, undescended testes, Beckwith-Wiedemann syndrome, WAGR syndrome: Wilms tumor, aniridia, genitourinary abnormalities, and mental retardation

Symptoms: painless abdominal or flank mass that **does not cross the midline**, fever, nausea, vomiting, hematuria, hypertension

Diagnosis:
- Abdominal ultrasound or CT shows intrarenal mass
- Biopsy is usually not done because of high risk abdominal seeding with malignant cells

Treatment:
- Total nephrectomy, chemotherapy and radiation
- Partial nephrectomy if both kidneys are involved

10. NEUROBLASTOMA

Neuroblastoma is a malignant tumor of the neural crest cell. It is usually seen in infants and children less than 2 years of age.

Location: most Neuroblastoma begins in adrenal gland, but they may occurs next to spinal cords or chest and spread to bones, face, skull, pelvic, shoulder, arms, legs, bone marrow, lymph node, eyes and skin

Si/Sx: opsoclonus-myoclonus syndrome also know as " **dancing eyes and dancing feet syndrome**", bone pain, flushed skin, tachycardia, profuse sweating

Diagnosis
- CBC, ESR, coagulation studies
- Urinary VMA and HMA
- Imaging: Abdominal and chest CT, bone scan
- BUN/Cr, LFTs

Treatment:
- Localized tumors are surgically resected
- Chemotherapy and radiation for metastatic tumors

11. TESTICULAR TORSION

Testicular torsion is the twisting of the spermatic cord, which blocks the testicle's blood supply

Si/Sx: sudden onset of testicular pain, nausea, vomiting, lightheadedness

Diagnosis:
- Physical exam shows **tender and high riding testes, and absent cremasteric reflex**
- Diagnoses can be confirmed with ultrasound, but it is rarely needed

Treatment: immediate surgical intervention

12. EPIDIDYMITIS
Epididymitis is characterized by inflammation of epididymis. It is common in young men between 19-35 years of age

Causes: gonorrhea and chlamydia are the most common cause, but other causes may include regular use of a urethral catheter, recent surgery of urinary tract

Si/Sx: testicular pain with fever, pyuria, painful scrotal swelling

Diagnosis:
- Physical exam shows **testes are at normal position**, tenderness around epididymis
- Urinalysis and urine culture

Treatment: bed rest and antibiotics

EAR INFECTION

1. OTITIS EXTERNA
Otitis Externa also know as swimmer's ear, is inflammation of the outer ear and ear canal

Si/Sx: severe pain with **manipulations of outer ear**

Cause: Excessive dryness, wetting

Diagnosis:
- Clinical diagnosis
- Ear exam may show thick otorrhea, edema, and erythema

Treatment:
- Combination of topical antibiotics **neomycin, polymyxin and topical steroids**
- If there is marked ear edema to the point that the ear canal is blocked and topical antibiotics may not penetrates far enough into the ear canal to be effective. Carefully place a **soaked wick** with **topical drops 3 times daily for 2 days to open the ear canal**, so that topical medicines will penetrate the canal

2. MALIGNANT OTITIS EXTERNA
Malignant otitis externa is a complication of otitis externa. **It affects and damages the bones of the ear canal, and base of the skull**

Risk factors: diabetes, chemotherapy week immune response

Cause: Pseudomonas, S. aureus, S. epidermis, Aspergillus

Diagnosis:
- Best initial diagnostic test is X-ray, CT or MRI of the head
- Most accurate test is biopsy

Treatment
- **Surgical debridement and IV ciprofloxacin**
- If **aspergillus is suspected**, then **add amphotericin** to the treatment. However, if patient has renal insufficiency, then give **lipophilic amphotericin**

3. OTITIS MEDIA

Otitis Media is an inflammation of the middle ear. It is common in children following upper respiratory infection (URI)

Cause: Eustachian tube drain fluid from the middle ear. Blockage of eustachian tube can lead to fluid buildup, which can cause ear infection

Risk factors: children between 6 months to 2 years are high risk due to short and straight eustachian tube, air pollution

Si/Sx: decreased hearing, ear pain, irritability fever, otorrhea

Diagnosis:
- Otoscope shows the followings:
  - **Loss of light reflex**
  - **Decreased mobility of tympanic membrane** (most sensitive and specific factor)

Management:
- Best initial treatment is **Amoxicillin**
  - If the patient is **allergic to penicillin**, then give **Azithromycin**
- If the patient is **not responding** to initial treatment **within 2-3 days**, then give **oral amoxicillin-clavulanate or IM ceftriaxone**
- If the patient is **still not responding**, then perform **Tympanocentesis or myringotomy**

Complication: Mastoiditis, meningitis

3a. ACUTE MASTOIDITIS

Acute Mastoiditis is complication of acute otitis media, which affects the mastoid bone

Diagnosis:
- Ear exam shows the followings:
  - Pinna is displaced inferior and anterior
  - Percussion of mastoid process causes pain

- CT of the temporal bone

Management: **depends on CT** of the temporal bone

- If CT of the temporal bone shows **inflammation,** then the treatment is **Myringotomy and IV antibiotics**
- If CT of temporal bone shows **inflammation and bone destruction,** then the treatment is **Mastoidectomy and**
- **IV antibiotics**

4.   OTITIS MEDIA WITH EFFUSION

Otitis media with effusion is characterized by a **non-purulent discharge in** the middle ear **without any symptoms of ear infection**

Diagnosis:

- Otoscope shows the fluid in the middle ear
- Audiometer or hearing test, but it is only performed if effusion is present for > 3 months

Management:

- Small effusion **do not require treatment** because they usually resolve spontaneously
- If effusion **does not resolve after three months, then** do **monthly hearing test**
- **Tympanostomy tube is placed if any of the following is present:**
  - **Effusion** is present for **4 months and patient has hearing loss**
  - **Bilateral** effusion is present for **6-12 months**

Complication of acute media: Acute Mastoiditis, Cholesteatoma

5.   CHOLESTEATOMA

Cholesteatoma is **abnormal squamous cell growth in the middle ear and** or **temporal bone**

Diagnosis:

- Ear exam shows **white opacity of tympanic membrane**
- Confirm with **CT of temporal bone**

Treatment: **Surgical resection**

ENDOCRINOLOGY

1. CONGENITAL HYPOTHYROIDISM

Congenital hypothyroidism is caused by decreased thyroid hormone production or agenesis of thyroid

Si/Sx: most infant have few or no symptoms, but infant with severe hypothyroidism may have **large tongue, hypotonia,** edema, mental retardation, umbilical hernia, widened anterior and posterior fontanels

Diagnosis: low T4 and increased TSH

Treatment: levothyroxine

Complications: Untreated or delayed treatment may lead to mental retardation and growth problems.

Note: it is mandated by the law to screen all newborn for hypothyroidism

2. CONGENITAL ADRENAL HYPERPLASIA (CAH)

Congenital adrenal hyperplasia is group of autosomal recessive disorders of adrenal gland

Types: three main types of CAH are: discussed below

Type	Characteristics	Treatment
21 -hydroxylase CAH	• **Hypotension and virilization** • **Diagnosis**: labs show **increased** K, ATCH and 17-hydroxyprogestrone, and **decreased** Na, aldosterone and cortisol	Prednisone, fluid and electrolytes replacement as needed
11-beta-hydroxylase CAH	• **Hypertension and virilization** • Diagnosis: **increased serum 11 -deoxycortisol**	Same as above
17alpha-hydroxylase CAH	• **Hypertension** • Diagnosis: labs shows **hypokalemia and metabolic alkalosis**	Same as above

NEWBORN JAUNDICE
Type: two main types of newborn jaundices are **physiologic** and
pathologic jaundice (discussed in below)

1. **PHYSIOLOGIC JAUNDICE**
Physiologic jaundice usually appears **2-4 days** after birth.
Mechanism: Before the baby is born and is growing inside the mother's
womb, placenta removes the bilirubin. After the baby is born, baby's liver
removes the bilirubin from the body via enzyme **glucuronosyltransferase.**
However, after birth it takes some time for the liver to gain its function, as
a result, unconjugated **bilirubin** increases, which results in physiologic
jaundice.
Cause:
   • Relative **glucuronosyltransferase** deficiency in newborn
   • Increased bilirubin production (In full-term newborn RBCs life
     span is 80-90 days, compare to adults 100-120 days)
Risk factors: factors that increase the risk of physiologic jaundice are
prematurity, polycythemia, breast feeding
Treatment: no treatment needed, physiologic jaundice usually clears on its
own

2. **PATHOLOGIC JAUNDICE**
Pathologic jaundice is caused by the factors that alter the bilirubin
metabolism in the liver
Characteristics of pathologic jaundice
   • If it appears in first 24 hours of life or after 14 days of life
   • Direct bilirubin> 2mg/dl/day
   • Total bilirubin increases > 5mg/dl/day
   • Total bilirubin > 12mg/dl/day in terms infant
Cause: Causes pathologic jaundice can be divided into conjugated and
unconjugated hyperbilirubinemia

Conjugated hyperbilirubinemia is caused by the followings:
   • **Infection:** TORCH infection, sepsis, hepatitis A & B, syphilis,
   • **Metabolic cause:** galactosemia, alpha -1 antitrypsin deficiency
   • **Heredity cause:** Rotor syndrome, Dubin-Johnson syndrome
   • **Other cause:** cystic fibrosis, hypothyroidism, **breastfeeding
     jaundice**

Unconjugated hyperbilirubinemia is caused by the followings:

- **Hemolytic** such as sickle cell disease, G6PD deficiency, Rh incompatibility, alpha-thalassemia
- **Congenital causes:** Crigler-Najjar syndrome, Gilbert syndrome
- **Other causes:** jaundice, polycythemia, hypothyroidism, **breast milk**

Complication: elevated unconjugated (indirect bilirubin) can cross the blood brain barrier and cause kernicterus (bilirubin encephalopathy)

Treatment:

- Treat the underlying cause
- When **unconjugated** bilirubin is **10-15 mg/dl,** start **phototherapy** to break down the bilirubin pigment
- If **phototherapy is ineffective** or patient has developed **bilirubin encephalopathy,** then do **exchange transfusion**

What is the difference between breastfeeding jaundice and breast milk jaundice?

Breastfeeding jaundice occurs in the **first week of life**. It is caused by insufficient breast milk intake, which results in dehydration or low caloric intake. Treatment: **Increase breastfeeding sessions to 8-10 time a day**

Breast milk jaundice occurs around **10-14 days of life**. There is no clear cause of breast milk jaundice. Substances in the maternal milk such as beta-glucuronidase and nonesterified fatty acid may inhibit the normal bilirubin metabolism, which increases the level of **unconjugated bilirubin.** Treatment: **phototherapy or exchange transfusion.** Breastfeeding it continued.

FAILURE TO THRIVE (FTT)

Failure to thrive as defined as **height and weight less than 5th percentile** for the age

Cause: FTT can be divided into three main types:

- **Organic factors**: when there is a mental or physical issue with the child himself. Such as GI disorders, inborn error of metabolism, cystic fibrosis, parasites, UTI
- **Inorganic factor**: when a caregiver is providing inadequate or improper feeding

- **Mixed** condition is caused when both organic and inorganic factors are present

Diagnosis:
- Plot height, weight and head circumference on growth chart
- Look for underlying condition
- Dietary history

Treatment: depends on cause
- Treat the underlying cause, if any
- Educate the parents about feeding infant and educate them about formula, food and liquids

GROWTH DISORDERS

1. SHORT STATURE
Short stature refers to any person whose height is significantly below, as compared to the people of same age and sex

Cause: it can be divided into three main types (discussed below)

1a. CONSTITUTIONAL GROWTH DELAY AND GENETIC SHORT STATURE
In both conditions **height & weight** are **equally decreased**

Patients are consistently growing on a growth curve, which is below the normal growth curve. For example: if their height was on 25-percentile growth curve, then they are consistently growing on the 25-percentile growth curve.

To differentiate between constitutional growth delay and genetic short stature look at the followings:
- **Check the bone age:**
  - o In **genetic** short stature **bone age** is **equal to the height age**
  - o In **constitutional** delay **bone age** is **delayed**
- **Puberty is delayed** in constitutional growth delay
- **Puberty** occurs **at normal time** in patients with genetic short stature

Treatment: reassurance

1b. GROWTH HORMONE DEFICIENCY
Patients have **normal weight gain,** but **length & height are decreased**

Patients in this group were growing consistently on the growth curve that is normal for their age and sex, but at some point they start to drop to lower and lower growth curve. Means, if they were growing on 75-percentile growth curve, then they dropped on 50-percentile growth curve and then to 25- percentile.
Diagnosis:
   •   IFG-1 & IGF-3
Treatment: GH injection

1c. MALNUTRIENT AND MALABSORPTION
Patient in this group have low weight, length and height, but the **weight is decreased more than length and height**
Diagnosis:
   •   Check the caloric intake
   •   Stool fat
   •   Sweat chloride
Treatment: Treat the underlying cause

Boards clue to get the diagnosis of tall stature patient:

   •   Tall patient with **a large head, ears and large testes** –Dx. **Fragile-X Syndrome**

   •   Tall patient with long limbs, **small testes, small penis and gynecomastia** –Dx. **Klinefelter syndrome** (XXY)

   •   Tall patient with a long face, long fingers, nodulocystic acne, **aggressive behavior** –Dx. **XYY male**

   •   Tall patient with the **long limbs and very long fingers** –Dx. **Marfan syndrome**

GENETIC DISORDERS

1. FRAGILE X SYNDROME
Cause: X-linked disorder associated with CGG trinucleotide repeats, affecting methylation and expression of Fragile X mental retardation protein (FMRP), which is required for normal neural development
Characteristics: elongated face with large jaw, large or everted ears, low muscle tone, hyperextensible ear, double-jointed thumbs, autism

2. DOUBLE Y MALES
Cause: genetic defect in which a male has an extra Y chromosome (XYY)
Characteristics: very tall height, nodulocystic acne, **antisocial behavior, aggressive**

3. KLINEFELTER SYNDROME
Cause: Genetic defect in which a male has an extra X chromosome (XXY)
Characteristic: tall height, **eunuchoid body shape** (long extremities, short trunk, shoulder equal to hip size)**, small testicles, gynecomastia, female type hair distribution**

4. DOWN SYNDOMRE
Cause: Down syndrome also known as trisomy 21, caused by presence of three copies of chromosome 21, instead of normal two copies
Characteristics: metal retardation (Down syndrome is the most common cause of mental retardation), **slanted palpebral fissure, epicanthal folds, transverse palmar crease**
Associated with endocardial cushion defect, VSD, ASD, duodenal atresia, hypothyroidism, increased risk of acute lymphocytic leukemia, Alzheimer's disease

5. EDWARDS' SYNDROME
Cause: Edwards' syndrome also known as trisomy 18, caused by presence of three copies of chromosome 18, instead of normal two copies
Characteristics: clenched fist with index finger **overlapping 3rd and** 4th fingers, **rocker bottom feet,** hammer toe, low set ears, hypoplastic mandible
Associated with VSD, ASD, Polycystic kidney disease
Life expectancy: patient usually dies within first year of life

6. PATAU'S SYNDROME

Cause: Patau's syndrome also known as trisomy 13, caused by presence of three copy of chromosome 13, instead of normal two copies

Characteristics: cleft lip, cleft palate, holoprosencephaly, small head, small eyes, polydactyly

Associated with VSD, ASD, Polycystic kidney disease

Life expectancy: patient usually dies within first year of life

7. TURNER SYNDROME

Cause: genetic defect in **females in which** one of the X chromosomes is missing (X0)

Characteristics: short stature, broad and flat chest, **wide spread nipples, sparse pubic hair, webbed neck, puffy hand and feet**

8. MARFAN SYNDROME

Cause: Autosomal dominant disorder, defect in folding of Fibrillin -1 protein

Characteristics: very tall height, slender limbs with long fingers and toes, flexible joints, **subluxation of lens in one or both eyes, scoliosis**

9. EHLERS-DANLOS SYNDROME

Cause: autosomal dominant defect in elastin gene

Characteristics: Hyperextensible skin, **blue sclera, easy scarring,** poor wound healing, increased joint mobility

10. PHENYLKETONURIA

Cause: autosomal recessive defect in phenylalanine hydroxylase, which is necessary to metabolize phenylalanine. Phenylalanine builds up and converts to phenylpyruvate

Characteristics: mental retardation, **fair skin, fair hair, eczema, fruity smell urine**

Treatment: diet modification, low phenylalanine and high tyrosine

11. GLACTOSEMIA

Cause: Galactose-1 phosphate uridyltransferase deficiency (most common types) impairs galactose metabolism

Characteristic: infant develops symptoms within few days after drinking formula or breast milk that contains lactose. Symptoms include irritability, lethargy, poor feeding, poor weight gain,

Treatment: lactose free milk

12. ANGELMAN SYNDROME
Cause: deletion of **maternal gene located on 15q13q11**
Characteristics: puppet-like movement, ataxia, inappropriate laughter and lack of speech

13. PRADER-WILLI SYNDROME
Cause: deletion of **paternal gene located on 15q13q11**
Characteristics: obese, **hyperphagia, short stature, small genitals,** small hands and feet

CHILDHOOD IMMUNODEFICIENCY

1. CHILDHOOD IMMUNODEFICIENCY

Condition	Characteristics	Treatment
Wiskott-Aldrich syndrome	• X-linked disease • Newborn with nonstop bleeding after circumcision • Triad consists of: **eczema, thrombocytopenia and recurrent infection** • Diagnosis: clinical and genetics	Bone marrow transplant
Chediak-Higashi syndrome	• Increased bleeding time, recurrent infection, albinism • Diagnosis: giant granules in leukocytosis	Bone marrow transplant
DiGeorge's syndrome	• New born with **tetany and seizure** (due to hypocalcemia) **within 24-48 hours of life** • Physical exam: wide set eyes and low set ears • Cause: congenital absent of 3rd and 4th pharyngeal pouch results in absent thymus and parathyroid • Diagnosis: clinical	Bone marrow transplant or thymus transplant
IgA deficiency	• Recurrent respiratory, **skin, GI, GU infection** • Anaphylaxis reaction during blood transfusion	Supportive care
Burton agammaglo-bulinemia	• Recurrent **sinopulmonary infection** starting around 6 months of age • **Small or absent lymph nodes, thymus and spleen** • Diagnosis: **B-cells are missing** and other **immunoglobulins are decreased**	IVIG
Severe combined immune deficiency	• Multiple viral, fungal and bacterial infections • Diagnosis: **Absence lymph nodes, thymus** and **spleen**	Bone marrow transplant
Chronic granulomatosis disease	• Recurrent **pneumonia, abscess formation** • Diagnostic test is **NBT or DHR test**	Bone marrow transplant

2. CHILDHOOD VIRAL ILLNESS

Virus	Characteristics	Treatment
Measles	• Maculopapular rash that starts on the face, then spreads down the body, and it fades in the similar pattern • **Cough, coryza, conjunctivitis** and **Koplik spots** (gray white spots on buccal mucosa) • Diagnosis: Clinical	Supportive and **oral vitamin A supplement**
Rubella	• Maculopapular rash that starts on the face, then spread down the body, and it fades in the similar pattern • **Retroauricular, posterior and occipital lymphadenitis, arthralgia** • Diagnosis: clinical	Supportive
Roseola (HHV-6)	• **High fever, up to 106°F or 41°C** and occipital lymphadenopathy. When **fever resolves** generalized **rose-colored** popular **rash appears** • Diagnosis: Clinical	**Supportive,** but if the patient is > **12 years of age or immunocom -promised,** then **IVIG and acyclovir**
Varicella	• **Pruritic rash** in **various stages**: macules, papules, vesicle and pustules • Diagnosis: Tzanck test, most accurate test is viral culture	Supportive and **topical ointment**
Erythema infectiosum (Parvovirus 19, fifth's disease)	• Fever, headache, malaise, **arthritis, lacy reticular rash** on extremities and over trunk, **"slapped cheek"** appearance on the face • Diagnosis: Clinical • Complication: aplastic anemia in a patient with sickle cell anemia	Supportive
Mumps	• Fever, headache, malaise **swelling of parotids** (unilateral or bilateral), **orchitis** • Diagnosis: Clinical diagnosis, **increased amylase** • Complication: infertility, but only if bilateral orchitis	Supportive and bed rest

3. HEREDITARY ANGIOEDEMA

Hereditary angioedema is a serious condition caused by hereditary deficiency of **C1 esterase inhibitor**

Si/Sx: **diffuse swelling** of face and airway, and abdominal cramping

Diagnosis: C1 inhibitor level, C1 inhibitor function, C2 and C4 complement pathway

Treatment:

- **Acute attack treatment: Fresh frozen plasma, it contains C1 inhibitor**
- Chronic treatment: androgen medication (danazol, or stanzol), these increasing the liver production of C1 esterase inhibitor, which reduces the frequency and severity of the attacks.

TORCH INFECTION

1. TOXOPLASMOSIS

Presentation: newborn with intracranial calcification, chorioretinitis, hydrocephalus

Cause: if during pregnancy mother consumes infected food (raw meat, drinking raw goat milk) or handles infected cat feces

Diagnosis: IgM serology,

Treatment: Pyrimethamine and sulfadiazine to mother

Prevention

- Mother should avoid above mention risk factor during pregnancy
- Spiramycin given to mother to prevent vertical transmission

2. VARICELLA-ZOSTER

Presentation: newborn with limb hypoplasia, " **zigzag**" skin lesions

Risk: Fetus or newborn is at risk of acquiring infection, if rash appears on mother 5 days before the delivery or 2 days after the delivery

Treatment: VariZIG to mother and neonate

Prevention: VZIG within 96 hours after exposure, but VZIG only decreases the effects of virus, it doesn't cures infection

Complication: Maternal pneumonia during varicella zoster infection is the leading cause of maternal death

3. SYPHILIS
Presentation: depends on time
- **Large edematous placenta** at birth
- Early (<2 years of age) presentation includes snuffles, failure to thrive, maculopapular rash
- Late (>2 years of age) presentation includes Mulberry molars, Hutchinson teeth, saber shins, saddle nose

Diagnosis:
- Best initial test is VDRL or RPR
- Most accurate test is FTA ABS or dark field microscope

Treatment: none

Prevention: Penicillin is only the medicine given to the pregnant mother with positive syphilis to prevent fetal transmission

4. RUBELLA
Presentation: newborn with deafness (most common presentation), congenital heart disease (e.g. PDA), **blueberry muffin rash, cataract**

Diagnosis: IgM serology

Treatment: None

5. CYTOMEGALOVIRUS (CMV)
Presentation: Newborn presents with **periventricular calcification, sensorineural hearing loss**

Diagnosis:
- Best initial test is neonate's urine or saliva titer
- Most accurate is urine or saliva PCR

Treatment: Ganciclovir. Advise parents that ganciclovir doesn't cure the infection; it prevents viral shedding and hearing loss

6. HERPES SYMPLEX VIRUS
Presentation: Newborn with **pneumonia, shock, petechiae on skin, eye and mucous membrane**

Diagnosis:
- Best initial test is Tzanck smear
- Most Accurate is PCR

Treatment: Acyclovir (to mother)

Prevention: If **active lesions** are present on mother genitals **during L&D,** then perform C-section

SCARLET FEVER

Scarlet fever is a bacterial illness caused by group A Streptococcus bacteria. It is common in children between 2 -10 years of age

Si/Sx: 5 main characteristic of scarlet fever are:

1. Strawberry tongue
2. Sandpaper like rash on the trunk
3. Cervical adenopathy
4. Pharyngitis
5. Fever

Diagnosis:

- Throat culture for group A strep
- Rapid antigen test

Treatment: penicillin, azithromycin or cephalosporin. Antibiotic is given to treat infection and **prevent rheumatic fever.**

RHEUMATIC FEVER

Rheumatic fever is an inflammatory disease that can affect heart, joints, skin and brain. It is common in children between 5-15 years of age

Cause: it usually develops 14-28 days after infection with groups A streptococcus bacteria such as strep throat or scarlet fever

Si/Sx: Sydenham chorea (uncoordinated jerky movements of face, hands and feet), chest pain, joint pain, joint swelling, skin rash, skin nodules, fever

Diagnosis: diagnosis of rheumatic fever depends on **two factors:**

1. Jones criteria (2 major and 1 minor)

Major criteria	
	• Migratory arthritis
	• Carditis
	• Subcutaneous skin nodules
	• Skin rash (Erythema marginatum)
	• Sydenham's chorea
Minor criteria	• Fever
	• High ESR
	• Arthralgia
	• Prolong PR interval on EKG

2. In addition, evidence of prior group A streptococcus infection by either a culture or positive antistreptolysin O (ASO) antibody titer

Treatment:
- For symptomatic relief – Tx. **Aspirin**
- Treatment for the Group B. strep – Tx. **Penicillin**

INFECTIOUS MONONUCLEOSIS

Infectious mononucleosis is infection caused by Ebstein-Barr virus. It spreads through saliva that is why it is sometime called" kissing disease"

Si/Sx: fever, sore throat, cervical lymphadenopathy

Diagnosis:
- Physical exam shows hepatomegaly, splenomegaly
- CBC shows atypical lymphocytosis
- Heterophil antibody test:
  - If this test is positive, then **treat the patient**
  - If this test is negative, then check **IgM antibody for viral capsid antigen**

Treatment:
- Advise patient **no contact sports until splenomegaly resolves** (~6 weeks)
- **Mild** disease - Tx. **Supportive care**
- **If patient has severe** disease or **airway obstruction** - Tx. **Steroids**

Complication: Nasopharyngeal carcinoma, Burkitt Lymphoma

2013 Recommended Immunizations for Children from Birth Through 6 Years Old

Birth	1 month	2 months	4 months	6 months	12 months	15 months	18 months	19–23 months	2–3 years	4–6 years
HepB	HepB			HepB						
		RV	RV	RV						
		DTaP	DTaP	DTaP		DTaP				DTaP
		Hib	Hib	Hib	Hib					
		PCV	PCV	PCV	PCV					
		IPV	IPV	IPV						IPV
				Influenza (Yearly)*						
				MMR						MMR
				Varicella						Varicella
				HepA§						

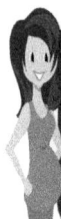

Is your family growing? To protect your new baby and yourself against whooping cough, get a Tdap vaccine towards the end of each pregnancy. Talk to your doctor for more details.

Shaded boxes indicate the vaccine can be given during shown age range.

NOTE: If your child misses a shot, you don't need to start over, just go back to your child's doctor for the next shot. Talk with your child's doctor if you have questions about vaccines.

FOOTNOTES: * Two doses given at least four weeks apart are recommended for children aged 6 months through 8 years of age who are getting a flu vaccine for the first time and for some other children in this age group.

§ Two doses of HepA vaccine are needed for lasting protection. The first dose of HepA vaccine should be given between 12 months and 23 months of age. The second dose should be given 6 to 18 months later. HepA vaccination may be given to any child 12 months and older to protect against HepA. Children and adolescents who did not receive the HepA vaccine and are at high-risk, should be vaccinated against HepA.

If your child has any medical conditions that put him at risk for infection or is traveling outside the United States, talk to your child's doctor about additional vaccines that he may need.

SEE BACK PAGE FOR MORE INFORMATION ON VACCINE-PREVENTABLE DISEASES AND THE VACCINES THAT PREVENT THEM

For more information, call toll free
1-800-CDC-INFO (1-800-232-4636)
or visit
http://www.cdc.gov/vaccines

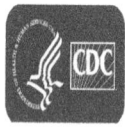

CDC

U.S. Department of Health and Human Services
Centers for Disease Control and Prevention

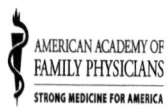

AMERICAN ACADEMY OF FAMILY PHYSICIANS
STRONG MEDICINE FOR AMERICA

American Academy of Pediatrics
DEDICATED TO THE HEALTH OF ALL CHILDREN

Vaccine-Preventable Diseases and the Vaccines that Prevent Them

Disease	Vaccine	Disease spread by	Disease symptoms	Disease complications
Chickenpox	Varicella vaccine protects against chickenpox.	Air, direct contact	Rash, tiredness, headache, fever	Infected blisters, bleeding disorders, encephalitis (brain swelling), pneumonia (infection in the lungs)
Diphtheria	DTaP* vaccine protects against diphtheria.	Air, direct contact	Sore throat, mild fever, weakness, swollen glands in neck	Swelling of the heart muscle, heart failure, coma, paralysis, death
Hib	Hib vaccine protects against *Haemophilus influenzae* type b.	Air, direct contact	May be no symptoms unless bacteria enter the blood	Meningitis (infection of the covering around the brain and spinal cord), intellectual disability, epiglottitis (life-threatening infection that can block the windpipe and lead to serious breathing problems), pneumonia (infection in the lungs), death
Hepatitis A	HepA vaccine protects against hepatitis A.	Direct contact, contaminated food or water	May be no symptoms, fever, stomach pain, loss of appetite, fatigue, vomiting, jaundice (yellowing of skin and eyes), dark urine	Liver failure, arthralgia (joint pain), kidney, pancreatic, and blood disorders
Hepatitis B	HepB vaccine protects against hepatitis B.	Contact with blood or body fluids	May be no symptoms, fever, headache, weakness, vomiting, jaundice (yellowing of skin and eyes), joint pain	Chronic liver infection, liver failure, liver cancer
Flu	Flu vaccine protects against influenza.	Air, direct contact	Fever, muscle pain, sore throat, cough, extreme fatigue	Pneumonia (infection in the lungs)
Measles	MMR** vaccine protects against measles.	Air, direct contact	Rash, fever, cough, runny nose, pinkeye	Encephalitis (brain swelling), pneumonia (infection in the lungs), death
Mumps	MMR** vaccine protects against mumps.	Air, direct contact	Swollen salivary glands (under the jaw), fever, headache, tiredness, muscle pain	Meningitis (infection of the covering around the brain and spinal cord), encephalitis (brain swelling), inflammation of testicles or ovaries, deafness
Pertussis	DTaP* vaccine protects against pertussis (whooping cough).	Air, direct contact	Severe cough, runny nose, apnea (a pause in breathing in infants)	Pneumonia (infection in the lungs), death
Polio	IPV vaccine protects against polio.	Air, direct contact, through the mouth	May be no symptoms, sore throat, fever, nausea, headache	Paralysis, death
Pneumococcal	PCV vaccine protects against pneumococcus.	Air, direct contact	May be no symptoms, pneumonia (infection in the lungs)	Bacteremia (blood infection), meningitis (infection of the covering around the brain and spinal cord), death
Rotavirus	RV vaccine protects against rotavirus.	Through the mouth	Diarrhea, fever, vomiting	Severe diarrhea, dehydration
Rubella	MMR** vaccine protects against rubella.	Air, direct contact	Children infected with rubella virus sometimes have a rash, fever, swollen lymph nodes	Very serious in pregnant women—can lead to miscarriage, stillbirth, premature delivery, birth defects
Tetanus	DTaP* vaccine protects against tetanus.	Exposure through cuts in skin	Stiffness in neck and abdominal muscles, difficulty swallowing, muscle spasms, fever	Broken bones, breathing difficulty, death

* DTaP combines protection against diphtheria, tetanus, and pertussis.
** MMR combines protection against measles, mumps, and rubella.

Last updated on 03/20/2013 • CS239274-A

2013 Recommended Immunizations for Children from 7 Through 18 Years Old

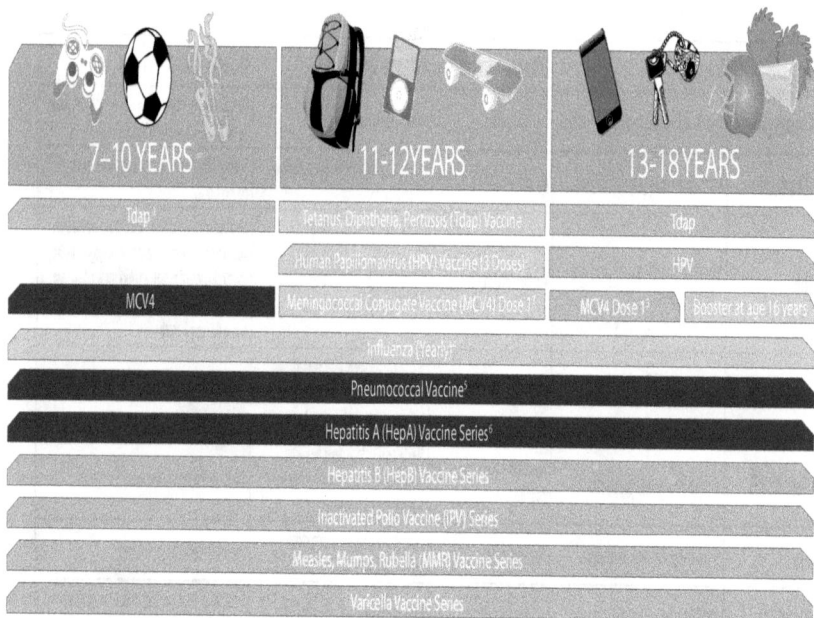

7–10 YEARS	11-12 YEARS	13-18 YEARS
Tdap¹	Tetanus, Diphtheria, Pertussis (Tdap) Vaccine	Tdap
	Human Papillomavirus (HPV) Vaccine (3 Doses)	HPV
MCV4	Meningococcal Conjugate Vaccine (MCV4) Dose 1³	MCV4 Dose 1³ — Booster at age 16 years
	Influenza (Yearly)	
	Pneumococcal Vaccine⁵	
	Hepatitis A (HepA) Vaccine Series⁶	
	Hepatitis B (HepB) Vaccine Series	
	Inactivated Polio Vaccine (IPV) Series	
	Measles, Mumps, Rubella (MMR) Vaccine Series	
	Varicella Vaccine Series	

These shaded boxes indicate when the vaccine is recommended for all children unless your doctor tells you that your child cannot safely receive the vaccine.

These shaded boxes indicate the vaccine should be given if a child is catching-up on missed vaccines.

These shaded boxes indicate the vaccine is recommended for children with certain health conditions that put them at high risk for serious diseases. Note that healthy children **can** get the HepA series⁶. See vaccine-specific recommendations at www.cdc.gov/vaccines/pubs/ACIP-list.htm.

FOOTNOTES

¹ Tdap vaccine is combination vaccine that is recommended at age 11 or 12 to protect against tetanus, diphtheria and pertussis. If your child has not received any or all of the DTaP vaccine series, or if you don't know if your child has received these shots, your child needs a single dose of Tdap when they are 7-10 years old. Talk to your child's health care provider to find out if they need additional catch-up vaccines.

² All 11 or 12 year olds – both girls *and* boys – should receive 3 doses of HPV vaccine to protect against HPV-related disease. Either HPV vaccine (Cervarix® or Gardasil®) can be given to girls and young women; only one HPV vaccine (Gardasil®) can be given to boys and young men.

³ Meningococcal conjugate vaccine (MCV) is recommended at age 11 or 12. A booster shot is recommended at age 16. Teens who received MCV for the first time at age 13 through 15 years will need a one-time booster dose between the ages of 16 and 18 years. If your teenager missed getting the vaccine altogether, ask their health care provider about getting it now, especially if your teenager is about to move into a college dorm or military barracks.

⁴ Everyone 6 months of age and older—including preteens and teens—should get a flu vaccine every year. Children under the age of 9 years may require more than one dose. Talk to your child's health care provider to find out if they need more than one dose.

⁵ A single dose of Pneumococcal Conjugate Vaccine (PCV13) is recommended for children who are 6 - 18 years old with certain medical conditions that place them at high risk. Talk to your healthcare provider about pneumococcal vaccine and what factors may place your child at high risk for pneumococcal disease.

⁶ Hepatitis A vaccination is recommended for older children with certain medical conditions that place them at high risk. HepA vaccine is licensed, safe, and effective for all children of all ages. Even if your child is not at high risk, you may decide you want your child protected against HepA. Talk to your healthcare provider about HepA vaccine and what factors may place your child at high risk for HepA.

For more information, call toll free 1-800-CDC-INFO (1-800-232-4636) or visit http://www.cdc.gov/vaccines/teens

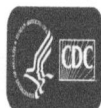

U.S. Department of Health and Human Services
Centers for Disease Control and Prevention

American Academy of Pediatrics
DEDICATED TO THE HEALTH OF ALL CHILDREN™

AMERICAN ACADEMY OF FAMILY PHYSICIANS
STRONG MEDICINE FOR AMERICA

Vaccine-Preventable Diseases and the Vaccines that Prevent Them

Diphtheria (Can be prevented by Tdap vaccine)

Diphtheria is a very contagious bacterial disease that affects the respiratory system, including the lungs. Diphtheria bacteria can be passed from person to person by direct contact with droplets from an infected person's cough or sneeze. When people are infected, the diphtheria bacteria produce a toxin (poison) in the body that can cause weakness, sore throat, low-grade fever, and swollen glands in the neck. Effects from this toxin can also lead to swelling of the heart muscle and, in some cases, heart failure. In severe cases, the illness can cause coma, paralysis, and even death.

Hepatitis A (Can be prevented by HepA vaccine)

Hepatitis A is an infection in the liver caused by hepatitis A virus. The virus is spread primarily person-to-person through the fecal-oral route. In other words, the virus is taken in by mouth from contact with objects, food, or drinks contaminated by the feces (stool) of an infected person. Symptoms include fever, tiredness, loss of appetite, nausea, abdominal discomfort, dark urine, and jaundice (yellowing of the skin and eyes). An infected person may have no symptoms, may have mild illness for a week or two, or may have severe illness for several months that requires hospitalization. In the U.S., about 100 people a year die from hepatitis A.

Hepatitis B (Can be prevented by HepB vaccine)

Hepatitis B is an infection of the liver caused by hepatitis B virus. The virus spreads through exchange of blood or other body fluids, for example, from sharing personal items, such as razors or during sex. Hepatitis B causes a flu-like illness with loss of appetite, nausea, vomiting, rashes, joint pain, and jaundice. The virus stays in the liver of some people for the rest of their lives and can result in severe liver diseases, including fatal cancer.

Human Papillomavirus (Can be prevented by HPV vaccine)

Human papillomavirus is a common virus. HPV is most common in people in their teens and early 20s. It is the major cause of cervical cancer in women and genital warts in women and men. The strains of HPV that cause cervical cancer and genital warts are spread during sex.

Influenza (Can be prevented by annual flu vaccine)

Influenza is a highly contagious viral infection of the nose, throat, and lungs. The virus spreads easily through droplets when an infected person coughs or sneezes and can cause mild to severe illness. Typical symptoms include a sudden high fever, chills, a dry cough, headache, runny nose, sore throat, and muscle and joint pain. Extreme fatigue can last from several days to weeks. Influenza may lead to hospitalization or even death, even among previously healthy children.

Measles (Can be prevented by MMR vaccine)

Measles is one of the most contagious viral diseases. Measles virus is spread by direct contact with the airborne respiratory droplets of an infected person. Measles is so contagious that just being in the same room after a person who has measles has already left can result in infection. Symptoms usually include a rash, fever, cough, and red, watery eyes. Fever can persist, rash can last for up to a week, and coughing can last about 10 days. Measles can also cause pneumonia, seizures, brain damage, or death.

Meningococcal Disease (Can be prevented by MCV vaccine)

Meningococcal disease is caused by bacteria and is a leading cause of bacterial meningitis (infection around the brain and spinal cord) in children. The bacteria are spread through the exchange of nose and throat droplets, such as when coughing, sneezing or kissing. Symptoms include nausea, vomiting, sensitivity to light, confusion and sleepiness. Meningococcal disease also causes blood infections. About one of every ten people who get the disease dies from it. Survivors of meningococcal disease may lose their arms or legs, become deaf, have problems with their nervous systems, become developmentally disabled, or suffer seizures or strokes.

Mumps (Can be prevented by MMR vaccine)

Mumps is an infectious disease caused by the mumps virus, which is spread in the air by a cough or sneeze from an infected person. A child can also get infected with mumps by coming in contact with a contaminated object, like a toy. The mumps virus causes fever, headaches, painful swelling of the salivary glands under the jaw, fever, muscle aches, tiredness, and loss of appetite. Severe complications for children who get mumps are uncommon, but can include meningitis (infection of the covering of the brain and spinal cord), encephalitis (inflammation of the brain), permanent hearing loss, or swelling of the testes, which rarely can lead to sterility in men.

Pertussis (Whooping Cough) (Can be prevented by Tdap vaccine)

Pertussis is caused by bacteria spread through direct contact with respiratory droplets when an infected person coughs or sneezes. In the beginning, symptoms of pertussis are similar to the common cold, including runny nose, sneezing, and cough. After 1-2 weeks, pertussis can cause spells of violent coughing and choking, making it hard to breathe, drink, or eat. This cough can last for weeks. Pertussis is most serious for babies, who can get pneumonia, have seizures, become brain damaged, or even die. About two-thirds of children under 1 year of age who get pertussis must be hospitalized.

Pneumococcal Disease

(Can be prevented by Pneumococcal vaccine)

Pneumonia is an infection of the lungs that can be caused by the bacteria called pneumococcus. This bacteria can cause other types of infections too, such as ear infections, sinus infections, meningitis (infection of the covering around the brain and spinal cord), bacteremia and sepsis (blood stream infection). Sinus and ear infections are usually mild and are much more common than the more severe forms of pneumococcal disease. However, in some cases pneumococcal disease can be fatal or result in long-term problems, like brain damage, hearing loss and limb loss. Pneumococcal disease spreads when people cough or sneeze. Many people have the bacteria in their nose or throat at one time or another without being ill—this is known as being a carrier.

Polio (Can be prevented by IPV vaccine)

Polio is caused by a virus that lives in an infected person's throat and intestines. It spreads through contact with the feces (stool) of an infected person and through droplets from a sneeze or cough. Symptoms typically include sudden fever, sore throat, headache, muscle weakness, and pain. In about 1% of cases, polio can cause paralysis. Among those who are paralyzed, up to 5% of children may die because they become unable to breathe.

Rubella (German Measles) (Can be prevented by MMR vaccine)

Rubella is caused by a virus that is spread through coughing and sneezing. In children rubella usually causes a mild illness with fever, swollen glands, and a rash that lasts about 3 days. Rubella rarely causes serious illness or complications in children, but can be very serious to a baby in the womb. If a pregnant woman is infected, the result to the baby can be devastating, including miscarriage, serious heart defects, mental retardation and loss of hearing and eye sight.

Tetanus (Lockjaw) (Can be prevented by Tdap vaccine)

Tetanus is caused by bacteria found in soil. The bacteria enters the body through a wound, such as a deep cut. When people are infected, the bacteria produce a toxin (poison) in the body that causes serious, painful spasms and stiffness of all muscles in the body. This can lead to "locking" of the jaw so a person cannot open his or her mouth, swallow, or breathe. Complete recovery from tetanus can take months. Three of ten people who get tetanus die from the disease.

Varicella (Chickenpox) (Can be prevented by varicella vaccine)

Chickenpox is caused by the varicella zoster virus. Chickenpox is very contagious and spreads very easily from infected people. The virus can spread from either a cough, sneeze. It can also spread from the blisters on the skin, either by touching them or by breathing in these viral particles. Typical symptoms of chickenpox include an itchy rash with blisters, tiredness, headache and fever. Chickenpox is usually mild, but it can lead to severe skin infections, pneumonia, encephalitis (brain swelling), or even death.

Last updated on 01/16/2013 • CS237027-A

PEDIATRICS CCS

CASE # 1

Case introduction
A 6-years-old male patient is brought to the ER by his parents because of continues blood oozing at the tooth extraction site after the tooth extraction

Initial vitals signs
Temperature: 38.6 degrees
Pulse: 78 beats/min, regular rhythm
Respiration rate: 16/ minutes

Blood pressure, systolic 126 mm Hg
Blood pressure, disystolic 74 mm Hg

Height: 48.0 inches
Weight: 70.0 lbs.
Body mass index: 21.4 Kg/m2

History of present illness (HPI)
A 6-years-old male patient is brought to the ER by his parents because of continues blood oozing at the tooth extraction site after the tooth extraction two hours ago. His parents are not aware of any disease in him. He has no history of bruising, hematuria, hemoptysis, and liver disease. He does not have petechia, purpura, and recent trauma. His appetite is good.

Past medical history
Hospitalization: none
Other medical conditions: none
Current medication: none
Allergies: none
Vaccination: up to date

Family history
Father and mother are healthy

Review of systems:
General: see HPI
Skin: see HPI
HEENT: see HPI
Musculoskeletal: see HPI
Cardiology: see HPI
Abdominal: see HPI
Genitourinary: see HPI

Please see pages 1-5 for general CCS cases approach

Step 1. None (patient is stable does not require any emergency measures)

Step 2. Order complete physical exam, and then move the clock forward
to get the results
Results show:
- Blood oozing from the extracted tooth site
- Rest of the physical exam is normal

Step 3. Order the labs, and then move the clock forward to get the results
- CBC
- UA
- BMP
- PT/INR
- PTT
- Bleeding time
- Blood type and Rh
- LFT

- Results show:
  o CBC shows 8,000 WBC with 65 % PMN & 16 %
    lymphocytes
  o PT/INR- 13 sec/ L,
  o PTT- 53 sec,
  o Bleeding time 5 minutes
  o A + blood type

Step 4. None

Step 5. Keep the patient in the ER

Step 6. Order
- NPO

Step 7. Order lab to confirm the diagnosis, and then move then clock
forward to get the results

- Factor 8 & 9
- Reticulocytes count

- Results show:
  o Factor 8 is 4%
  o Factor 9 is WNL
  o Reticulocyte count is - 2 %

Step 8. May order hematology consultation

Step 9. Medicine: give Factor 8 therapy and do interval follows up:
- Follow PTT and factor 8 until they are normalize
- Send patient home and make a follow- up appointment after a week

Case usually ends here

Step 10. Counsel
- No Aspirin
- Seat belt
- Counsel parents

Diagnosis: Hemophilia A

Case # 2

Case introduction
A 4 month-old white male is brought to the ER by his parents because of 3 day history of cough, runny nose and wheezing

Initial vitals signs
Temperature: 37.8 degrees
Pulse: 148 beats/min, regular rhythm
Respiration rate: 30/ minutes

Blood pressure, systolic 88 mm Hg
Blood pressure, disystolic 52 mm Hg

Height: 24.0 inches
Weight: 14.0 lbs.
Body mass index: 17.0 Kg/m2

History of present illness (HPI)
A 4 month-old white male is brought to the ER by his parents because of 3 day history of cough, runny nose and wheezing. He was born at 40 weeks with normal vaginal delivery. He attends day care and has no known sick contacts. He is on formula diet and has not been eating well from last three days. He is coughing frequently, has vomited twice. He has no diarrhea. He is up to date with vaccination.

Past medical history
Hospitalization: none
Other medical conditions: none
Current medication: none
Allergies: none
Vaccination: up to date

Family history
Father and mother are healthy

Review of systems:
General: see HPI
Skin: see HPI
HEENT: see HPI
Musculoskeletal: see HPI
Cardiology: see HPI
Abdominal: see HPI
Genitourinary: see HPI

Please see pages 1-5 for general CCS cases approach

Step 1. Oder pulse oxygen saturation, and then move the clock forward to get the results

- Results shows:
- o   Oxygen saturation is 96%

Step 2. Order complete physical exam, and then move the clock forward to get the results

- Results show:
- o   Lung exam shows bilateral wheezing in all areas
- o   Rest of the physical exam is normal

Step 3. Order the labs, and then move the clock forward to get the results

- CBC
- UA
- BMP
- Chest x-ray
- ABG

- Results show
- o   WBC shows 14,00. ABG PaO2- 57mm Hg, PaCO2- 41mmHg, pH 7.35
- o   Chest x-ray shows focal atelectasis, hyperinflation of lungs

Step 4. Medicine

- Nebulized albuterol, ribavirin, epinephrine
- IV access and IV normal saline
- Humidified oxygen

Step 5. Admit the patent in wards

Step 6. Oder

- NPO

Step 7. Order labs

- Nasopharyngeal swab for RSV

Step 8. None

Step 9. Interval follow-ups every 1-2 hour until oxygen normalizes and patient feels better
- Discharge the patient and make a follow-up appointment after 2-4 days

Step 10. Counsel
- Wear seat belt
- Parents education- no smoking

Diagnosis: Bronchiolitis

OBSTETRICS

Gravida is total number of pregnancies, whether or not they were carried to terms, including the current pregnancy
Parity is total number of pregnancies carried > 20 weeks, including viable and non-viable
Term delivery is delivery of an infant after 37 weeks of gestation
Premature delivery or preterm delivery is delivery of an infant before 37 weeks of gestation

Estimated delivery date by Nagele rule = Last menstrual period (LMN) + 7 days – 3 months + 1 years
For example: if LMP began 04/20/ 2014, delivery date is 01/27/2015

PREGNANCY
Diagnosis: Pregnancy is diagnosed based on the followings:
- **Best initial test is urine β-HCG**
- Then, confirm the diagnosis with **transvaginal ultrasound**. It usually shows a gestational sac within first 4-5 weeks if β-HCG is ≥ 1,500 mIU/ml.

FIRST TRIMESTER PRENATAL TESTING

1. ANEMIA
Best initial test is CBC (normal hemoglobin (Hb) is 10-12 g/dl)
- If **Hb < 10 g/dl,** then **check MCV**
  - o If MCV**< 80** –Dx. **Iron deficiency anemia.** Treat it with **iron sulfate**
  - - If iron sulfate fails to raise Hb levels, then do hemoglobin electrophoresis to check if the patient has **thalassemia**
- If MCV**> 100**
  - o Most **common cause** of macrocytic anemia (MCV > 100) in pregnant women is **folic acid deficiency.** Treat it with **folate replacement**
  - o If the patient with macrocytic anemia (MCV > 100) and has **peripheral neuropathy**, then the **Dx. is B12 deficiency** and treat it with **Vitamin B12 replacement**

2. BLOOD TYPE, RH STATUS AND ANTIBODY SCREENING
- If the mother is **Rh-positive**, then there is **no need to give RhoGAM**
- If the mother is **Rh-negative**, then check **anti-D antibodies**
  - **If she has anti-D antibodies,** then there is **no use of giving** RhoGAM because she has already formed anti-D antibodies
  - If she **does not have anti-D antibodies,** then **give her RhoGAM at 28 weeks of gestation** and **within 72 hours after delivery**

Rh-negative mother with **no anti-D antibodies** should receive RhoGAM with any of the following:
- At 28 weeks of gestation and within 72 hours of the followings:
  - After delivery
  - **Miscarriage**
  - **Elective or spontaneous abortion**
  - **Amniocentesis**
  - **Placenta abruption**
  - **Placenta previa**
  - **Vaginal bleeding**

3. PLATELET COUNT
Thrombocytopenia is considered when platelet count is < 150,000

To distinguish gestational thrombocytopenia from other disorder such as HELLP syndrome, check the other values:
- Gestational thrombocytopenia shows isolated low platelet count
- HELLP syndrome shows low platelet, low RBCs, increase AST and ALT

4. SYPHILIS
- Best initial screening test is VDRL or RPR
- If it is positive, then make to sure to confirm it with FTA or MHA-TP before initiating the treatment because VDRL or RPR is positive in other disease as well

Treatment: IM penicillin. If the patient is allergic to penicillin, then desensitize her with oral penicillin and then still treat her with penicillin. It prevents transplacental transmission.

5. HIV

Make sure to **get patient consent** prior to performing any HIV tests
Diagnosis:

- Best initial test is ELISA
- Then, confirm the diagnosis with Western blot test
- CD 4 cell count

Treatment: Start HAART in pregnant women:

- If CD4 count is <500, then start HAART right away regardless of gestational age
- If CD4 count is > 500, then start HAART in 2nd trimester

Note: HAART treatment regimen in pregnant women must include ZDV and ZDV should be given intrapartum as well

HAART medicines that are **contraindicated** in pregnancy are:

- Nevirapine – side effects: fetal hepatotoxicity
- Efavirenz- side effects: neural tube defect
- Didanosine and stavudine – side effects: fetal lactic acidosis

Delivery options for a HIV-positive mothers are following:

- Women should be offered to have a C-section before 38 weeks of gestation, before the rupture of membrane
- Near-term women can have **elective C-section,** if she has high CD 4 T cells count and viral load <1,000 copies/ml
- Near–term pregnant women with **viral loads > 1,000 copies/ml** should have a C-section at 38 weeks gestation, before the rupture of membrane

1. What is the most common mode of fetal HIV transmission?
Answer. Vertical transmission to fetus with infected vaginal secretion during vaginal delivery

6. RUBELLA IgG ANTIBODIES
Check Rubella IgG antibodies
- If woman **does not have IgG Rubella antibodies**, then **do not give her rubella immunization** during pregnancy; advise her to stay away from a person who is known to have rubella infection, and give rubella immunization after the delivery

Important: If rubella immunoglobulin is given to a non-pregnant woman, then she should be advised to avoid conceiving for at least for 4 weeks after receiving rubella immunoglobulin

7. URINALYSIS AND URINE CULTURE
It is usually done to see if a pregnant woman has asymptomatic bacteriuria
Asymptomatic bacteriuria is characterized by presence of significant number **of bacteria (> 10,000 mL) in the urine**, but **no UTIs symptoms** are present
Treatment: pregnant woman is usually treated with Amoxicillin or nitrofurantoin otherwise she may develop pyelonephritis

8. GONORRHEA AND CHLAMYDIA
Symptoms: purulent discharge, urgency, frequency, burning while urinating,
Diagnosis:
- Best initial test is urethral swab **(gram stain and culture)**
- Diagnosis is confirmed with DNA Probe

Treatment:
- **If gonorrhea** is found on the culture, then treat the patient with **IM ceftriaxone and** single dose of **oral azithromycin**
- **Chlamydia** is treated with single dose of **oral azithromycin**

9. TRICHOMONAS
Trichomonas is a non-viral STD, it can cause premature labor in a pregnant woman
Diagnosis:
- Wet mount prep, which shows motile organism

Treatment: Metronidazole

10. BACTERIAL VAGINOSIS

Bacterial vaginosis is a normal vaginal flora it is only treated in symptomatic patients

11. TUBERCULOSIS (TB)

Diagnosis and treatment: As per TB

Note: Streptomycin is not given to pregnant woman because it causes ototoxicity in fetus

12. GLUCOSE SCREENING

Glucose screening is done at first visit only if the patients has risk factors for diabetes, such as obesity, family history, age >30, personal history of diabetes. Otherwise, glucose screening is performed between 24- 28 weeks of gestation

NORMAL WEIGHT GAIN DURING PREGNANCY

- Average weight gain during the pregnancy is approximately 28 lbs.

FETAL HEART TONE

- Between 10-12 weeks of gestation, fetal heart tones can be heard with Doppler ultrasound
- Between 16-20 weeks of gestation, fetal heart tones can be heard with normal stethoscope

UTERUS LOCATION AND SIZE

- Uterus enter the abdomen at 12th week of gestation
- Uterus reaches the umbilicus approximately at 20th week of gestation
- Uterine size is measured in centimeters, from the pubic symphysis to the top of the fundus. Approximately 20-35 weeks of gestation uterus size should be equal to the number of gestation weeks. Any difference more than 2-3 cm, between the uterine size and gestation week is called size and date discrepancy, which should be further evaluated with ultrasound.

Biparietal diameter is measured with ultrasound between 16-20 weeks of gestation. It is the **most accurate way to measure fetal age**

SECOND AND THIRD TRIMESTER SCREENING

1. ORAL GLUCOSE TOLERANCE TEST (OGTT)

Oral glucose tolerance test is performed to screen for gestational diabetes. It is usually performed between **24-28 weeks** of gestation, but in a **high-risk** patient, it should be performed at the **first prenatal visit**.

High risk: obesity, >30 years of age, family history of diabetes mellitus, previous fetal macrosomia, stillbirth or neonatal death.

OGTT work-up includes two tests, **1-hour 5g OGGT**, and **3-hour 100g**. OGTT is done in a following manner:

1-hour oral 50g OGGT

A patient is given 50 grams of oral glucose, and then blood sample is taken from a **vein of the arm after 60 minutes** and results are interpreted as follow:

- If blood glucose level is < 140 mg/dl, then it is considered a **normal response,** no additional glucose testing is required
- If blood glucose level is more than > 185 mg/dl, then it is diagnosed as a **gestational diabetes,** and the patient should be **started on insulin,** no additional glucose test is required
- If blood glucose is between 140mg/dl -185 mg/dl, then it requires further confirmation with **3-hour 100g glucose tolerance test**

3-hours 100 g OGGT

Overnight fasting is required before this test is performed, and patient's fasting blood glucose is checked before the test

- If patient's **fasting blood** glucose is **>126 mg/dl**, then this is considered as **gestational diabetes**. No additional OGGT test is needed, start the patient on **treatment.**
- If patient's **blood sugar is <126 mg/dl, then perform a 3-hour 100g OGTT.** 100 g oral glucose is given to the patient, and blood sample is taken from a vein of the arm at **3-hour intervals**. Results are interpreted as follows:

- Pregnant woman with one abnormal value (see table on the side) is diagnosed with **impaired glucose tolerance**
- Pregnant woman with 2 or more impaired values is diagnosed with **gestational diabetes**

> - **Normal values:**
> - Fasting glucose <95 mg/dl
> - 1-hr glucose < 180 mg/dl
> - 2-hrs glucose < 155 mg/dl
> - 3-hrs glucose < 140 mg/dl

Management:
- Mother with impaired glucose tolerance and gestational diabetes is treated as follow:
  - Tight glucose control
  - ADA diet and regular exercise
  - Insulin
- **Mode of delivery**
  - If fetus is **< 4,500 g,** then **labor may be induced**
  - If fetus is **> 4,500 g,** then **C-section delivery** is performed to prevent the vaginal delivery compilations
- During delivery, maternal blood glucose should be maintained between 80- 100 mg/dl with dextrose and insulin
- Maternal insulin requirement decrease after the delivery due to decreased hPL level
- Maternal diabetes is the most common cause of fetal macrosomia

POSTPARTUM ORAL GLUCOSE TOLERANCE TEST
Women with GDM are at increased risk of developing **overt diabetes.** Therefore, women with GDM should **have 2-hour 75g OGTT 3-4 weeks after the delivery**

SUMMARY OF ORAL GLUCOSE TOLERANCE TEST

Nonfasting 1-hr 50-gram OGTT

If blood glucose **<140/mg/dl-** Dx. **No gestational** DM

between 140-185mg/dl – **confirm with 3 hrs 100 g**

If blood glucose **> 185 mg/dl-** Dx. **Gestational** DM

Check **fasting blood** sugar **before** 3-hrs 100 OGGT

If **fasting** blood glucose **> 126** – Dx. **Gestational DM**, 3 hrs 100 OGGT is **not needed**

If **fasting** blood glucose **< 126mg/dl-** preform **fasting 3 hrs 100 OGGT.** Interpretation as follow

- Normal values:
- Fasting glucose <95-mg/dl
- 1-hr glucose < 180-mg/dl
- 2-hrs glucose< 155-mg/dl
- 3-hrs glucose< 140-mg/dl

- If one value is abnormal – Dx. **Impaired glucose tolerance**
- If 2 or more is abnormal value- Dx. **Gestational diabetes (GDM)**

2. GROUP B BETA-HEMOLYTIC STREPTOCOCCI (GBS) SCREENING

All pregnant women should get vaginal swab between **37-38 weeks** of gestation to check for GBS. If it is found, then manage it as follow:

Management:
- **Intrapartum** IV **penicillin** is given to prevent neonatal sepsis and endometritis. Treatment **given before labor and delivery is ineffective** because GBS re-grows during labor and delivery.
- If patient is allergic to penicillin, then give IV clindamycin, erythromycin or cefazolin

In addition treatment for GBS is also given, if patient has any of the followings:
- Labor < 37 weeks
- Rupture of membrane >18 hours
- Maternal fever during labor
- Positive GBS culture any time during your pregnancy
- Previous baby with GBS

3. MATERNAL SERUM ALPHA-FETOPROTEIN (MS-AFP)

Purpose: purpose of this test is to determine, if a fetus have trisomy (trisomy21 or trisomy 18), neural tube defect, intrauterine growth retardation (IUGR) or fetal demise

Screening criteria: MS-AFP is offered to all pregnant women, but it is recommended for a pregnant woman with the family history of birth defects, age>35 during the time of pregnancy, use of harmful drugs during pregnancy

Best performed: MS-AFP is most accurate, if it is measured between **16-20** weeks' of gestation (**Normal MS-ASP values: .85 - 2.5 MoM**)

Cause: The most common cause of abnormal MS-AFP level is incorrect **gestation date.**
- If MS-AFP level is abnormal (lower or higher than normal range), then get **an ultrasound to confirm the gestation dates.**
  - If gestation **date is not correct**, then **repeat the MS-AFP**, but only if pregnancy is within 15-20 weeks of gestation.
  - If gestation **date is correct**, then **check MS-ASP level** (results are discussed on the next page)

1. MS-ASP < .85 MoM signifies trisomy: get **amniocenteses, to check**
   karyotype **abnormalities and serum markers** (MS-AFP, estriol, beta-
   hCG and inhibin-A). Results are as follow:

Karyotype	MS-AFP	Estriol	Beta-HCG	Inhibin-A
Trisomy 21	Low	Low	High	High
Trisomy 18	Low	Low	Low	N/A

2. **MS-ASP >2.5MoM** usually signifies **neural tube defects, fetal demise
   or IUGR**. To distinguish between them, get **amniotic fluid-AFP and
   acetylcholinesterase levels**
   - If both are increased, then the Dx. **Neural tube defects.**
   - If only acetylcholinesterase is increased, then the Dx. IUGR **or
     stillbirth.**

SUMMARY OF MS-AFP TEST

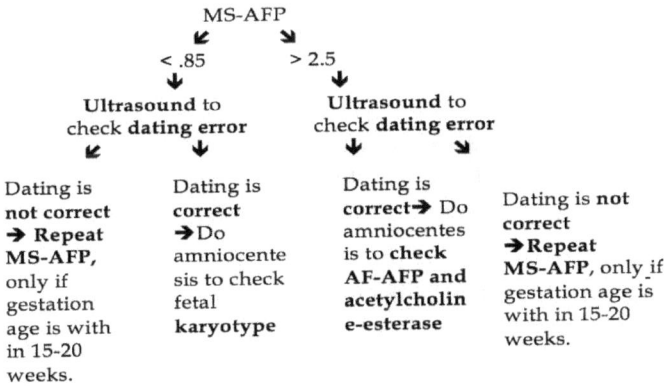

```
                          MS-AFP
                       ↙       ↘
                   < .85        > 2.5
                     ↓            ↓
              Ultrasound to   Ultrasound to
            check dating error  check dating error
                 ↙    ↓          ↓        ↘
```

Dating is not correct → **Repeat MS-AFP,** only if gestation age is with in 15-20 weeks.	Dating is correct → **Do** amniocentesis to check fetal **karyotype**	Dating is correct → Do amniocentesis is to check **AF-AFP and acetylcholin e-esterase**	Dating is **not correct** → **Repeat MS-AFP,** only if gestation age is with in 15-20 weeks.

- **FETAL KARYOTYPE**
  - **Down syndrome (Trisomy 21)**
    - ↓ MS-AFP   ↓ Estriol   ↑ β-HCG   ↑ Inhibin-A
  - **Trisomy 18**
    - ↓ MS-AFP   ↓ Estriol   ↓ β-HCG
- **AF-AFP and Acetylcholinesterase**
  - ↑ AF-AFP and ↑ Acetylcholinesterase – Dx. **Neural tube defect**
  - **Normal** AF-AFP and ↑ Acetylcholinesterase – Dx. **IUGR or still birth**

PRENATAL DIAGNOSTIC TESTING

1. AMNIOCENTESES
Amniocentesis is a prenatal test in which a small amount of amniotic fluid is removed using ultrasound-guided needle, and then fluid is sent for chromosomal analysis. It is performed after 15 weeks of gestation. **Recommended** to woman with the followings:
- Abnormal abdominal ultrasound
- Family history of certain birth defects, previous pregnancy or child with birth defect
- Mothers age 35 or more at the time of delivery

Complications miscarriage risk **0.06 %**, infection, preterm labor

2. CHORIONIC VILLUS SAMPLING (CVS)
Chorionic villus sampling is a prenatal test, which can be done earlier than the amniocentesis, in the first trimester (10-12 weeks of gestation). This test is performed to detect certain birth defects. In this test, ultrasound-guided needle is used to take a tissue sample of chorionic villus.
Compilations: miscarriage risk **1%**, **limb defect** if CVS is performed before 9 weeks of gestation

3. PERCUTANEOUS UMBILICAL BLOOD SAMPLING (PUBS)
PUBS is a prenatal test, in which fetus' blood is drawn from the fetal umbilical cord, and then that blood is used to detect birth defects. It is performed after 17 weeks of gestation
Complication: miscarriage **1-2%**, infection, premature rupture of membrane

NON-STRESS TEST (NST)
Non-stress test is performed in pregnancies over > 28 weeks gestation. This test checks if the fetus is well-being. Doppler is used to monitor fetal heart rate, and how fetal heart rate responds to the fetal movements. Results are interpreted as a **reactive NST or non-reactive NST**
- **A reactive NST** means that the fetus shows at least two heart accelerations 15 bpm above baseline for at least 15-20 seconds within 20 minutes. This indicates that fetus is doing well

- **Nonreactive NST** means that the fetus is not showing results that are seen in reactive stress test. It could mean that the fetus is **either sleeping or in jeopardy**. Vibroacoustic stimulation can help to distinguish them. **Vibroacoustic test** wakes up a sleeping baby and test may show reactive stress test. However, if the fetus is still showing nonreactive test, then do the **biophysical profile.**

BIOPHYSICAL PROFILE
Biophysical profile has 5 components and score is assigned based on these components, which are:
1. Fetal movement
2. Fetal breathing
3. Fetal tone
4. Amniotic fluid volume
5. Fetal heart rate

All components are measured with ultrasound. A score 8-10 means fetus is well, and 0-2 scores worrisome. 0-2 score required future testing with contraction stress test

CONTRACTION STRESS TEST (CST)
In a contraction stress test, oxytocin is given to the mother to induce uterine contractions and fetal heart strip is monitored.
- A positive CST is defined as late deceleration with each contraction; it implies that the fetus is in jeopardy and in most cases C-section is performed.

OLIGOHYDROMONA
Oligohydromona is characterized by amniotic fluid < 500 ml or amniotic fluid index less than 5 cm
Cause: renal agenesis, IUGR, premature rupture of membrane
Diagnosis: Ultrasound
Treatment: treat the underlying cause
Complication: pulmonary hypoplasia, limb deformity, musculoskeletal abnormalities, cord compression,

POLYHYDRAMNIOS
Polyhydramnios is characterized by amniotic fluid more than 2 L or amniotic fluid index >25 cm

Cause: GI disorders (duodenal atresia, esophageal atresia, gastroschisis and diaphragmatic hernia), CNS disorders (anencephaly and myotonic dystrophy), achondroplasia, maternal causes (DM, intrauterine infection), and Rh incompatibility

Diagnosis: ultrasound, Rh typing, maternal DM

Treatment: treat the underlying cause

Complications: Cord prolapse, placental abruption, premature death, perinatal death

INTRAUTERINE GROWTH RETARDATION (IUGR)

Intrauterine growth retardation is characterized as a developing baby weighs less than 90% of other babies of the same gestational cause.

Types: two main types of IUGR are symmetric and asymmetric IUGR, which are based on 4 parameters that are measured with ultrasound. Results are following:

Parameters	Symmetric	Asymmetric
Abdominal circumference	Decreased	Decreased
Biparietal diameter	Decreased	**Normal**
Head circumference	Decreased	**Normal**
Femur length	Decreased	**Normal**

Cause: maternal (smoking, alcohol, drugs abuse or SLE), **fetal** (TORCH infection, chromosomal abnormalities, congenital abnormalities) and **placental** (preeclampsia, infarction, abruption).

Note: Maternal and placental factors usually give asymmetric IUGR, and fetal factors usually give symmetric IUGR

Diagnosis:
- Ultrasound
- NST, BPP, CST
- Doppler flow of umbilical artery

Treatment: give IM betamethasone to enhance lung development and delivery the baby

SAFE DRUGS DURING PREGNANCY

Condition	Medicine
Pain, fever, minor aches, headache	Acetaminophen
Heartburn	Antacids
Morning sickness, vomiting	Phenergan, scopolamine, Reglan
Constipation	Stool softener and laxative (Metamucil, Dulcolax, Colace)
Allergies	Antihistamine (Benadryl, Claritin)
Infection	Antibiotics: penicillin, ampicillin, amoxicillin, cephalosporins, erythromycin and nitrofurantoin
Antihypertensive	Hydralazine, methyldopa, labetalol
Diabetes	Insulin
Coagulopathy	Heparin

TERATOGEN DRUGS AND SIDE EFFECTS

DRUG	SIDE EFFECTS
Alcohol	Fetal alcohol syndrome (flat mid face, smooth philtrum, short palpebral fissures, thin vermillion borders of lips)
Angiotensin converting enzyme inhibitors (ACEIs)	**Renal** anomalies, craniofacial abnormalities
Anesthetics	**Respiratory** depression, CNS depression
Aminoglycosides	Deafness
Barbiturates	Respiratory depression, CNS depression
Cigarettes	**Prematurity**, intrauterine growth retardation
Carbamazepine	Neural tube defect
Diethylstilbestrol (DES)	**Adenocarcinoma** of vagina, clear cell vaginal cancer, cervical incompetence
Iodine	Cretinism
Lithium	Cardiac (Ebstein) anomaly
NSAIDs	Premature ductus arteriosus closure
Oral contraceptives (OCPs)	VACTERL syndrome
Phenobarbital	Vitamin K deficiency
Phenytoin	Hypoplastic nails, Intrauterine growth retardation, typical face
Tetracycline	**Yellow** or brown colored teeth
Valproate	Neural tube defect
Warfarin	Craniofacial defect, chondrodysplasia

ABORTION

INDUCED ABORTIONS

1. If **gestation age is < 49 days**
- Treatment: Misoprostol and mifepristone
    - Follow-up with beta hCG and transvaginal ultrasound because some patients may require D&C, if they had incomplete abortion
    - Complications: sepsis from clostridium sordelli

2. If gestation age is **< 20 weeks** of gestation –Tx. **D&C**

3. If gestation age is **> 20 weeks** of gestation - Tx. **D& E**
- Complications of D& E
    - Immediate complication is retained placenta
    - Delayed complications are cervical trauma and cervical insufficiency

FETAL DEMISE
Fetal demise also known as fetal death is unintentionally loss of pregnancy after 20th week of gestation

SPONTANEOUS ABORTION
Spontaneous abortion is also known, as miscarriage is unintentionally loss of pregnancy before 20th week of gestation

Diagnosis:
- Beta-hCG
- CBC to determine the need for blood transfusion
- Rh blood type screening
- Pelvic exam
- Doppler ultrasound to check the fetal heartbeat
- Ultrasound to see if **all or some parts of the fetus are present.** This helps determine the type of abortion

Differential diagnosis of abortion

Types of abortion	Characteristics	Treatment
Threatened abortion	• Vaginal bleeding • Pelvic exam shows **no cervical dilation** • **Fetal heart tones** are present on doppler ultrasound • Ultrasound shows **intact product of conception**	Bed rest, Pelvic rest
Inevitable abortion	• Vaginal bleeding • Pelvic exam shows **cervical dilation** • **Fetal heart tones** are present on doppler ultrasound • Ultrasound shows **intact product of conception**	D& C
Complete abortion	• Vaginal bleeding • Pelvic exam shows no cervical dilation • **No fetal heart tones** are present on doppler ultrasound • Ultrasound shows **no product of conception**	Follow beta-hCG until it becomes zero
Incomplete abortion	• Vaginal bleeding • Pelvic exam shows no cervical dilation • **No fetal heart tones** are present on doppler ultrasound • Ultrasound shows **some** product of conception	D& C
Missed abortion	• Vaginal bleeding • Pelvic exam shows no cervical dilation • **No fetal heart tones** are present on doppler ultrasound • Ultrasound shows **product of conception**	Induce the labor

ECTOPIC PREGNANCY

Ectopic pregnancy is an obstetric condition in which embryo implants outside the uterus. Most of the ectopic pregnancies occurs in fallopian tube (tubal-pregnancy), but can also occur in cervix, ovaries or abdomen

Risk factors: pelvic inflammatory disease, Intrauterine device in place while getting pregnant, tubal surgery, tubal ligation,

Si/Sx: lower abdominal pain, vaginal bleeding

Diagnosis:

- Beta-hCG
- Ultrasound
- Laparoscopy

Management:

- If patient is unstable, then do **laparotomy**
- If the patient is stable, then **check β-hCG level and perform transvaginal ultrasound**:

  - If **β-hCG> 1,500** mIU and transvaginal ultrasound shows intrauterine pregnancy, then treat the patient as follow:
  - **Methotrexate is given, only if beta-hCG < 6,000 mIU, ectopic mass < 3.5 cm, no fetal heart motion, and no history of folic acid use.**
  - If a patient does not meet the criteria for methotrexate, then perform **laparoscopy** to determine the size of ectopic pregnancy
    - If it is **< 3 cm, then do salpingostomy.** Fallopian tube is left open to heal on its own to maintain fertility.
    - If it is **> 3 cm, then do salpingectomy**

  Note: Beta-hCG is followed weekly, until it reaches zero to ensure complete resolution

  - If **β-CG is < 1,500mIU** and **transvaginal** ultrasound shows **no intrauterine** pregnancy, then **repeat β- hCG and transvaginal ultrasound after 72 hours**

  - If **β-hCG doubles after 72 hours** - Dx. normal pregnancy, and manage the patient as per pregnant woman
  - If **β-hCG does not double after 72 hours** -Dx. Tubal pregnancy-Tx. **Laparoscopy**

FETAL HEART RATE
- Normal fetal heart rate is between 110- 160bpm
- Normal fetal heart rate has following characteristics: beat-to-beat variability, has accelerations and no decelerations

1. **Early decelerations** are decreased fetal heart rate below the baseline, but soon returns to baseline. These decelerations **coincide with uterine contraction;** means that the decelerations begin and end approximately the same time of the uterine contraction. Early deceleration usually signifies fetal **head compression.**
   Treatment: no treatment is required because these are not harmful

2. **Late decelerations** are gradual decrease in fetal heart rate that occurs **after the uterine contractions.** Late decelerations are worrisome and signify **uteroplacental insufficiency.**
   Treatment:
   o Place the mother in lateral decubitus position, give oxygen and stop oxytocin, if applicable. Give IV fluids and tocolytic such as ritodrine or magnesium sulfate to relax the uterus.
   o If decelerations are still present, then deliver the baby.

3. **Variable decelerations** have **no relation to uterine contraction.** It often signifies **umbilical cord prolapse.**
   o Treatment: Place the mother in **lateral decubitus position, give oxygen and stop oxytocin, if applicable. Give IV fluids and check out umbilical cord prolapse.**

UMBILICAL CORD PROLAPSE
Umbilical cord prolapse is obstetrics emergency in which umbilical cord comes out of the cervix.
Boards tip: Look for fetus with severe bradycardia or severe variable acceleration during delivery
Treatment:
- Put mother in knee-to-chest position, elevate the presenting parts, give terbutaline, and perform urgent C-section

THIRD TRIMESTER BLEEDING

1. ABRUPTIO PLACENTA

Abruptio placenta is a premature (before the baby is delivered) separation of the placenta from the uterus. It occurs 1 out of 100 deliveries
Risk factors:

- Abdominal trauma (hit to the abdomen, fall, or automobile accidents)
- Cocaine use
- HTN
- Previous abruption placenta
- Increased uterine distention (multiple pregnancies or large volume of amniotic fluid)

Si/Sx: painful vaginal bleeding, abdominal pain, uterine tenderness, hyperactive uterine contraction
Diagnosis:

- Clinical diagnosis
- Transvaginal or transabdominal ultrasound can be used, but it may not be reliable because ultrasound detects only a small percentage of abruptio placenta

Treatment:

- If the mother or fetus is in **distress,** then stabilize the mother, and then do **emergency C-section**
- **Vaginal delivery may be induced,** if bleeding is heavy but controlled, fetus is dead, or pregnancy is > 36 weeks of gestation with mother and fetus stable
- If pregnancy is far-term (<32 weeks) and mother and fetus are stable or mild abruption, then **manage the pregnancy expectantly;** hospital observation, bed rest, fetal monitoring, IV fluids and blood products, as needed

Complication: DIC, hemorrhagic shock, fetal hypoxia, fetal death

2. UTERINE RUPTURE

Uterine rupture is a tear in the wall of the uterus. It is a life-threatening condition for the mother and fetus, and may occur before or during the labor

Risk factors:
- Prior classic uterine incision
- Myomectomy
- Grand multiparity
- Excessive oxytocin stimulation

Si/Sx: painful vaginal bleeding, abdomen pain, chest pain, loss of fetal electronic fetal heart rate signals, maternal hypotension, may be able to palpate fetal part in maternal abdomen

Treatment:
- Immediate laparotomy with delivery of the fetus. A C-section is not done because baby is in abdomen instead of uterus
- Further management depends on the severity of rupture and condition of the patient.
  - If the patient is unstable or does not desire any more children, then uterus is removed (hysterectomy).
  - If the patient is stable or desires more pregnancies, then uterus is usually repaired to preserve fertility.

Compilation: Those patients who have had uterus repair should have C-section delivery at 36 weeks for the subsequent pregnancies to reduce the risk of uterus re-rupture

3. PLACENTA PREVIA

Placenta Previa is an obstetric condition in which placenta grows on the lower part of the uterus and covers all or some part of the cervical opening.

Risk factors:
- Previous placenta previa
- Advance maternal age
- Grand multiparous
- Multiple gestations
- Abnormal uterus shape

Si/Sx: Painless vaginal bleeding, which may stop on its own in 1-2 hours and starts again in days or weeks. Fetus is usually normal

Diagnosis: transabdominal ultrasound

Type: type of placenta previa depends on placenta's proximity to cervical os. (Discussed in the table in the table below)

Type of Placenta Previa

Type	Characteristics
Marginal	Placenta is next to cervix but is not covering internal os
Partial	Placenta is covering some part of internal os
Complete	Placenta is covering all of the cervical os opening

Treatment:
- If the mother or fetus is **unstable,** then do **emergency C-section**
- If the **pregnancy is remote term and mother and fetus are stable or mild abruption,** then pregnancy can be **managed expectantly**: hospital observation, bed rest, fetal monitoring, IV fluids and blood products as needed.
  - Corticosteroids (betamethasone) is also given to the mothers, who is < 32 weeks of gestation, to enhance the fetal lung maturity
- Stable mother with term pregnancy should have **C-section delivery. Vaginal delivery** can only be tried **if placenta is > 2 cm away** from cervical os.

Complication: placenta accreta, placenta incerta, and placenta percreta

4. VASA PREVIA

Vasa previa is an obstetrics condition in which fetal vessels are crossing or running close to inner cervical os. These vessels are at increased risk of rupture when membrane ruptures and can cause fetal death

Risk factors:
- Multiple gestations
- Accessory lobe
- Velamentous insertion of umbilical cord

Si/Sx: classic triad - painless vaginal bleeding, membranes rupture and fetal bradycardia

Diagnosis:
- Clinical diagnosis (classic triad)
- Ultrasound with color-flow Doppler, rarely needed to confirm the diagnosis, it shows fetal vessels crossing the membranes over the internal cervical os

Treatment: immediate c- section otherwise fetus may die

HYPERTENSION

Hypertension is a common medical problem, which may also be present during pregnancy. Two main types of hypertension seen during pregnancy are chronic hypertension and gestational hypertension

1. CHRONIC HYPERTENSION

Chronic hypertension is defined as BP > 140/90 mm Hg that is **present before the conception or < 20 weeks of gestation.**
Complication: it may progress to pre-eclampsia.
Treatment: oral methyldopa, labetalol or Nifedipine

2. GESTATIONAL HYPERTENSION

Gestational hypertension is defined as BP > 140/90 mmHg, which **develops > 20 weeks of gestation.**
Complication: may progress to pre-eclampsia.
Treatment: close follow-ups and treatment with oral methyldopa, labetalol or Nifedipine

Note:

- ACEs and ARBs are not used to treat HTN during pregnancy because both of them are teratogen
- Anytime a pregnant woman presents with elevated blood pressure, make sure to check urine protein because hypertension during pregnancy may progress to pre-eclampsia

PRE-ECLAMPSIA

Pre-eclampsia is a characterized by BP > 140/90 mmHG and proteinuria developing after 20 weeks of gestation. Pre-eclampsia is subdivided into mild and severe pre-eclampsia. If it is left untreated, it may progress to eclampsia. (Discussed in the table on next page)

Differential diagnosis of pre-eclampsia

Type	Physical symptoms	Lab value
Mild pre-eclampsia	• Edema of hands, feet and face	• BP> 140/90 mmHg • Proteinuria: 1 -2 + on urine dipstick or 300 mg in 24 hours
Severe pre-eclampsia	• Generalized edema • **Headaches** • **Visual changes** • **RUQ epigastric pain**	• BP > 160/100 mmHg • Proteinuria: 3-4 + on urine dipstick or 5 g in 24 hours
Eclampsia	• Same as severe pre-eclampsia • **New onset seizure**	• Same as severe pre-eclampsia

Management:

Mild pre-eclampsia:

- If mother is near-term, then **stabilize the mother and induce delivery**
- If mother is far-term, then manage as follow:
  - Bed rest and expectant management
  - Lower the acutely elevate BP with IV hydralazine or labetalol, and then maintain the lower blood pressure with oral methyldopa

Severe pre-eclampsia and eclampsia

- Stabilize the mother;
  - Lower BP with **IV hydralazine or labetalol** (goal: systolic BP 160-110 and diastolic BP 90-100, to maintain fetal blood flow)
  - Give **IV MgSO4** to control the seizure and as a seizure prophylaxis
- Then **induce the vaginal delivery** regardless of gestation age
- Betamethasone is given to the mother with gestational age < 32 weeks to enhance the fetal lung maturity

HELLP Syndrome

HELLP syndrome is a life-threatening obstetrics complication. It is usually considered variant of pre-eclampsia. HELLP is the abbreviation of the main features of the condition:

- Hemolysis
- Elevated liver enzymes (AST & ALT)
- Lower platelets

Si/Sx: same as mild or severe pre-eclampsia

Labs: same as mild or severe pre-eclampsia **plus hemolysis, low platelet and high liver enzymes**

Treatment:

- Stabilize the mother:
  - Lower the BP with IV **hydralazine or labetalol**
  - Give **IV MgSO4** to control the seizure and as a seizure prophylaxis
  - Platelet transfusion if platelets are < 20, 000 or if platelets are < 50,000 mm and C-section is planned,
- Then deliver the baby regardless of gestational age
- Betamethasone is given to the mother with gestational age < 32 weeks to enhance the fetal lung maturity

LIVER DISEASES

1. ACUTE FATTY LIVER

This condition is caused by **impaired fatty acid metabolism by fetus mitochondria**

Si/Sx: Look for a pregnant woman with signs of pre-eclampsia, sever-eclampsia or HELLP + **hypoglycemia, increased ammonia and hyperbilirubinemia**

Management: Admit the patient ICU, IV fluids and prompt delivery

Frequently asked

INTRAHEPATIC CHOLESTASIS OF PREGNANCY

Si/Sx: mild pruritus that begins on the extremity, and then moves to trunk, but **no skin lesions**

Diagnosis: Markedly elevated bile acids

Management:
- For symptomatic relief –Tx. Antihistamines
- For Intrahepatic cholestasis –Tx. Ursodeoxycholic acid

Complications: Fetal prematurity, fetal distress, and fetal loss

PRURITIC URTICARIAL PAPULES AND PLAQUES OF PREGNANCY
Symptoms: itching and urticarial papules and plaques rash that begins on abdomen, and then later spread to extremities
Treatment: Topical steroids and antihistamines

HERPES GESTATIONIS
It is not associated with herpes simplex virus
Si/Sx: **intense pruritus, small vesicles** and **tense bullae** that starts on the limbs first, and then later spread on trunk
Diagnosis :Immunofluorescent stain of biopsy
Treatment: Oral corticosteroids
Complication: Stillbirth and intrauterine growth retardation

URINARY TRACT INFECTIONS

1. ASYMPTOMATIC BACTERIURIA
Asymptomatic bacteriuria is characterized by presence of significant number **of bacteria (> 10,000 mL) in the urine**, but **no UTIs symptoms** are present
Treatment:
- 1st line of treatment is oral nitrofurantoin
- 2nd line treatment is amoxicillin or Cephalexin

2. ACUTE CYSTITIS
Si/Sx: urgency, **frequency, burning, suprapubic tenderness**, hematuria
Diagnosis:
- **Urine analysis** shows increased urinary nitrites, increased leukocyte esterase, pyuria, bacteriuria
- **Urine culture:** positive for offending bacteria with colony count exceeding 10 x 5/ml

Treatment:
- 1st line of treatment is oral nitrofurantoin
- 2nd line treatment is amoxicillin or Cephalexin

3. PYELONEPHRITIS
Si/Sx: urgency, frequency, dysuria, fever, chills, **flank pain, costovertebral angle (CVA) tenderness**
Diagnosis:
- **Best initial test is urine analysis**
- **Most accurate test is urine culture**
- Renal ultrasound or CT, it is usually done to check for stones or other source of obstruction

Treatment:
- **Admit** and **give IV 3rd generation cephalosporin and tocolytic** (to prevent premature delivery)
- If a patient is not responding after 48 -72 hours of treatment, then get **ultrasound** of abdomen and pelvis to check for abscess or UTI obstruction
  - If ultrasound shows abscess - Tx. Percutaneous drainage
  - If ultrasound shows stone - Tx Nephrostomy

THYROID

Remember during pregnancy, TIBG and total T4 are increased, **but** free T4 and TSH are normal
- If a pregnant women presents with symptoms of hyperthyroidism, then check **free T4 (fT4)**:
  - If fT4 is **increased,** then the diagnosis is **hyperthyroidism**
  - If fT4 is within **normal range**, then the diagnosis is **anxiety**

Graves' disease management during pregnancy
- **PTU is given during the first trimester,** and **subtotal thyroidectomy is performed** during 2nd **trimester.** Methimazole should not be given to pregnant women because it causes congenital aplasia cutis.

Hypothyroidism management during pregnancy

- Levothyroxine dose may need to be **increased** in **pregnant woman** or if woman is taking **oral contraceptive containing estrogen** because in these thyroxine-binding globulin (TBG) is increased, which reduces the absorption of **levothyroxine**

HYPERCOAGULABE STATE

- If a pregnant mother has history of DVT, pulmonary embolism or any other hypercoagulable condition, then manage her as follow:
  - Through out the pregnancy – Tx. Low molecular weight heparin
  - During labor and delivery switch LMWH to heparin and warfarin

FIBRONECTIN TEST

Fibronectin is a protein produced by fetal cells. It begins to break down and can be detected in vaginal discharge after 35 weeks of gestation. However, if it is present between 22-34 weeks of **gestation, then it indicates preterm delivery is likely to occur.**
Management: Give tocolytic and IM betamethasone to hasten the fetal lung maturity

TOCOLYTICS CONTRAINDICATIONS

- Ritodrine or terbutaline is not used in patients with severe cardiac disease, hyperthyroidism and uncontrolled diabetes
- IV Magnesium sulfate is not used in patients with myasthenia gravis and end-stage renal disease
- NSAIDs are not used if gestation > 32 weeks because it may cause premature closure of ductus

CERVICAL INSUFFICIENCY

Cervical insufficiency is a serious obstetrics condition in which pregnant woman has painless cervical dilation during the second trimester
Cause

- **Cervical trauma** that usually occurs during D& E
- **Cervical laceration** that usually occurs during previous pregnancy
- **Deep cone biopsy** that usually occurs during abnormal Pap smear
- **Anatomic anomalies** that usually occurs due to DES exposure in-utero

Management:

- If any of the followings are **present,** then give **antibiotics and allow labor**
  - Chorioamnionitis
  - Membrane has ruptured
  - Labor has started
- If any of the above is **not present,** then place **emergent cervical cerclage**

Electives cervical cerclage

- Electives cervical cerclage are placed 13-16 weeks of gestation in women with repeated unexplained pregnancy loss
- These are removed at 36-37 weeks of gestation after confirming fetal lung maturity

LABOR

True labor is defined as uterine contraction occurring every 2-3 minutes, lasting 45-60 seconds with the intensity of 50 mmHg

PRETERM LABOR

Preterm labor is defined as

- Labor that occurs between 20-27 weeks of gestation
- Has at least 3 contraction in 30 minutes
- Cervical dilation > 2 cm or serial exams show change in cervical dilation or effacement

Risk factors: maternal smoking, previous preterm pregnancy, multiple pregnancy, pyelonephritis, chorioamnionitis, premature rupture of membrane

Symptoms: lower abdominal or backache, abdominal cramping or menstrual-like cramping, fluid leak from vagina, increased pressure in pelvis or vagina

Diagnosis:

- **Pelvic exam shows** at least 3 contractions in 30 minutes, and cervical dilation > 2 cm or serial exams show change in cervical dilation or effacement
- **Nitrazine paper** test shows that the **paper turns blue** when a small amount of vaginal fluid is placed on it

- **Fern test shows** " fern-like" pattern on a slide, when a small amount of vaginal fluid is placed on a slide and viewed under microscope
- **Ultrasound**

Treatment:

- Place the mother in lateral decubitus position, pelvic rest, bed rest, IV fluids and oxygen. If contraction still continues, then give tocolytic such as beta2 agonists (terbutaline, ritodrine), calcium channel blockers (Nifedipine) or magnesium sulfate
- IM betamethasone is given to mother < 32 weeks of gestation
- Stable patient < 24 weeks gestation can be managed outpatient with tocolytic and bed rest

Contraindication for tocolytic: fetal demise, lethal fetal anomaly, advances cervical dilation; severe preeclampsia, eclampsia, abruption placenta, chorioamnionitis

PREMATURE RUPTURE OF MEMBRANE (PROM)

Premature rupture of membrane is defined as **rupture of membrane before the onset of labor**

Risk factors: most common cause is ascending infection from lower genital tract, other risk factors include smoking, STDs, young maternal age

Diagnosis:

PROM is diagnosed by sterile speculum exam to evaluate cervical dilation and effacement and following

- Amniotic fluid pooling in posterior vaginal fornix (most useful and definitive diagnostic test)
- **Nitrazine paper** test shows paper turn blue when a small amount of vaginal fluid is placed on it
- **Fern test shows** " fern-like" pattern on slide, when a small amount of vaginal fluid is placed on slide and viewed under microscope
- Ultrasound

Treatment:

If **chorioamnionitis is present,** then obtain cervical culture, give broad-spectrum antibiotics and induce delivery

If **chorioamnionitis is not present,** then management depends on the gestational age, which is as follow:

- Patient **< 24 of gestation** has poor outcomes. **Baby can be delivered or send patient home and advise bed rest**
- Patients between **24- 33 weeks of gestation** should be hospitalized; get cervical culture, and give prophylactic ampicillin and erythromycin. Additionally, give IM betamethasone if mother is < 32 week of gestation
- Prompt delivery if patient >**34 weeks** of gestation

Chorioamnionitis is an inflammation of the fetal membranes (chorion and amnion). It is caused by ascending bacterial infection from lower genital tract. Chorioamnionitis is a **clinical diagnosis,** based on the following symptoms:

- PROM
- Uterine tenderness and maternal fever
- Absence of UTI or URI

LABOR

Order of fetal positions during normal labor and delivery (L&D)
During normal L&D fetus goes through the following 6 step-wise positions:

1. Descent
2. Flexion
3. Internal rotation
4. Extension
5. External rotation
6. Expulsion

STAGES AND DURATION OF LABOR

Labor	Definition	Progression	Abnormality
Stage 1 – latent phase: effacement	• From 0 to 3-4 cm cervical dilation	• < 20 hours in primipara • < 14 hour in multipara	• Prolongation phase: no cervical change in 20 hours in primipara or 14 in multipara

- **Cause: analgesia** is the most common cause of **prolongation of latent phase**
- **Treatment: rest and sedation**

Labor	Definition	Progression	Abnormality
Stage 1- Active phase: Dilation	• Begins at cervical dilation at 3cm • Ends at 10 cm cervical dilation	• In nulliparous woman 1.2cm/hour • In multipara women 1.5 cm/hour	• **Arrest phase** is no cervical change in > 2 hours • **Prolongation phase:** taking more than normal time

- **Causes of active stage abnormalities:** three p's: **passenger** (fetal size or abnormal presentation), **power** (inadequate contractions), and **pelvic**

- Management:
  - If the patient has **hypotonic uterine contractions**- Tx. **IV oxytocin**
  - If the patient has **hypertonic contractions** – Tx. **Morphine**
  - If the patient has **adequate contraction**-Tx. **Emergency C-section**

Labor	Definition	Progression	Abnormality
Stage 2 – Descent of fetus	• **Begins at 10 cm** dilation of cervix • Ends with **delivery of the baby**	• < 2 hour in nulliparous or < 3 hours if nulliparous is **with epidural** • <1 hour in multipara or < 2 hours in multipara without epidural	• **Arrest:** Failure to deliver < 2 hour in nulliparous or < 1 hours multipara ○ +1 hour for epidural

- **Causes of descent stage abnormalities:** three p's: **passenger** (fetal size or abnormal presentation), **power** (inadequate contractions), and **pelvic**

- **Management:**
  - ○ If the patient has **hypotonic uterine contractions**- Tx. **IV oxytocin**
  - ○ If the patient has **hypertonic contractions** – Tx. **Morphine**
  - ○ If the patient has **adequate contraction**, then the management depends on fetal head
    - If fetal head is **not engaged**-Tx. **Emergency C-section**
    - If fetal head is **engaged**-Tx. **Do vacuum extraction or obstetrics forceps**

- In addition C-section may be performed in this stage if any of the following is present:
  - ○ Membrane has not ruptured
  - ○ Cervix is not fully dilated to 10 cm
  - ○ Mother has small pelvic
  - ○ Fetal head is not engaged
  - ○ Fetal head orientation is not known

- If patient does not have any of the above – Do vacuum extraction or obstetrics forceps

Labor	Definition	Progression	Abnormality
Stage 3 – Expulsion	• After the delivery of baby to delivery of placenta • Ends with delivery of placenta	• < 30 minutes	• **Failure to delivery placenta within 30 minutes after the delivery**

Cause: possibly placenta accrete, incerta and percreta

Management:
- Initial treatment is **IV oxytocin**
- If IV oxytocin is ineffective- Tx. **Manuel removal** of placenta
- If both are ineffective- Tx. **Hysterectomy**

BREECH PRESENTATION
Breech presentation is defined as fetal lie with the buttocks or feet close to the cervix, opposed to head (cephalic presentation)

Types: Three main types of breech presentations are:
- **Frank breech,** in which fetus' hips are flexed and knees are extended
- **Complete breech,** in which fetus's both hips and knees are flexed
- **Footling or incomplete breech,** in which one or both feet or knees are prolapsed into the maternal vagina

Treatment: external cephalic version is performed in women **after 36 weeks** of gestation. In this maneuver pressure is applied to mother's abdomen to achieve cephalic (head down) presentation. It is **not recommended before 36 week of gestation** because sometimes fetus maneuver itself into cephalic presentation

SHOULDER DYSTOCIA
Shoulder dystocia is an obstetrics emergency that occurs when, after the delivery of the fetal head, the baby's anterior shoulder gets stuck behind mother pubic bone.

Management: is as follow:

Initial maneuver:

- **McRobert's maneuver:** this is **best initial maneuver.** Have the mother hyperflex her thighs tightly to her abdomen. This maneuver widens the pelvis and flattens the spine in the lumbar region. It is effective in 42 % of the cases
- **Suprapubic pressure:** apply pressure over the bladder. It decreases fetal shoulder breadth
- **Rubin II maneuver:** place two fingers behind anterior shoulder; apply pressure downward and rotate fetus shoulder
- **Wood-Screw maneuver:** place two fingers behind posterior shoulder; apply pressure upward and rotate fetus shoulder

Last resorts are:

- **Zavanelli's maneuver:** push the fetal head back and perform C-section
- **Intentional fetal clavicular fracture**

INDICATIONS OF C-SECTION

Fetal factors	• Abnormal heart rate • Fetal malposition such as transverse lie, incomplete breech, • Big baby • Cephalopelvic disproportion (head is too large to pass through birth canal)
Maternal factors	• Active genital herpes • HIV • Previous C-section with classic incision • Uterine surgery • Cervical carcinoma • Large uterine fibroids
Placenta or umbilical cord factors	• Umbilical cord prolapse • Placenta previa • Placenta abruption

POSTPARTUM HEMORRHAGE

Postpartum hemorrhage is defined as a loss of blood > 500 ml during vaginal delivery or > 1,000 ml during C-section.

1. UTERINE ATONY

This is the most common cause of postpartum hemorrhage
Management:
- Uterine massage
- If uterine massage is ineffective, then give Oxytocin, carboprost or methylergonovine

Contraindication for methylergonovine
- Methylergonovine is contraindicated if patient has hypertension
- Carboprost should is contraindicated if patient has asthma

2. VAGINAL LACERATIONS

This is the second most common cause of postpartum hemorrhage
Degree:
- First-degree: laceration is limited to superficial perineal skin
- Second-degree: laceration involves perineal muscles and fascia
- Third-degree: lacerations involves anal sphincter
- Fourth-degree: perineal muscles, anal sphincter and rectal mucosa

Management:
- 1st and 2nd degree lacerations- Tx. No treatment required
- 3rd and 4th degree lacerations –Tx. Surgical suturing

3. RETAINED PLACENTA

This is caused by retained part of the placenta. Inspection of placenta shows **missing cotyledon**
Management: Manual removal or D& C

4. UTERINE INVERSION

This is caused by pulling too hard on the cord, uterus comes out of vagina and appears" **red beefy mass"**
Management:
- If uterus is **relaxed**- Tx. **Manual replacement of uterus followed by oxytocin**

- If uterus is **contracted**, then first **relax the uterus with halothane or terbutaline, and** then manual replacement of uterus followed by oxytocin

LOCHIA
Lochia is the vaginal discharge, which is seen in a woman **4-6 weeks after giving birth**. It contains blood, mucus, and uterine tissue. For first 3-5 days, it is **red** in color due to blood and uterine tissue, as it thins it gradually turns **brownish pink** and **eventually white or yellowish-white**. It has an **odor similar to that of normal menstrual fluid**, but if it is **foul smelly,** then one should suspect **endometritis**.

ENDOMETRITIS
Endometritis is irritation or inflammation of the endometrium of the uterus. It is the most common cause **of fever 2-3 days postpartum**
Risk factors: miscarriage, childbirth, prolong labor, C-section, PID, D& C
Si/Sx: fever, abdominal distention, pelvic pain
Diagnosis:
- WBCs count
- ESR
- Endometrial, vaginal, urine and blood culture

Treatment:
- Empiric treatment with IV gentamicin and clindamycin or broad-spectrum antibiotics until culture and sensitivity is known
- If fever persists despite treatment, then get CT of abdomen and pelvis
  - If **abscess** is found on CT - Tx. Percutaneous drainage
  - If **no abscess** is found on CT - Dx. **Septic thrombophlebitis, it is treated with IV heparin for 7 -10 days**

Complication: infertility, peritonitis, abscess, and septicemia

POSTPARTUM CONTRACEPTION
- Contraception in breast-feeding mothers maybe **deferred for three months** because prolactin inhibits the ovulation by suppressing the LH and FSH surge

- **Progestin** is the only contraception that can be safely used during breast-feeding (estrogen component are avoided because it increases the hypercoagulable state, and diminishes lactation)

BREASTFEEDING

Benefits of breastfeeding for a mother:
- It helps them **lose weight faster**
- **Increases** the **bone density**
- **Decreases** the risk of **breast cancer and ovarian cancer**
- **Decreases** the risk of **developing diabetes**

Benefits of breastfeeding for a **neonate**
- Prevents GI infections, GERD,
- It has IgG antibody, which lowers respiratory tract infection
- Decreases the risk of otitis media

Contraindications for breastfeeding
- **HIV**
- **HSV**, only if lesions present on breast
- **HBV**, only until neonates receives HBV vaccine
- **CMV**
- **Substance abuse**
- **Breast cancer**

POSTPARTUM BREAST MASS

1. GALACTOCELE
This condition is caused by **blockage of a milk duct**
Symptoms: **fluctuating nonerythematous** breast mass
Treatment: None, most of the galactocele resolves spontaneously

2. MASTITIS
This condition is caused by **S. aureus, transmitted from infant's throat or nose**
Si/Sx: **non-fluctuating erythematous** breast mass, **fever and chills**
Treatment:
- **Dicloxacillin** and advice patient to **continue breast-feeding from the affected side of the breast,** otherwise it will lead to **breast abscess**

3. BREAST ABSCESS

This condition is a complication of mastitis

Symptoms: fluctuating erythematous breast mass, **fever and chills**

Diagnosis: clinical diagnosis, but confirm it with **ultrasound** (not mammogram)

Treatment: Surgical drainage

POSTPARTUM MOOD DISORDERS

Postpartum mood disorders are mental health disorder that affects women within first year after giving birth

Disorder	Characteristic	Treatment
Postpartum blue	Mother is tearful, but she **continues to take care** of herself and her child	None
Postpartum depression	Mother is tearful, and she **does not take care** of herself and her child	SSRIs
Postpartum psychosis	Mother experience **delusions, hallucinations**, and may have thought about hurting her child	Hospitalization and separate her from her child until she is better

POST TERM PREGNANCY

Post term pregnancy is defined as pregnancy that continues more than 42 weeks of gestation

Complication: post term pregnancy increases the risk of perinatal morbidity and mortality

Diagnosis:
- Clinical diagnosis
- Ultrasound is usually done to confirm the pregnancy dates

Management:
- If dates are sure and cervix is favorable, then induce the labor with IV oxytocin and artificial rupture of membrane

- If dates are sure, but the cervix is unfavorable, then labor can be induced by prostaglandin E2, followed by IV oxytocin. Other option is to do twice-weekly NSTs and AFIs to ensure fetal well-being
- If dates are unsure preform twice-weekly NSTs and AFIs. If fetal is not doing well at any time during the exam, then deliver the baby

Rh INCOMPATIBILITY

Rh incompatibility (also known as rhesus isoimmunization) causes hemolytic anemia in newborn. It is usually seen in second or subsequent pregnancy

Cause: Rh-negative mother and Rh-positive father have a Rh-positive baby. During the first pregnancy mother may get exposed to fetus' blood, and forms antibodies against Rh-positive blood. As a result this reaction is seen second or subsequent pregnancy

Diagnosis:

- Kleihauer-Batke test, this test measures the amount of fetal hemoglobin in mother's blood
- PUBS, it directly measures fetal hematocrit and degree of anemia
- Ultrasound doppler is performed to measure the blood flow through the fetal middle cerebral artery

Treatment: if fetus has severe anemia and is < 34 weeks gestation, then perform intrauterine intravascular transfusion. However, if a fetus with severe anemia is > 34 weeks of gestation, then delivery is usually performed.

Prevention

- Rh-negative mother should receive RhoGAM at 28 weeks of gestation and within 72 hours of **delivery**
- RhoGAM within 72 hours of **miscarriage, elective or spontaneous abortion, amniocentesis, placenta abruption, placenta previa or vaginal bleeding**

Note: If both of the parents are Rh-negative, or if the mother is Rh-positive and father is Rh-negative, then there is no need to give RhoGAM

GYNECOLOGY

VAGINAL DISCHARGE
Some vaginal discharge is normal, but a sudden change in color, odor or significant increase or decrease in the amount, may indicate infection.

Vaginal discharge differential diagnosis

1. PHYSIOLOGICAL VAGINAL DISCHARGE
Physiological vaginal discharge is normal in healthy reproductive age women. It is caused by high estrogen and is **usually seen during ovulation**
Chief complaint: **thin watery** discharge
Diagnosis:
- Vaginal speculum exam shows **clear watery discharge**, normal vaginal epithelium
- Vaginal **pH < 4.5**

Treatment: Progestin

2. CANDIDA VAGINITIS
Candida vaginitis is a fungal infection of vaginal mucosa caused by candida albicans
Risk factors: diabetic women, someone on antibiotics, pregnant, HIV-positive women
Chief complaint: vaginal itching, burning and **thick curdy white** discharge
Diagnosis:
- Vaginal speculum exam shows thick **curdy white discharge**, inflamed vaginal epithelium
- Vaginal **pH< 4.5**
- Wet mount test: microscopic examination of KOH prep shows **pseudohyphae**

Treatment:
- Single dose of oral fluconazole or any " azole", other **than metronidazole**
- If single dose of oral fluconazole was ineffective –Tx. **7 days course of fluconazole**

Boards Tip:
- If a patient keeps coming back with recurrent candida vaginitis despite medicine compliance, then **get HIV test**

3. BACTERIAL VAGINOSIS

Bacterial vaginosis is caused by overgrowth of normal vaginal bacteria known as Gardnerella

Chief complaint: **fishy odor vaginal** discharge, **gray white discharge**

Diagnosis:
- Vaginal speculum exam shows **gray white discharge**
- Vaginal **pH > 5.0**
- Wet mount: Microscopy with saline wet mount shows " **clue cells"**
- **Whiff test**: vaginal discharge gives **fishy odor** when it is placed on KOH prep

Treatment: Oral Metronidazole. It is also safe in pregnant women in all trimesters

4. TRICHOMONAS VAGINITIS

Trichomonas vaginitis is the most common **non-viral sexual transmitted** disease (STD), caused by Trichomonas vaginalis (**pear-shaped flagellated** protozoa). It can stay asymptomatic in male's seminal fluid

Chief complaint: **Green frothy discharge**, burning and pain with intercourse

Diagnosis:
- Vaginal speculum exam shows **green discharge and strawberry** appearance of cervix
- Vaginal **pH >5.0**
- Wet mount: Microscopy with saline wet mount shows **motile organism**

Treatment:
- Metronidazole for **patient** and **sexual partner**

Important: if metronidazole is given to a breastfeeding mother, then advice her to not to breastfeed for 24 hours after taking metronidazole

PELVIC INFLAMMATROY DISEASE (PID)

Pelvic inflammatory disease is a general term used for infection of the upper genital tract.

Cause: most common causes are **chlamydia and gonorrhea,** but other cause may include trichomoniasis, herpes virus, HPV, systemic inflammation, radiation, local trauma

Differential diagnosis of PID

1. CERVICITIS

Cervicitis is inflammation of cervix, a lower end of uterus that opens into the vagina

Si/Sx: most of the patients are asymptomatic, but symptoms may include **yellow-green mucopurulent discharge,** painful urination, pain during intercourse, vaginal bleeding after intercourse

Diagnosis:
- Pelvic exam may show redness of cervix, inflammation of the vaginal walls, discharge from cervix
- Beta-HCG to **rule out pregnancy**
- **Best initial diagnostic test is cervical swab for gram stain**
- **Most accurate diagnostic test** includes urethral culture, DNA probe or nucleic acid amplification test
- **WBCs and ESR are usually normal**

Treatment: outpatient treatment with single dose of oral azithromycin and cefixime or ceftriaxone

2. ACUTE SALPINGO-OPHORITIS

Si/Sx: mucopurulent cervical discharge, **cervical motion tenderness, bilateral pelvic pain and fever**

Diagnosis:
- Pelvic exam shows cervical motion tenderness, bilateral lower abdominal-pelvic tenderness
- Beta-HCG to **rule out pregnancy**
- Cervical culture for **gram stain and sensitivity**
- **ESR and WBCs are usually increased**
- Ultrasound may show pelvic abscess

Management:
- **Outpatient** treatment with **ofloxacin and metronidazole**

- **Inpatient** treatment with **IV cefotetan or cefoxitin and doxycycline or clindamycin and gentamicin.** Inpatient treatment is given if patient has any of the followings:
  - Fever **>102.2 F**
  - Pregnant
  - Nulligravida
  - Adolescent
  - **IUD** in place
  - Outpatient management **failure**
  - Ultrasound shows **pelvic abscess**

Complication: Untreated acute salpingo-oophoritis can:
- Gets worse and leads to **tubo-ovarian abscess**
          Or
- Heals with scar that causes **chronic PID**

3.   TUBO-OVARIAN ABSCESS
Si/Sx: Toxic appearing patient, severe lower abdominal pain, back pain, rectal pain, high fever
Diagnosis:
- Beta-HCG to **rule out pregnancy**
- Cervical culture for gram stain and sensitivity
- Blood culture
- **ESR and WBCs are usually increased**
- Ultrasound may show **bilateral complex pelvic abscess**

Management:
- **Inpatient** treatment with **IV clindamycin and gentamycin**
- If patient is **not responding to treatment** within **72 hours** – Tx. **Exploratory laparotomy with or without TAH and BSO or percutaneous drainage**

4.   CHRONIC PID
Si/Sx: chronic lower abdominal pain, cervical motion tenderness, or infertility. Discharge and fever are usually not absent

Diagnosis:
- Cervical culture is usually negative
- **WBCs and ESR are usually normal**
- Ultrasound shows complex bilateral cystic mass

Management:
- If the patient complain of pain, then give **analgesics**
- **Lysis of tubal adhesion may help restore fertility**
- If the patient has severe unremitting pelvic pain – Tx. TAH-BSO

PAP SMEAR

1. PAP SMEAR SCREENING
Pap smear screening begins at the **age of 21 or 3 years after the first intercourse**, whichever comes first
Frequency of screening:
- If the patient is < 30 years of age:
  - If **conventional methods** is used, then do screening **very year**
  - If **liquid base** (thin prep) is used, then do screening **every 2 years**
- If the patient is > 30 years old and has **3 consecutive negative pap smear**, then do screening **very 3 years**

Note: Pap screening for **homosexual females** is same as heterosexual females, even though they are at low-risk of HPV infection

2. ABNORMAL PAP SMEAR WORK UP

2a. If the pap smear shows **low** or **high grade** squamous cell carcinoma or **cervical cancer, then** next step is to get **colposcopy & ectocervical biopsy**

2b. If pap smear shows **atypical squamous cell of undetermined significance (ASCUS)**, then manage the patient as follow:
- If **conventional method** was used, next step:
  - If the patient is unreliable, then do **colposcopy and biopsy**
  - If the patient is reliable patient, then repeat Pap smear after 6 months:
    - If Pap smear is still abnormal after 6 months, then do **Colposcopy & ectocervical biopsy**

- If Pap smear is normal after 6 months, then **repeat Pap until 2 consecutive negative Pap smears**

- If **liquid base method** was used, then do *DNA* **testing**
  o If DNA testing shows **HPV 16 or 18**, then do **colposcopy and biopsy**

Note:
- HPV 16, 18,31,33 and 35 associated with cervical cancer
- HPV 6, and 11 are benign cause venereal warts

2c. All **non-pregnant** women should also have **endocervical curettage** (ECC)

Note:
- Endocervical curettage is **not performed in pregnant women** because it increases the risk of bleeding and membrane rupture

2d. **Cone biopsy** is performed after ECC, if patient has any of the followings:
- Pap smear worse than histology
- Abnormal ECC histology
- Endocervical lesion
- Biopsy show micro-invasive cervix cancer

- Complications of cone biopsy
  o Incompetent cervix
  o Cervical stenosis

PREVENTION OF CERVICAL DYSPLASIA

Gardasil® vaccine
- Recommended to all females between 9- 26 years of age
- It protects against HPV 6, 11, 16 and 18
- Three doses are given: 0, 2 and 6 months
- Women should get regular Pap smear despite vaccination
- It not recommended not pregnant, lactating, immunosuppressed females
- It does not affect the efficacy of oral contraceptives

- Women with previous abnormal cervical pathology may still receive vaccine

CERVICAL CANCER

Cervical cancer is the cancer of the cervix. It mostly affects women < 40 years of age

Risk factors:

- Human papillomavirus (HPV) infection
- Smoking
- Family history of cervical cancer
- Sexual activity at an early age
- Multiple sexual partners
-

Note: HPV 16, 18, 31, 33, and 35 are associated with **cervical cancer. HPV 6 and 11** are associated with **venereal warts**

Si/Sx: abnormal vaginal bleeding between periods, bleeding after intercourse, pelvic pain and vaginal discharge. Patient with advanced stages may have urine incontinence, fecal incontinence, back pain, bone pain or fractures

Diagnosis:

- Pap smear
- Visible lesion should be followed up with **colposcopy and endocervical biopsy**
- **Check distance metastasis with** x-ray, sigmoidoscopy and cystoscopy
- Staging is clinical, usually based on pelvic exam and may include intravenous pyelogram (IVP)

Management:

- Localized disease is managed based on colposcopy findings, which is as follow:

Type of localized cancer	Management

CIN 1	• Observation and follow-up:
	  o Pap smear every 6 months
	     Or
	• Pap+ colposcopy or HPV-DNA every 12 months

CIN 2 or 3	• Loop-electrosurgical excision procedure (LEEP), it is preferred due to low risk of bleeding and infection rate
	     Or
	• Cold-knife conization
	
	  o After LEEP or cold-knife conization patient should is managed as CN1 follow-ups

Recurrent CIN 2 or 3	• Hysterectomy

- **Invasive tumors' management is based on the tumor spread in the cervix:**

Stage	Spread to the cervix	Management
Ia 1.	≤ 3 mm deep	Simple hysterectomy
Ia 2.	> 3mm but ≤ 5mm deep	Modified hysterectomy
Ib.	> 5mm deep	Radical hysterectomy
IIb.	Distance metastasis	Radiation and chemotherapy

- Management of cervical cancer **during pregnancy**

Stage	Management
CIN/Dysplasia	• Pap smear and colposcopy every 3 months • Then repeat Pap and colposcopy 2 months after the delivery. If patient still has lesions, then do radical hysterectomy or radiation o Mode of delivery: vaginal delivery
Micro –invasive cervical cancer	• Cone biopsy is performed to ensure that there is no frank invasion (>5mm depth), o If no frank invasion is seen then manage the patient as CIN/Dysplasia
Invasive cancer	• Depends on gestational age o < 24 weeks of gestation-Tx. radical hysterectomy or radiation o > 24 weeks of gestation- Tx. conservative management till 32-33 weeks, then perform C-section and hysterectomy

Cervical cancer prevention:
- Pap smear screening starting at age 21, or 3 years after first intercourse, whichever comes first
- Safe sex to prevent HPV infection
- HPV vaccine to all females between 9-26 years of age

VULVAR CANCER
Vulvar cancer is a cancer that affects outer surface of female genitalia such as labia, skin folds outside the vagina, clitoris, or the glands outside of the vaginal opening

Cause: most common vulvar cancer is squamous cell carcinoma, other causes include adenocarcinoma, basal cell carcinoma, melanoma, sarcoma, Paget's disease, malignant melanoma

Risk factors: HPV infection, obesity, diabetes, hypertension

Si/Sx: Pruritus, irritation, raised lesions

Diagnosis:

- Biopsy
- Staging is surgically done
    - Stage I: Tumor confined to vulva with size < 2 cm
    - Stage II: Tumor confined to vulva with size > 2 cm
    - Stage III: tumor spreads to lower urethra, vagina or anus

Treatment: Local excision for stage I and II cancer, and wide excision for stage III cancer. Radiation for metastatic tumors

VAGINAL BLEEDING

1. **PREMENARCHAL VAGINAL BLEEDING**

- Causes
    - Foreign body (most common cause)
    - Sexual abuse
    - Sarcoma botryoides
    - Precocious puberty

Management:

- **Perform pelvic exam under sedation** to look for **foreign body**, and treat appropriately
- If no foreign body is found, then do **CT or MRI of the head and pelvis** to rule out pituitary tumor or pelvic tumor, and treat appropriately
- If pelvic exam and imaging are negative, then the diagnosis is **precocious puberty**

2. **VAGINAL BLEEDING IN REPRODUCTIVE AGE WOMEN**

Important: if a reproductive age women present with vaginal bleeding, then the first step in management is to rule out pregnancy with urine beta-hCG

2a. UTERINE LEIOMYOMA

Uterine leiomyoma refers to benign neoplasm that arises from **smooth muscle of the uterus**. Uterine leiomyoma is **estrogen–dependent**, they show rapid growth during pregnancy or with estrogen-progesterone combined OCPs, and shrinks after menopause.

Types and symptoms:
- **Intramural:** most common type, and is usually asymptomatic
- **Submucosal:** located in endometrial side of the uterus
  - Symptoms: Menorrhagia and intermenstrual bleeding
  - Complication: infertility and recurrent abortion
- **Subserosal:** located outside uterus
  - Complications: compression of bladder, rectum or ureter

Diagnosis:
- Pelvic exam shows **asymmetric** and **nontender** uterus
- **Ultrasound** for **intramural** and **subserosal leiomyoma**
- **Ultrasound** with **saline infusion** for **submucosal leiomyoma**

Management:
- **GnRH analog** are used before surgery to decrease the size
- If a patient wants to **preserve fertility** - Tx. **Myomectomy**
  - Advise patient to have C-section deliveries after myomectomy because of increased risk of uterine rupture
- If a patient wants to **preserve uterus** – Tx. **Embolization of uterine artery**
  - This is not done in woman, who wants to be pregnant in the future because it increases the risk of placental abnormalities
- **Definitive therapy or when fertility is completed** - Tx. **Hysterectomy**

2b. ADENOMYOSIS

Adenomyosis is an ectopic endometrial gland **within the myometrium** of uterus

Cause: there is no known cause

Si/Sx: most of the patients are asymptomatic, but symptoms may include dysmenorrhea, menorrhagia, dyspareunia

Diagnosis:
- Pelvic exam shows **symmetric and tender uterus**
- Ultrasound shows ectopic endometrial gland and stroma within the myometrium of the uterus

Treatment: intrauterine levonorgestrel

3. VAGINAL BLEEDING IN POSTMENOPAUSAL WOMEN

Vaginal bleeding in a postmenopausal woman is **endometrial carcinoma,** until proven otherwise. But other cause may include **endometrial atrophy, vaginal atrophy**

Cause: there is no exact known cause of endometrial cancer, but increased level of estrogen seems to have a significant role. Estrogen stimulates the endometrial lining of the uterus

Risk factors:
- Diabetes
- Obesity
- Infertility
- Polycystic ovarian syndrome
- Early mensuration (before age 12)
- Menopause starting after age 50

Diagnosis:
- Endometrial biopsy
- Vaginal ultrasound, to measure the endometrial thickness, in postmenopausal women **normal endometrial thickness is < 5mm**

Management: depends on biopsy
- If endometrial **biopsy is normal,** then get **hysteroscopy,** to check if bleeding is caused by endometrial hyperplasia or ovarian polyp
- If endometrial **biopsy** shows **atrophy–** Tx. **Estrogen + progesterone.** Estrogen is always combined with progesterone because unopposed estrogen increases the risk of endometrial carcinoma
- If endometrial **biopsy** shows **adenocarcinoma, then get staging of the cancer and treatment depends on stages** (see below)

Stages	Management
Limited to uterus	TAH & BSO
Extension to cervix	TAH & BSO + Radiation
Metastatic disease	TAH& BSO + Radiation + Chemotherapy

TAH: Total abdominal hysterectomy. BSO: Bilateral salpingo - oophorectomy

o   **Radiation therapy** is performed in patients with poor prognosis, such as positive surgical margin, poorly differentiated tumor, lymph node metastasis or >50% myometrium invasion

DYSFUNCTIONAL UTERINE BLEEDING (DUB)

Dysfunctional uterine bleeding is abnormal bleeding from the uterus due to change in hormonal level

Cause: anovulatory cycle (unopposed estrogen), estrogen producing tumor, infection, vWF factor deficiency, and endocrine disorder such as thyroid, adrenal

Si/Sx: Menorrhagia (bleeding between periods), menorrhagia (heavy bleeding), oligomenorrhea (period lasting 35- 90 days),

Diagnosis:

- DUB is diagnosis of exclusion
- Rule out bleeding disorder, endocrine disorder, renal disorder, pregnancy
- Rule out anatomic lesions, endometrial cancer, polyps

Management:

- If a patient is **unstable,** then put a **Foley catheter to tamponade bleeding, give high dose IV estrogen, and perform D&C.**
- **If the patient** is stable, then **check the hemoglobin level** and manage the patient as follow:
  - o   If hemoglobin is **>12g/dl** – Tx. **Iron supplement**
  - o   If hemoglobin is **9-12g/dl** – Tx. **Iron + monophasic OCP**
  - o   If hemoglobin is **<9 g/dl** –Tx. **Transfusion+ IV estrogen** and **OCP**
  - o   If bleeding continues – Tx. D&C

PRIMARY DYSMENORRHEA

Primary dysmenorrhea is characterized by cramping pain in the lower abdomen that occurs just before the periods. It **usually begins 2-5 years after the menarche**

Cause: Excessive production of **prostaglandin F2- alpha**

Si/Sx: aching pain in the abdomen, feeling of pressure in the abdomen, nausea, vomiting

Treatment:
- **Best initial treatment is NSAIDs,** which relieves the symptom by inhibiting the prostaglandin synthesis.
- Estrogen and progesterone **OCPs is the second-line** treatment

ENDOMETRIOSIS

Endometriosis is an abnormal growth of endometrial cells outside of the uterus. It is the **most common cause of infertility in women more than 30 years of age.** Ovaries are the most common location of ectopic endometrial gland.

Endometriosis is most **common cause of secondary dysmenorrhea**

Si/Sx: dysmenorrhea (painful periods), **dyspareunia** (painful intercourse), **dyschezia** (painful bowel movement), pelvic or low back pain during menstrual cycle

Diagnosis:
- Pelvic exam may show uterosacral nodularity
- Laparoscopy is used to visualize the ectopic gland

Treatment:
- Best initial treatment is **continuous dose of progesterone or OCPs.**
- Second-line treatment is testosterone derivatives (danazol or Danocrine) or GnRH analogs (Lupron or leuprolide)
- Surgery is reserved for **refractory cases;**
  - Laparoscopy lysis adhesion is done if the patient **desires the fertility.**
  - If the patient **does not want to preserve fertility or is an older patient,** then consider total hysterectomy and bilateral salpingoopherectomy (TAH/BSO)

PRECOCIOUS PUBERTY
Precocious puberty refers to the development of secondary sexual characteristics and growth, before age 8 in females and 9 in males.

Normal puberty landmarks

Normal puberty landmarks	Age
Thelarche (Breast development)	9-10 years
Adrenarche (pubic and axillary hair)	10-11 years
Growth spurt	11-12 years
Menarche (onset of first menses)	12-13 years

Cause: there is no known specific cause, but some known causes include, transient hormonal change, CNS tumors, genetic disorder, ovarian tumor
Types: two main types of precocious puberty are **incomplete** and **complete** isosexual precocious puberty

1. **Incomplete isosexual precocious puberty** refers to early development of **one puberty landmark** such as thelarche, adrenarche or menarche. This condition is caused by either transient hormone spike or increased end-organ sensitivity. Treatment: **conservative management**
2. **Complete isosexual precocious puberty** refers to early development of **all puberty landmarks**. This condition is caused by CNS pathology, McCune-Albert syndrome, granulosa cell tumor or idiopathic (discussed below)

2a. **McCune-Albert syndrome**
   Si/Sx: precocious puberty, **Cafe-au-lait spots**, multiple bone fractures
   Diagnosis: labs show increased aromatase enzyme activity, increased estrogen
   Treatment: Aromatase enzyme inhibitor

2b. **Granulosa cell tumor**
   Si/Sx: precocious puberty, pelvic mass
   Diagnosis: labs show increased estrogen. Pelvic ultrasound shows a mass
   Treatment: Surgery

2c. CNS etiology

Cause: CNS etiology such as tumor, meningitis, encephalitis, hydrocephalus

Si/Sx: complete precious puberty, other symptoms depend on the cause

Diagnosis: labs show increased GnRH and increased FSH

Treatment: treat the underlying cause

2d. Idiopathic

Idiopathic precious precocious puberty accounts for majority of the precocious puberty cases

Si/Sx: no specific symptoms

Diagnosis: diagnosis of exclusion

Treatment: GnRH antagonist

PRIMARY AMENORRHEA

Primary amenorrhea is a condition in which menstrual bleeding never occurred

Diagnosis: it is diagnosed by presence of one of the following:

- Absence of menses, plus **no signs of secondary sexual** developments (growth, breast development, pubic hair and axillary hair) **at age 14**
- Absence of menses, but **presence of secondary sexual developments at age 16**

Cause: lots of causes can cause primary amenorrhea, but the primary causes can be divided into three main type based on presence or absence of breast and uterus. Which are as follow:

1. **Both uterus and breasts are present** (discussed on the next page)
2. **Breasts are present, but uterus is absent** (discussed on the next page)
3. **Breasts are absent, but uterus is present** (discussed on the next page)

Note: Pregnancy is the **most common cause of primary amenorrhea.** Therefore, it is necessary to rule out pregnancy first with the urine pregnancy test.

Diagnostic workup:

- Rule out pregnancy

- **Physical exam to check for breath development** (normal breast development suggest adequate estrogen production)
- Get abdominal **ultrasound to check if uterus is present**

1. Differential diagnosis of primary amenorrhea, **when both uterus and breasts are present**

Diagnosis	Characteristic	Treatment
Imperforate hymen	• Patients usually complain of cyclic pelvic pain • Genital exam shows **red-purple bulging membrane** at introitus	Surgical opening of imperforate hymen
Transverse vaginal pouch	• Patient usually complain of cyclic pain • Genital exam shows **blind vaginal pouch**	Surgical repair
Physical stress such as anorexic, athletes, Excessive exercise	• Patient's history and physical exam is usually helpful	OCP

2. Differential diagnosis primary amenorrhea, when **breasts are present, but uterus is absent**

Diagnosis	Characteristic	Treatment
Androgen insensitivity syndrome	• Physical exam shows **no pubic and axillary hair** • Karyotype shows **XY** chromosomes • Ultrasound **shows internal testes**	**Surgical removal of internal testes**, otherwise patient may develop testicular cancer. **Estrogen replacement** after the surgery
Müllerian agenesis	• **Normal pubic and axillary hair** • Karyotype show **XX** chromosome • Ultrasound shows **absence of mullerian duct derivatives**: fallopian tube, uterus, and upper vagina.	**Surgical elongation of vagina**

Note: In Müllerian agenesis, ovaries and lower vagina are present because these are not derived from Müllerian duct.

3. **Differential diagnosis** for primary amenorrhea, when **breasts are absent** but **uterus is present**

Diagnosis	Characteristic	Treatment
Turner syndrome	• Physical exam shows **short stature female, broad nipple, no secondary sexual** characters • **Increased FSH** level • Karyotypes shows X0 chromosome • Ultrasound shows streak ovaries	Estrogen and progesterone replacement
Hypothalamic-pituitary failure	• **Low FSH** • Karyotype shows XX chromosome • Heat CT to rule out tumor	Estrogen and progesterone replacement
Kallmann syndrome	• Anosmia **(loss of smell)** • Rest of the characteristics are same as hypothalamic- pituitary failure	Estrogen and progesterone replacement

SECONDARY AMENORRHEA

Secondary amenorrhea is absence of menstruation in a women who has been having normal menstrual cycles before

Diagnosis: it is diagnosed by the presence of one of the followings:

- Absence of menses for **3 months** if **previous regular menses**
- Absence of menses for **6 months** if **previous irregular menses**

Cause: pregnancy, hypothyroidism, elevated prolactin level, outflow obstruction, PCOS, brain tumor, estrogen deficiency, ovarian failure, brain tumors, change in LH and FSH levels

Diagnosis: diagnosing the exact cause of secondary amenorrhea can be challenging. Follow the approach below to narrow down a diagnosis.

1. **Pregnancy test:** pregnancy is the **most common cause of the secondary amenorrhea**. Therefore, it is important to rule out pregnancy before doing any tests

2. **TSH:** after ruling out the pregnancy check TSH. Low TSH level leads to increased TRH, which can further lead to increased prolactin level. Prolactin suppresses the LH and FSH and causes amenorrhea. If patient has **hypothyroidism,** then treat the patient with **levothyroxine**

3. **Prolactin level:** after ruling out hypothyroidism. Check prolactin levels. **Anti-psychotics or brain tumors** can cause high prolactin.

   - If a patient is taking anti-psychotics, then **switch the medicine.**
   - If the patient is not taking anti-psychotics, then get CT head to look for a pituitary tumor. **Pituitary tumor less than 1 cm** is treated with **bromocriptine.** Tumor **more than 1 cm is surgically removed.**

4. **Progesterone challenge test** (PCT) is performed after excluding pregnancy, THS and prolactin level. In this test patient is given one IM progesterone shot or oral 7 days medroxyprogesterone, and then follow-up with patient after 2-7 days to check if patient has withdrawal bleeding

4a. If patient experiences **withdrawal bleeding,** it means she is not ovulating **(anovulation).** Treatment: **Cyclic progesterone** is given to prevent endometrial hyperplasia, and add clomiphene if pregnancy is desired

4b. If **no bleeding occurs,** then either this patient has **low estrogen** or there is **outflow obstruction** such as adhesions or cervical stenosis.
   - If an **obstruction** is found, then it is **surgically relieved.**
   - If no obstruction is found, then it is likely due to **low estrogen** levels and that should be further evaluated with **estrogen progesterone challenge test**

5. **Estrogen progesterone challenge test** is performed after PCT. In this test patient is given estrogen for 21 days followed by progesterone for 7 days, and is checked for withdrawal bleeding

5a. If **no bleeding** occurs, then either this patient has **Asherman syndrome** or there is outflow tract obstruction such as adhesions or cervical stenosis.
   - If an **obstruction** is found, then it is **surgically relieved.**

- If no obstruction is found, then it means the patient has **Asherman syndrome,** which is further diagnosed with **hysterosalpingogram,** and treated with **adhesion lysis and estrogen replacement.** Stents are usually left in place to prevent re-adhesion

5b. If the **bleeding occurs,** then **check FSH levels**
- Low FSH (< 40 mIU/mL) means **gonadal failure,**
- FSH > 40 mIU/mL means **hypothalamus-pituitary dysfunction,** get head CT to rule out tumor.

Treatment: Regardless of the FHS levels, give patient **estrogen and progesterone.** Estrogen replacement is given to prevent osteoporosis and estrogen deficiency. Cyclic progesterone is also required to prevent endometrial hyperplasia. If the tumor is found, then surgically remove the tumor, and give estrogen and progesterone replacement

URINE INCONTINENCE

Urine incontinence is involuntary urine loss

Types and causes: the most common types are:
- **Stress incontinence** that is usually caused by **weakness of pelvic floor** muscles that support the bladder and urethra
- **Overflow incontinence** is usually seen in patient with nerve denervation such as diabetic neuropathy, multiple sclerosis or patients taking anticholinergic medicine. In this conditions patients **do not sense bladder fullness and, urine leaks** when bladder pressure exceeds the urethral pressure
- **Urge incontinence** is seen in patients with **involuntary contractions** of detrusor muscles
- **Bypass fistula is** seen in patients with obstetric and gynecology trauma or injury. Two most common fistulas are vesicovaginal fistula and uterovaginal fistula.

Diagnosis:
- UA and urine culture should be done to exclude UTI
- BUN/Cr, to exclude renal dysfunction
- Specific diagnosis depends on the specific cause (discussed below)

Symptoms, diagnosis and treatment of urine incontinence

Diagnosis	Symptoms	Diagnostic tests	Treatment
Stress incontinence	**Small volume** of urine loss during physical movement such as **cough, sneezing exercising**	Q-tip test	Pelvic strengthening exercises and estrogen. Surgery is reserved for refractory cases
Overflow incontinence	**Small volume** of urine loss, pelvic fullness present **during day and night**	Cytometric studies show residual bladder volume > 200 cc	Discontinue offending medicine, intermittent catheterization
Urge incontinence	**Large volume** of urine loss **without any warning,** present during day and night	Cytometric studies show residual bladder volume < 50 cc, and involuntary detrusor muscle contractions	Oxybutynin
Bypass fistula	**Continues** small amount of urine lost during day and at night	Intravenous pyelogram shows dye leaking from the urinary tract fistula	Surgery

PELVIC ORGAN PROLAPSE

Pelvic organ prolapse is a disorder in which muscles and ligaments supporting women's pelvic organs weaken and pelvic organs drop from their normal positions.

Cause: Childbirth, heavy lifting, obesity, normal aging, menopause

Si/Sx: pelvic pressure, sensation that something is falling out of vagina, urine incontinence, difficulty with bowel movement,

Types: four main types of pelvic organ prolapse are (discussed below)

Types of pelvic organ prolapse

Type	Location	Common symptoms
Uterine prolapse	Cervix descends in the **vagina**	Urinary incontinence, urgency and/or frequency
Cystocele	Bladder bulges into the **anterior wall of vagina**	Urine incontinence, urgency and/or frequency
Rectocele	Rectum bulges into the **posterior wall of vagina**	Constipation
Enterocele	Loop of bowel bulges into the **posterior vaginal wall**	Constipation

Treatment:

- **Best initial treatment** is pelvic **strengthening exercises** such as Kegel exercise. However, if symptoms are **affecting patient's** daily living, then **vaginal pessary device** may be used to support uterus, bladder and rectum.

- **Surgery** is a **last resort**. However, it is also the first-line of treatment in patients **with procidentia** (entire uterus outside the introitus).

OVARIAN TUMOR

Ovarian tumors are tumors that arise from the ovaries. These can be benign or malignant

Types: Three main types of ovarian tumors are:

- **Epithelial cell tumors** arise from the cells on the surface of the ovaries. Epithelial cell tumors account for 70 % of all ovarian tumors. **Most common epithelial tumors as serous, mucinous, clear ell and endometrioid**

- **Germ cell tumors** arise from the reproductive cells of the ovaries. Germ cell tumors account for < 2% of ovarian tumors. **Most common germ cell tumors are dysgerminoma, choriocarcinoma, teratomas, yolk sac tumor**

- **Stromal cell tumors** arise from supporting tissues within the ovaries. Stromal cell tumors account for 5-8% of ovarian tumors. **Most common stromal cell tumors are granulosa-stromal tumors and Sertoli-Leydig cell tumor**

Risk factors for ovarian cancer	Protective factors for ovarian cancer
<ul><li>Increased number ovulations</li><li>Nulliparity</li><li>Infertility</li><li>BRCA 1 gene</li><li>Use of talc powder</li><li>Family history of ovarian, breast and colorectal cancer</li></ul>	<ul><li>OCP</li><li>Breast-feeding</li><li>Chronic anovulation</li><li>Short reproductive life</li></ul>

Si/Sx: depends on the stage
- Patient in **early stages** of ovarian cancer may be asymptomatic or may have palpable adnexal mass, vague abdominal symptoms
- Patients in **late stages** of ovarian cancer usually have palpable **abdominal mass, increased abdominal girth, distention and pain**

Diagnosis:
- Abdominal ultrasound
- Tumor markers (discussed below)

Ovarian cancer tumor markers

Tumor marker	Ovarian tumor
CA-125, CEA	Epithelial tumor
Estrogen	Granulosa-stromal tumor
Testosterone	Sertoli-Leydig tumor
LDH	Dysgerminoma
HCG	Choriocarcinoma
AFP	Endodermal sinus tumor
HCG, AFP	Embryonal carcinoma

Treatment:
- Benign tumors are surgically removed
- Malignant tumor: TAH/BSO plus postoperative chemotherapy

OVARIAN CYSTS

Ovarian cysts are fluid-filled sacs in the ovaries. These are **common in reproductive aged women**

Cause: cysts forms during the menstrual cycle from follicles. These follicles produce estrogen and progesterone hormones and releases egg during the ovulation. Some times follicles keep growing and become functional cysts

Si/Sx: menstrual irregularities, pelvic pain, and pelvic pressure. Ruptured cysts causes sudden severe abdominal or pelvic pain, fever

Diagnosis:

- Beta-HCG to exclude pregnancy or ectopic pregnancy
- Diagnosis is confirmed with ultrasound

Management:

- If ultrasound shows **fluid filled simple cyst**, then manage as follow:
  - Cysts **< 7 cm** are treated with **OCPs and follow-up in 6-8 weeks to ensure resolution**
  - Cysts **> 7 cm** are removed by **laparoscopic**
- If ultrasound shows **complex cyst**, then manage as follow:
  - If the patient wants to **preserve fertility**, then do **cystectomy**
  - If the patient **does not want to preserve fertility**, then do **oophorectomy**

OVARIAN TORSION

Ovarian torsion refers to twisting of ovaries that may occlude the ovarian artery and or vein

Si/Sx: sudden onset of severe lower abdominal pain, fever, vomiting

Diagnosis:

- Initial step is to do urine Beta-hCG to rule out pregnancy
- Ultrasound - shows ovarian mass twisted around its axis

Management:

- **Laparoscopy:** untwist the ovaries and observe for perfusion:
  - If ovaries shows **adequate perfusion** –Tx. **Cystectomy**
  - If ovaries becomes **necrotic** –Tx. **Oophorectomy**

GESTATIONAL TROPHOBLASTIC TUMOR (GTT)

Gestational trophoblastic tumor is a form of tumor that is derived from abnormal placental tissue, inside women's uterus (womb).

Types: Two main types of gestational trophoblastic tumor are hydatidiform mole and choriocarcinoma

1. **Hydatidiform mole** (also known as **molar pregnancy**) accounts for about 80% GTT. It rarely spreads outside of the uterus. Sub-type of hydatidiform moles are:

    1a. **Complete molar pregnancy** occurs when **a sperm fertilizes an abnormal egg**. Instead of forming embryo, the cell forms a **"grape-like"** cysts, it has chromosomal pattern of **46, XX**.

    1b. **Partial mole** occurs when **two sperms fertilize an egg**. Some fetal parts are formed, it has chromosomal pattern of **69, XXY**.

2. **Choriocarcinoma** accounts for about 5% of GTT. It can spread outside of the uterus.

Si/Sx: irregular vaginal bleeding that usually occurs in early second trimester, **hyperemesis gravidarum, uterus size more than gestational dates**

Diagnosis:
- Physical exam shows **uterus size more than gestational dates**, missing fetal heart tone
- Serum Beta-HCG, which is usually markedly high (>100,000 mIU/mL)
- Chest X-ray to rule out metastasis
- Pelvic ultrasound may show " snowstorm" ultrasound

Management:
- Get baseline β-hCG
- Chest X-ray to rule out metastasis
- D & C and tissue pathology

Treat as follow:
- If **no metastasis**, but pathology and karyotype shows:
    - **Absent fetus** and **46XX** – Tx. **1 year OCP**
    - **Nonviable fetus** and **69 XXY**- Tx. **1 year OCP**
- If **metastasis** to **pelvic** or **lungs** or **limited to the uterus**
    - Give methotrexate or actinomycin D until β-hCG is zero,
        - Continue follow β-hCG **for 3 weeks**
        - Then, keep patient on **OCP for 1 year**: check β-hCG every month for 1year

- If **metastasis to the brain or liver**
  - Give methotrexate + Actinomycin D+ Cyclophosphamide **until β-hCG is zero**
    - Continue follow **β-hCG for 3 weeks**
    - Then **OCP for 5 year**: check β-hCG every 2 months for the first 2 years, and then every 3 months for the next 3 year

Prognosis:
- If tumor is limited to the uterus, then there is 100% cure rate
- If tumor is metastasis to pelvic or lung, then there is >95% cure rate
- If tumor is metastasis to brain or liver, then there is 65% cure rate

HIRSUTISM AND VIRILIZATION
Hirsutism is excessive body hair. Virilization is a hyperandrogenism state (clitoromegaly, temporal balding, voice deepening, increased muscle mass, and amenorrhea).

Si/Sx: women usually present with excessive hair growth on chest, abdomen, chins, upper lips and virilization

Causes: most common causes of hirsutism and virilization are adrenal tumor, congenital adrenal hyperplasia, ovarian cancer and polycystic ovarian syndrome (disused in table below)

Differential diagnosis of hirsutism and virilization

Disease	Diagnosis	Treatment
Adrenal tumor	• Labs shows **increased DHEAS** • Abdominal CT or ultrasound	Surgery
Congenital adrenal hyperplasia	• Usually due to 21-alpha-hydroxylase defect • Labs shows **increased 17-hydroxyprogestrone,**	Glucocorticoids
Ovarian cancer	• Labs shows very high **testosterone level (> 200 ng/dL)** • Pelvic CT or ultrasound	Surgery
Polycystic ovarian syndrome (PCOS)	• Labs shows **LH: FHS ratio 3:1** • Pelvic ultrasound shows **" Pearl necklace sign"**	Treatment of PCOS is discussed on the next page

Treatment for PCOS:

- Weight loss may help ovulation and spare the fertility
- Clomiphene citrate to induce ovulation
- Metformin for diabetes
- Spironolactone to treat facial hair growth
- OCPs are given to prevent endometrial hyperplasia and endometrial carcinoma

INFERTILITY

Infertility is defined as failure to conceive **after 12 months of unprotected** intercourse

Cause: abnormal sperm production accounts for 40 % of the infertility, anovulation 30%, anatomic defect of the female reproductive tracts 20 % and 10 % of cases have no known cause

Diagnosis:

Abnormal sperm factor accounts for most of the cases of infertility, so it necessary to rule out male conditions first

1. **Male workup** usually involves checking semen for any abnormalities. Normal semen has the following characteristics:
   - Ejaculation volume > 2 ml
   - Sperm pH 7.2 - 7.8
   - Sperm density > 20 million/ml,
   - Initial sperm forward motility > 50 %
   - Normal sperm morphology > 50%

1a If semen meets the normal **criteria,** then we can move to **female** workup

1b If the semen **does not meet** the normal criteria, then **repeat the semen test** in 2-3 days. If results **come back normal,** then proceed to **female testing.** However, if **results are still abnormal,** then the following treatment options may be tried

Treatment: if the male has semen abnormalities, then treatment **depends** on severity of **semen abnormalities:**

- If **sperm is minimal abnormal,** then **intrauterine insemination** may be tried
- If sperm is **severely abnormal,** then **intracytoplasmic sperm injection with in vitro fertilization** may be tried
- If **sperm is not viable** or if **above discussed options fail,** then the **sperm donor is needed**

2. **Female work-up** should be performed after semen test is normal. Do the tests in the following order:

    2a. Elevation of body temperature

    2b. Check endocrine disorders such as hypothyroidism,

    2c. Prolactinoma

    2d. Check anovulation history (menstrual regularities)

    2e. Check uterine cavity with hysterosalpingogram

    2f. Laparoscopy

Treatment:

- If any endocrine disorder is found, then treat the disorder
- Anovulation is treated with **clomiphene citrate** (first choice) **or HMG.**
- **Laparoscopy** may be tried to fix tubal damage and restore fertility, but if tubal damage is severe, then **In-vitro fertilization** should be planned

BREAST MASS

1. FIBROCYSTIC DISEASE

Fibrocystic breast disease is a benign breast disease, characterized by painful lump in the breast. It is common in women, in her 30s.

Cause: there is no known cause, but symptoms are **related to woman's hormones levels**, which occur just before and during menstruation

Si/Sx: breast pain, multiple, bilateral cysts that are tender to touch, cysts usually resolve within a few weeks

Diagnosis: usually no work-up is needed, ultrasound is done if cyst does not disappear in few weeks

Treatment: OCPs and **follow-up patient** in 6 weeks

2. FIBROADENOMA

Fibroadenoma is the most common benign tumor of the breast; it is composed of **fibrous and glandular tissue**

Cause: fibroadenoma is estrogen dependent tumor that grows during pregnancy and OCPs use, and gets smaller after the menopause

Si/Sx: lump that may be painless, rubbery, moves easily under the skin

Diagnosis:
- Ultrasound
- Fine needle biopsy

Treatment: Excision

3. MASTITIS

Mastitis is an infection of the breast that causes breast inflammation, erythema, and pain. It is usually seen in **postpartum breastfeeding women**

Cause: S. Aureus, which is transferred from infant's throat or nose, during breastfeeding

Treatment:
- **Anti-staphylococcal medicine** such as dicloxacillin or cephalexin and advice the patient to **continue breast feeding** from the affected side of the breast to prevent duct blockage, otherwise it may progress to breast abscess

Compilation: Breast abscess: it is a painful collection of pus in the breast. Most breast abscesses develop secondary to bacterial infection such as S.Aureus. Patient develops a painful fluctuating mass. Diagnosis is usually confirmed with ultrasound, and treated by **draining the abscess**

BREAST CANCER

1. **Ductal carcinoma in situ** (DCIS) is the most common noninvasive breast cancer, which develops in milk ducts. It may progress to invasive ductal carcinoma
2. **Lobular carcinoma in situ** (LCIS) is the second most common noninvasive breast cancer, which develops in the lobules of the breast. It may progress to invasive lobular carcinoma.
3. **Inflammatory breast disease** is very aggressive form of breast malignancy. In this condition cancer cells blocks the lymph vessels of the skin of the breast, and breast skin appears as skin of an orange **"Peau d' orange"**
4. **Paget disease of breast / nipples** is a rare breast malignancy, which affects the nipple and breast. It gives breast **eczema-like appearance:** red, scaly, itchy and inflamed. **Nipples may become inverted and may have straw-colored or bloody discharge.**

Stages of breast cancer

Stage	Area involved
Stage 0	Carcinoma in situ
Stage 1	Tumor size < 2cm
Stage 2	Tumor size > 2 cm but < 5 cm
Stage 3	Tumor > 5 cm plus lymph nodes involvement
Stage 4	Distance metastasis

Risk factors for breast cancer:
- Female gender
- Family history of breast cancer
- Personal history of breast cancer
- BRCA 1 or BRCA 2 gene
- Radiation exposure
- Having first child after age 35
- Nulliparity
- Postmenopausal hormone therapy
- Alcohol
- High fat and low fiber diet

Diagnosis:
- Breast **ultrasound for woman < 30 years** of age
  - If ultrasound shows **simple cyst**, then get **needle aspiration**
  - If ultrasound shows **complex cyst**, then get **ultrasound guided core biopsy**
- **Mammogram** for woman **> 30 years of** age
- Breast lump biopsy
- Lymph node biopsy
- Estrogen and progesterone receptors
- HER2 receptor
- Bone scan, alkaline phosphate, chest x-ray, CT scan

Treatment:
- Stage 1 and 2 cancers are treated with lumpectomy, axillary lymph node dissection, and radiation therapy.
- Moderate to high risk cancer are treated with chemotherapy followed by radiation therapy
- Women with ER or PR positive receptor should be treated tamoxifen and chemotherapy

- Trastuzumab is given to patient with positive HER2 receptors

CONTRACEPTIONS

1. **Barrier methods advantages and disadvantages**
   - Male condoms are protective against STDs
   - Female diaphragm needs to insert in vagina an hour prior to planned intercourse. However, they do not provide any protection against STDs

2. **Progestin only contraceptives:** three main types of progestin only modalities are:
   - Progestin only **oral** pill are called " **minipill,**" it needs to be taken **daily and continuously. It can be safely given to a breast-feeding mother**
   - Progestin-only **intramuscular** also known as **Depo-Provera**, has to be administered **every three months**. It is the only **safe contraceptive** that can be used in patients with **sickle-cell disease, epilepsy or iron deficiency anemia**
   - Progestin only **subcutaneous patch** is a slow release and it works **continuously for 3 years**

3. **Estrogen- progesterone combined contraceptives:** main types of combined contraceptive are:
   - Oral form also known as **YAZ**, is 24 days of active pill followed by 7 days of placebos
   - Vaginal ring also known as **NuvaRing**, it is inserted into the vagina for 3 weeks, and then removed for 1 week to allow withdrawal bleeding
   - Transdermal patch also known as **Ortho Evra** is placed for 3 weeks, and then removed for 1 week to allow withdrawal bleeding

Contra-indication and benefits of combined OCPs

Absolute contraindication	Relative contraindication	Benefits

• Pregnancy
• DM with vascular disease
• Migraines with aura
• Uncontrolled HTN
• Liver disease
• Known hypercoagulable state
• Previous DVT or PE
• Hormone dependent cancer
• Smoker>35 years
	• **DM**
	• **Migraine**
	• **Choric HTN**
	• Depression
		• Decreases
		  ○ Dysfunctional uterine bleeding
		  ○ Dysmenorrhea
		  ○ Endometrial cancer
		  ○ Ovarian cancer
		  ○ Ectopic pregnancy

4. **Intrauterine device (IUD):** two main types of IUDs are:
    - **Levonorgestrel IUD** also known as **Marina**, it releases hormones **over 5-year period**. It may also **lower the bleeding and cramping**
    - **Copper T band** also known as **Paraguard**, it releases hormones **over 10-years period**. It may **increase the bleeding and cramping**

    Absolute contraindications for IUDs:
    - Pregnancy
    - Previous PID
    - Pelvic malignancy
    - Active pelvic infection

5. **Permanent sterilization** is irreversible; it is a best option for those who do not desire any more children
    - Vasectomy: it is a removal of segment of vas deference in men
    - In female, permanent sterilization options include cutting, clipping or ligation of fallopian tubes

MENOPAUSE

Menopause is the cessation of woman's menstrual cycles. In US average age of menopause 51 years

Si/Sx: Menstrual periods that occur less often and eventually stop, hot flashes and sweating, skin flushing, insomnia,

Diagnosis: increased FSH (**FSH to LH ratio 3:1**)

Treatment: Hormone replacement therapy (HRT) is a **combination of estrogen and progesterone.** Estrogen controls the **vasomotor symptoms** (e.g. hot flashes, palpitations) and progesterone is added to the treatment because unopposed estrogen can cause endometrial hyperplasia and increase the risk of endometrial cancer.

Risks and benefits of HRT therapy

Benefits of HRTs	Reduces the risk of colorectal cancer and osteoporotic fractures
Risks of HRT	Increases the risk of DVT and heart attack. Risk of breast cancer increases if HRT is used for > 4 years

- Guidelines for HRT:
    - Only for vasomotor symptoms (Hot Flashes)
    - Use the lowest dose
    - Use for shortest duration, and reevaluate every year
    - Never use for cardiovascular disease
    - Do not use them for more than 4 years

- Contraindication for HRT therapy:
    - Estrogen-sensitive cancer
    - Liver disease
    - Unexplained bleeding
    - Active thrombosis

OSTEOPOROSIS

In osteoporosis bones become fragile, weak and more easily to break

Risk factors: thin white female with family history (most common cause), smoking, alcohol, sedentary lifestyle, low calcium intake and steroids

Diagnosis:
- Spine x-ray
- Bone density testing with DEXA scan; DEXA $\geq$ - 2.5 signifies osteoporosis

Treatment:
- First-line of treatment is bisphosphonate (alendronate, risedronate), these inhibits the osteoclast cell
- Second-line treatment is raloxifene, these increases the bone density
- Estrogen replacement is the last resort because estrogen increases the hypercoagulable states

Lifestyle modifications
- Vitamin D and calcium supplement
- Weight bearing exercises, as tolerated
- Smoking cessation
- Stop alcohol consumption

Osteoporosis screening with DEXA:
- In postmenopausal **women:**
  - **Without** risk factors start at > 65 years of age
  - **With risk** factors start 60-64 years of age
- In men
  - **With risk** factors start > 65 years of age
  - **Without** risk factor start> **80 years of age**

OBSTETRICS /GYNECOLOGY CCS

Case # 1

Case introduction
A 28-years-old woman comes to the clinic to get her OCPs refills before she goes to Italy for vacation for two weeks

Initial vitals signs
Temperature: 37.2 degrees
Pulse: 68 beats/ min, regular rhythm
Respiration rate: 18/ minutes

Blood pressure, systolic 123 mm Hg
Blood pressure, disystolic 75 mm Hg

Height: 62.0 inches
Weight: 135.0 lbs.
Body mass index: 24.7 Kg/ m2

History of present illness (HPI)
A 28-years-old woman comes to the clinic to get her OCPs refills before she goes to Italy for vacation for two weeks. She is sexually active with her husband and she uses OCPs to prevent pregnancy. She denies any weight gain. She says she has not had her period in last two months and lately been experiencing nausea and vomiting in the morning. She did not do any home pregnancy test. She denies vaginal discharge, painful urination or previous STDs.

Past medical history
Hospitalization: None
Other medical condition: None
Current medication: None
Allergies: latex
Vaccination: up to date

Family history
Father has osteoarthritis and mother is healthy.

Social history
Marital history: Married; 1 child
Occupation: Flight attendant
Recreational: Cooking, travel
Personal habits: She smokes 6 cigarettes a day and drinks socially. She
denies drugs

Review of system:
General: see HPI
Skin: see HPI
HEENT: see HPI
Musculoskeletal: see HPI
Cardiology: see HPI
Abdominal: see HPI
Genitourinary: see HPI

Please see pages 1-5 for general CCS cases approach

Step 1. None (patient is stable does not require any emergency measures)

Step 2. Order complete physical exam including genitals, and then move the clock forward to get the results
- Results show:
- o Genitals exam shows dark blue vagina and vulva
- o Rest of the exam is normal

Step 3. Order labs, and then move the clock forward to get the results
- Urine pregnancy test " stat "
- CBC
- UA
- BMP

- Results shows:
- o Positive pregnancy test

Step 4. None

Step 5. Office

Step 6. None

Step 7. Order first-trimester pregnancy labs, and then move the clock forward to get the results
- Urine culture and sensitivity
- BMP
- Transvaginal ultrasound
- RPR
- Rubella antibody
- PPD test
- HIV
- Blood type and Rh
- Hepatitis B Ag

- Gonorrhea
- Chlamydia
- PAP Smear

- Result shows:
  o Ultrasound shows intrauterine pregnancy
  o Blood type A+
  o Rubella antibody is positive
  o RPR, HIV and Hepatitis B Ag is negative
  o CBC and BMP is WNL

Step 8. None

Step 9. Pre-natal vitamins, folic acid

Step 10. Counseling, screening and follow-up in 4 weeks or refer to OB/GYN

- No smoking, alcohol, illegal drugs
- Seat belts
- Pregnancy education,
- Diet high in iron

Diagnosis: Pregnancy

CASE # 2

Case introduction
A 24-year-old woman comes to clinic because of vaginal itching, burning
and thick curdy white discharge.

Initial vitals signs
Temperature: 37.2 degrees
Pulse: 68 beats/min, regular rhythm
Respiration rate: 18/ minutes

Blood pressure, systolic 123 mm Hg
Blood pressure, disystolic, 75 mm Hg

Height: 62.0 inches
Weight: 135.0 lbs.
Body mass index: 24.7 Kg/m2

History of present illness (HPI)
A 24-year-old woman comes to clinic because of vaginal itching, burning
and thick curdy white discharge. She says she noticed the some itchiness 2
weeks ago, and then it progressed to burning and curdy discharge. She
also has pain during intercourse. She denies burning sensation during
urination and frequent urination. She is sexually active with her husband
and they use condoms for birth control. She dines any history of STDs. She
was diagnosed with diabetes II 5 years age and taking metformin.

Past medical history
Hospitalization: None
Other medical condition: Diabetes type 2
Current medication: Metformin
Allergies: latex
Vaccination: up to date

Family history
Father and mother are healthy.

Social history

Marital history: Married; 1 child

Occupation: Schoolteacher

Recreational: travel, reading

Personal habits: She does not smoke, drink alcohol or use drugs

Review of system:

General: see HPI

Skin: see HPI

HEENT: see HPI

Musculoskeletal: see HPI

Cardiology: see HPI

Abdominal: see HPI

Genitourinary: see HPI

Please see pages 1-5 for general CCS cases approach

Step 1. None (patient is stable does not require any emergency measures)

Step 2. Order complete physical exam including genitourinary, and then
move the clock forward to get the results
- Results show:
  o Vagina is covered with white patches
  o Rest of the physical exam is norma

Step 3. Order labs, and then move the clock forward to get the results
- Urine pregnancy test
- CBC
- UA
- BMP
- Wet mount
- Vaginal pH
- Vaginal discharge culture and sensitivity

- Results show:
  o Pregnancy test is negative
  o Vaginal pH: 4.9
  o Wet mount prep shows mycelia
  o Vaginal culture is positive for Candida

Step 4. Single dose oral fluconazole

Step 5. Make a follow-up appointment after a week, and then move the
send then patient home

Step 6. None

Step 7. Move the clock to next follow-up appointment
- Patient usually feels better

Step 8. None

Step 9. Make a next follow-up appointment after a month

Case usually ends here

Step 10. Counsel and screening
- No smoking, alcohol, illegal drugs
- Safe sex
- Wear seat belt while driving
- PAP smear
- Age appropriate screening

Follow up in a week

Diagnosis: **Vaginal candida**

Case # 3

Case introduction
A 27-year-old female comes to the ER with abdominal pain, cramping, slight fever, and dysuria of 3 days.

Initial vitals signs
Temperature: 38.7 degrees
Pulse: 84 beats/min, regular rhythm
Respiration rate: 21/ minutes

Blood pressure, systolic 110 mm Hg
Blood pressure, disystolic, 75 mm Hg

Height: 62.0 inches
Weight: 135.0 lbs.
Body mass index: 24.7 Kg/m2

History of present illness (HPI)
A 27-year-old female comes to the ER with abdominal pain, cramping, slight fever, and dysuria of 3 days. She says she noticed green vaginal discharge 4 days ago. She has also been experiencing nausea and vomiting and has vomited 3 times. She denies vaginal bleeding, blood in the urine or previous vaginal discharge. She is sexually active with multiple partners and uses condoms for birth control. She denies any history of STDs

Past medical history
Hospitalization: None
Other medical condition: None
Current medication: None
Allergies: latex
Vaccination: up to date

Family history
Father and mother are healthy.

Social history
Marital history: Single
Occupation: Bartender
Recreational: travel
Personal habits: She smokes 6 cigarettes a da, drinks socially, and uses drugs

Review of system:
General: see HPI
Skin: see HPI
HEENT: see HPI
Musculoskeletal: see HPI
Cardiology: see HPI
Abdominal: see HPI
Genitourinary: see HPI

Please see pages 1-5 for general CCS cases approach

Step 1.
- IV access
- IV normal saline
- IV morphine

Step 2. Order complete physical exam, and then move the clock forward to get the results
- Results show:
- o Abdominal shows lower abdominal tenderness, bilateral adnexal & cervical motion tenderness
- o Rest of the physical is normal

Step 3. Order labs, and then move the clock forward to get the results
- Urine pregnancy test (under stat option)
- UA
- BMP
- CBC
- Urine culture and sensitivity
- Cervical culture and gram stain

- Results show:
- o Urine pregnancy test is negative
- o CBC shows 18,000 WBC with 80% PMN & 12% lymphocytes
- o Culture and sensitivity is pending

Step 4. Medicine
- IV promethazine, IV ceftriaxone, IV doxycycline and acetaminophen

Step 5. Admit the patient in wards

Step 6: Order the followings
- NPO
- Bed rest with bathroom privilege

Step 7. Order labs

- Order STD tests such as HIV, RPR, Gonorrhea, etc.

Step 8. None

Step 9. Interval follow-ups every 8 - 12 hours
- Patients usually get better in 48-72 hours
- Discharge the patients
- Follow-up appoint in a week

Case usually ends here

Step 10. Counseling and screening
- No alcohol, smoking, illegal drugs
- Safe sex
- Wear seat belt while driving
- Contraception use
- PAP smear
- Other age specific screening can be ordered for later date

Diagnosis: **Pelvic Inflammatory Diagnosis**

ETHICS

AUTONOMY
An adult patient with a **sound mind** has right to refuse treatment, blood products, or surgery. Frequently asked question in boards, a Jehovah's Witness: who was just involved in a motor vehicle accident and now requires a blood transfusion. However, patient is refusing the blood transfusion. In this case, respect the patient decision; just give him IV fluids, or whatever else is acceptable to the patient.

Pregnant women with a sound mind have right to refuse treatment to **her** and **her unborn child**, regardless of the gestation age. However, once the infant is born, then it becomes physician's responsibility to provide the treatment in newborn's best interest.

Exception: **Incompetent or delirious** patients can be **restrained** or **hospitalized against their will,** if they are a danger to themselves or others.

INFORMED CONSENT
Informed consent is based on patient's autonomy. It can be in **writing or oral.** For the consent to be informed, patient should be informed about **risks, benefits, and alternative treatment or procedures.** It should be in the **language patient can understand** and must be **given for each particular procedure.** Patient should be allowed to make his own decision

DO NOT RESUSCITATE (DNR) ORDER
DNR order is a medical order, which instructs health care providers to not to perform endotracheal intubation and CPR, in the event patient's breathing stops or heart stops beating.

FUTILE CARE
Futile care means that a physician has no obligation to continue providing treatment, if the treatment has no health benefits to the patient.

MEDICAL EMERGENCY PROCEDURES

A competent patient has right to refuse any treatment, tests or procedures

If a patient is not capable of making medical decision because of **impaired cognitive function**, then the decision-making process is followed in a following **stepwise manner:**
1. Health care proxy
2. Living will
3. **Previously stated wish** to family, close neighbor or close friends
4. Spouse
5. Patients children who is 18 years of age or older
6. Patient's mother or father
7. Siblings who is 18 years of age or older
8. A close friend, if patient has no family

WITHHOLDING INFORMATION FROM PATIENT

- A patient should always be told about his diagnosis
- If a patient does not want to know the diagnosis, then a physician should ask the patient about the reason for his request and try to resolve the issue. However, if patient is still refusing to know his diagnosis, then have the patient sign the document and withhold the information until patient wants
- If patient's family requests a physician to withhold the diagnosis from the patient, then the physician should first ask the family for the reason of their request. Physician may temporarily hold the information from the patient, but ultimately, patient should always be told about his diagnosis

WITHHOLDING AND WITHDRAWING THE TREATMENT

A competent adult patient has right to withhold and withdraw from any treatment at any time during the treatment

BRAIN DEATH
Brain death is defined as irreversible end of brain activity. The characteristics of brain death are:
- No corneal reflex
- No cortical reflex
- No brain reflex
- **Positive** apnea test

CONFIDENTIALITY
Patient has full right to have his medical information confidential, but **confidentially can be broken in the following situations:**
- Danger to others
- Transmissible disease
- Duty to warn and protect (if patient says that he is going to kill someone, then it is a physician's responsibility to inform the person in danger and the authorities, or both)
- Court mandate
- Suspected child abuse

Frequently test confidentially question
Q. A 25 years old male just been diagnosed with HIV. He is very upset and requests that you do not disclose his HIV status to his wife. What is the next step in management?
A. Encourage the patient to talk to his wife

DOCTOR-PATIENT RELATIONSHIP
A Physician has **no obligation to accept** a patient. However, **once** physician **accepts** the patient, and then physician **cannot abandon** the patient, **until a substitute** physician is found

Physician has right to refuse treatment to a HIV positive patient

SEXUAL CONTACT WITH PATIENT
Sexual contact between a **psychiatrist and patient** is **never acceptable.** However, sexual contact between **other physicians and patient** is **acceptable,** but only after they **end their doctor-patient relationship**

GIFTS
Small gifts that are **not given with the intensions of specific** treatment, procedures or tests, are **acceptable**. Any gift tied to a **specific treatment, procedure or test, is not acceptable**

PHYSICIAN ASSISTED SUICIDE
Physician assisted suicide is always wrong. However, physician may give a pain reliever with **the primary goal to reduce the pain,** which may also shorten the patient's life span.

ORGAN DONATION
Even if person's driver license says that he is an organ donor, a physician is still required to get that person's family or health care proxy's approval for organ donation

IMPAIRED PHYSICIAN
Impaired physician should be reported to a higher authority. Impaired physician means, that a physician, who is a danger to the medical care. A physician drinking, getting in fights or stealing outside his hospital, is not considered impaired physician and is not reportable. Impaired physician can be reported to the following authorities:

- **Residents or physician in training** should be reported to the program **director** or department **chair**
- **Faculty** should be reported to the **dean** or department **chair**
- **A physician in practice should be** reported to the **state medical board**

REPORTING ABUSE
All health care providers are **obligated to report child abuse and elderly** abuse. Even if the claim is found to be false, health care provider **has immunity by the court,** as long as, the report was made in good faith.

Health care providers **cannot report** domestic violence or spousal abuse without **patient's wish.**

PATIENT'S MEDICAL RECORDS

A physician cannot release patient's medical records to anyone without patient's consent. However, physician can release patient's medical records without patient's consent, if court orders or subpoena

A physician cannot obtain patient's medical records from patient's previous physician or other current physicians without patient's consent

MINORS

Patients under 18 years of age do not have capacity to understand their medical condition; they need parents or guardian to make their medical decisions

Exception: In a life-threatening situation, physician can ignore parent or guardian refusal of intervention and proceed to treat a minor. For example, if Jehovah's Witness parents or guardian is refusing lifesaving blood transfusion to the **minor, then physician can overrule their wish** and proceed to blood transfusion

EMANCIPATED MINOR

Emancipated minor is a legal term by which minor who is < 18 years of age is free from control of his or her parents or guardian, moreover, parents or guardian are also free from any obligation towards that minor. Minors are considered emancipated minors, if they are:
- Married
- Living independently and financially independent
- Serving in the military
- Raising their own children

Partial emancipation is a legal term in which minors are emancipated for particular purpose such as:
- Obtaining OCPs
- STD treatment
- Seeking treatment or intervention for substance abuse
- Seeking treatment for psychiatric illness

Notes:

DERMATOLOGY

YEAST SKIN INFECTION

TINEA
Tinea is a superficial skin infection caused by fungus. It is common in children, and thrives in warm moist areas
Specific name depends on the body area it affects:
- Tinea **corporis** affects the skin of the body. It appears **red-colored, raised** border that **clears centrally as it expands**
- Tinea **versicolor** is chronic fungal infection of the skin caused by Pityrosporum (also known as Malassezia furfur). Patient usually present with hypopigmented macules on face and trunk in summers
- Onychomycosis affects the nail, and causes **brittle and yellow discolored nails**
- Tinea **cruris** affects **groins area**
- Tinea **capitis** affects the **head**
- **Tinea pedis** affects the **feet**

Diagnosis:
- Best initial test is KOH prep
- **Note:** KOH prep of tenia versicolor shows classic spaghetti-meatballs appearance
- Most accurate test is fungus culture

Treatment: most of the tinea infections are treated with **topical azoles** such as ketoconazole, clotrimazole, with the exception of followings:
- Tinea versicolor is treated with **selenium sulfide, ketoconazole is the 2nd choice**
- **Nail infection is treated with oral itraconazole or terbinafine**
- Tinea capitis **is treated with griseofulvin**

BACTERIAL SKIN INFECTION

1. IMPETIGO

Impetigo is a superficial skin infection caused **by Staphylococcus aureus** (most common cause) **and Streptococcus pyogenes**. It spreads either by direct contact with skin-to-skin either or auto-inoculates in nose or mouth
Si/S: Red sores, which breaks **open, oozes fluid, and honey colored crusts**
Diagnosis: clinical diagnosis
Treatment:

- **Local** skin infection is treated with **topical mupirocin**
- **Bullous or extensive** disease is treated with **oral** dicloxacillin, or cephalexin

2. ERYSIPELAS

Erysipelas is a dermis and epidermis infection caused by **group A-beta-hemolytic streptococcus** (Pyogenes)
Si/Sx: bright red appearance of face, high fever, chills, vomiting, and headaches, which starts within 48 hours of infection
Diagnosis: clinical diagnosis
Treatment:

- **Stable patient** is treated with **oral** dicloxacillin or cephalexin
- **Serve disease** or **unstable** patient is treated empirically with IV Nafcillin or oxacillin, until the sensitivity is known.

3. CELLULITIS

Cellulitis is a severe inflammation of **dermis** and **subcutaneous tissues** caused by **staphylococcus aureus or streptococcus pyogenes**
Diagnosis: clinical diagnosis
Treatment:

- **Stable patient** is treated with **oral** dicloxacillin, or cephalexin
- **Serve disease** or **unstable** patient is treated empirically with IV Nafcillin or oxacillin, until the sensitivity is known

4. NECROTIZING FASCIITIS

Necrotizing fasciitis is a life-threatening condition, which begins with a traumatic injury to the skin, and then quickly spreads into the fascial planes of the skin.

Cause: **Staphylococcus aureus, clostridium perfringens**
Si/Sx: high fever, pain out of proportion, crepitus, local inflammation may be absent
Diagnosis: X-ray, MRI or CT shows air in tissues
Treatment: Immediate surgical debridement plus antibiotics clindamycin and penicillin to keep the infection from spreading

HAIR FOLLICLE INFECTION
Three most common hair follicle infections are folliculitis, furuncles and carbuncles. Folliculitis leads to furuncle that further leads to carbuncles
Cause:
- Most common cause is **Staph. Aureus**
- Hot tub folliculitis caused by **Pseudomonas aeruginosa**

1. FOLLICULITIS
Folliculitis is inflammation and infection of the hair follicles of the skin. Folliculitis may look like a red pimple with pus in it
Treatment:
- 1st line treatment is warm compress
- 2nd line treatment is topical mupirocin (2nd choice)

2. FURUNCLES
Furuncle is a **deep folliculitis** that causes painful swollen area. It is full of pus and dead tissue
Treatment: Warm compression, incision and drainage, oral dicloxacillin or cephalexin

3. CARBUNCLES
Carbuncles is a **cluster of furuncles** that fused to become a single lesion
Treatment: Incision and drainage, oral dicloxacillin or cephalexin

ALOPECIA AREATA
Alopecia areata is an unknown etiology condition that cause hair loss usually form scalp
Symptoms: patchy hair loss with **smooth edges**
Treatment: intralesional corticosteroids

AUTOIMMUNE SKIN DISEASES

1. BULLOUS PEMPHIGOID

Bullous pemphigoid is an autoimmune skin disease that causes the formation of bullae between dermis and epidermis

Si/Sx: **thick walled bullae that do not rupture easily**

Diagnosis: **Biopsy** with **immunofluorescent antibody** shows IgG **antibodies** and **complement deposit along the basement membrane**

Treatment: Oral corticosteroids

2. PEMPHIGUS VULGARIS

Pemphigus is an autoimmune disease that causes the formation of **blisters on the skin** and **oral mucosa.**

Si/Sx: **thin and fragile** blisters, **painful oral ulcers, Nikolsky sign**

Diagnosis: Most accurate test is **biopsy**

Treatment: **Oral corticosteroids.** If corticosteroids are ineffective, then give cyclophosphamide, azathioprine or IVIG

MALIGNANT AND PREMALIGNANT LESIONS

1. SEBORRHEIC KERATOSIS

Seborrheic keratosis usually appears as a **greasy hyperpigmented crusty lesions** that appear to be **stuck onto skin** surface. It is commonly seen in elderly

Diagnosis: shave biopsy

Treatment: liquid nitrogen or excision

2. ACTINIC KERATOSIS

Actinic keratosis is a **non-tender** erythematous macule that develops on the **sun-exposed areas.** It is a premalignant skin condition that can progress to squamous cell carcinoma

Diagnosis: local **excision**

Treatment: cryotherapy, topical 5-fluorouracil

3. SQUAMOUS CELL CARCINOMA

Squamous cell carcinoma of the skin appears **as an ulcerated nodular mass** that develops on the **sun-exposed** areas such as lips, ears, neck, arm or hands.

Diagnosis: biopsy
Treatment: surgical excision

4. BASAL CELL CARCINOMA

Basal cell carcinoma is the most common form of cancer in the US. It develops on sun-exposed areas. It looks like **pearly papules** on the skin
Diagnosis: shaves or **punch biopsy**
Treatment: Moh's surgery

5. MALIGNANT MELANOMA

Malignant melanoma is the leading cause of death from skin disease. It usually starts as a simple mole, which later **develops** into cancer.
Common **characteristics** of melanoma are: Mnemonic **ABCDE**

- **A**symmetric
- **I**rregular Border
- **C**hange in colors
- **D**iameter > 6 mm
- **E**nlarging or growing

Diagnosis: Full thickness biopsy
Management: Excision and Interferon. Interferon appears to reduce the recurrence
Prognosis depends on the depth of melanoma

6. KAPOSI'S SARCOMA

Kaposi's sarcoma is caused by **human herpesvirus 8.** It is common in immunocompromised patients or **HIV positive** patient with **CD 4 counts < 100.** Patients have **purplish lesion on the skin**
Treatment:

- Best initial treatment for HIV-related Kaposi's sarcoma is HAART treatment, which can help raise CD4 count. Patients usually show complete resolution of the skin lesions while on HAART.
- Specific treatment for Kaposi's sarcoma is liposomal Adriamycin and vinblastine

SEBORRHEIC DERMATITIS

Seborrheic dermatitis **is an erythematous greasy patch** with white flaking **(dandruff).** It is usually found around eyebrows, nasolabial folds, or scalp
Treatment: Topical **ketoconazole or selenium sulfide**

CONTACT DERMATITIS

Contact dermatitis is a **linear pruritic rash** that appears at the site of contact with irritant such as belt buckle site, wristwatch area, or a body part that came in contact with poison ivy

Diagnosis: Definitive diagnosis is **skin patch testing**

Treatment:
- Identifying and remove the source
- **Mild** contact dermatitis is treated with **topical steroids**
- **Extensive** contact dermatitis is treated with high dose **oral steroids for 2-3 weeks, and then steroids are gradually tapered** to prevent the relapse

PITYRIASIS ROSEA

Pityriasis Rosea is a pruritic skin eruption **that starts as a herald patch, and** then **spreads in a " Christmas tree distribution"**, but **palms and soles are spared**

Treatment: **no treatment is required, it usually resolves** in 1-3 months

ROSACEA

Rosacea is a chronic skin condition characterized by **flushing and redness** on **nose, cheeks, chin, and forehead**. It **exacerbates** with food, exercise, sun exposure, hot weather, stress, spicy foods, alcohol, or hot baths. It usually coexists with **blepharitis**

Treatment: Topical metronidazole, but If eyes are involved, then treat it with **oral doxycycline**

ATOPIC DERMATITIS

Itchy inflammatory skin condition that affects the flexor surface of the skin

Treatment:
- **Avoid hot water, drying soaps and other irritants**
- **Keep the skin moist** with creams or emollients

PSORIASIS

Psoriasis is a chronic remitting immune–mediated skin disease. It is characterized by red skin with flaky **silvery scales on the extensor surface**, other symptoms: fingernail pitting, **Auspitz sign** (pinpoint bleeding after removal of overlying scales) and **Köbner's phenomenon** (lesions appear at the site of skin injury)

Treatment:

- Mild disease. Tx. **Topical salicylic** acid is used initially to remove the collection of scaly material, and then apply **emollient**
- Moderate disease –Tx. **Topical vitamin D derivative** (calcipotriene) **vitamin A** (tazarotene)
- If >30% body is involved – **Tx. UV light therapy**
- Systemic disease – **Tx. DMARDS** (Methotrexate, cyclosporine)

HERPES ZOSTER

Herpes zoster **is also known, as shingles is the** reactivation of chicken pox virus in **sensory nerve ganglion**, which causes painful skin rash with blisters and burning sensation over the affected dermatomes. It is often seen in elderly and immunocompromised patients

Diagnosis:

- Clinical diagnosis
- Most accurate test is Tzanck test, but it is rarely needed

Treatment:

- Steroid
- Most effective treatment is oral acyclovir or famciclovir
- **Gabapentin** is used to control pain in post-herpetic neuralgia. But, if gabapentin is ineffective, then use **TCAs (amitriptyline or Nortriptyline) or topical capsaicin**

SCABIES

Scabies is a contagious skin condition caused by mites. It usually causes **intense pruritus and burrows** between the fingers and toe, genital area or breast creases

Diagnosis: scrape test: apply mineral oil to burrow, and then scrape the organism out

Treatment: Topical permethrin cream, but if topical permethrin cream is ineffective, then give single dose of oral ivermectin

PEDICULOSIS

Pediculosis is an infection caused by lice. It is easily transmitted from person-to-person during the direct contact

Types: two common types of pediculosis are:

- Pediculosis capitis, which infests head hair
- Pediculosis pubis (crabs), which infests pubic hair

Si/Sx: most common symptom is pruritus

Diagnosis: direct visual inspection with fine-toothed comb

Treatment: Topical permethrin cream, but if topical permethrin cream is ineffective, then give single dose of oral ivermectin

ERYTHEMA NODOSUM

Erythema nodosum is **inflammatory condition of the fat cells,** under the skin that results in **painful, tender nodules.** It is usually seen on anterior surface of the lower legs with smooth and shinny appearance

Cause:

- OCP
- IBD
- Pregnancy
- Sarcoidosis, streptococcal infection, sarcoidosis, syphilis
- Hepatitis, histoplasmosis

Treatment: treat underlying cause and NSAIDs

ERYTHEMA MULTIFORME

Erythema multiforme is a hypersensitive reaction in response to an infection or medicine

Si/Sx: "target" or "iris" like lesions on **palms and soles,** itching, fever, joint aches

Cause:

- HSV or Mycoplasma
- Penicillin, Phenytoin
- Sulfa drugs
- NSAIDs

Treatment: **Antihistamine and treat underlying cause**

MORIBILLIFORM RASH

Moribilliform rash **is a hypersensitive drug reaction that looks like measles** (rash first appears on the trunk, and then spreads to the limbs and neck) and **blanches with pressure.** It may develop few days after starting the medicine or after completing the course of the medicine

Treatment: **Stop offending** medicine **and topical or oral antihistamines**

STEVEN -JOHNSON SYNDROME

Steven -Johnson syndrome is a life-threatening hypersensitivity drug reaction that involves the **skin (<10-15%)** and **mucous membrane**

Cause:
- Penicillin, phenobarbital, phenytoin,
- Sulfa drugs
- NSAIDs

Si/Sx: symptoms begin as flu-like symptoms, then painful red or purplish lesions appears that spreads and blisters, and eventually epidermis layer separates from dermis and sheds

Diagnosis: Skin biopsy

Treatment:
- Stop the offending drug
- IVIG and analgesics
- **Intubate the patient,** if respiratory tract is involved
- Transfer the patient in **ICU or burn unit** care

Complication: Most common cause of death is combination of infection, dehydration and malnutrition

TOXIC EPIDERMAL NECROLYSIS (TEN)

Toxic epidermal necrolysis is a life-threatening hypersensitivity drug reaction. It is a severe form of Steven -Johnson syndrome, involving **> 30% body surface area.** Other characteristic feature of TEN is Nikolsky's sign (top layers of the skin sloughs off with gentle rub)

Cause:
- Phenobarbital, phenytoin,
- NSAIDs
- Allopurinol

Diagnosis: skin biopsy

Management:
- Stop the offending drug
- Transfer the patient in **burn unit care or ICU unit, supportive management and nutritional support**

Complication: Most common cause of **death** is **sepsis**

ACNE

Acne is a skin condition that starts with blockage of the hair follicle, filled with keratin and sebum material, followed by infection of lipophilic bacteria *Propionibacterium acnes*, which breaks down the sebum and causing inflammatory reaction and rupture the cysts

Open comedones are called blackheads and closed comedones are called whiteheads

Diagnosis: clinical diagnosis

Treatment:
- **Mild** acne is treated with **topical benzoyl peroxide**. If benzoyl peroxide is ineffective, then **add topical erythromycin or clindamycin**
- **Moderate** acne is treated with **topical antibiotics** (topical benzyl peroxide or topical erythromycin or clindamycin) and **topical tretinoin**
- **Severe** acne is treated with **oral tetracycline**. If tetracycline is ineffective, then give **oral isotretinoin**

NOTE: oral isotretinoin is teratogenic, **a reproductive age woman** must have **pregnancy test** before starting oral isotretinoin, and then she should be put on **2 forms of contraception's:** one barrier method and an another form of contraceptive

PORPHYRIA CUTANEA TARDA

Porphyria cutanea tarda is autosomal dominant defect in heme synthesis (low activity (<50%) of uroporphyrinogen decarboxylase enzyme in RBC and liver)

Si/Sx: non-healing blisters on sun exposed area, hyperpigmentation of skin, and increased hair growth

Exacerbating factors:
- Alcoholism
- Liver disease, hepatitis C
- **Estrogen containing** oral contraceptives
- Iron overload and diabetes

Diagnosis: Wood lamp urine test of urinary uroporphyrin
Treatment: best initial treatment is phlebotomy. If phlebotomy is not possible, then give deferoxamine
Prevention: stop drinking alcohol, stop estrogen containing OCPs and use sun protection barriers

TOXIC SHOCK SYNDROME

Toxic shock syndrome is a life-threatening condition caused by Staphylococcus aureus
Risk factors: tampons use in menstruating women, surgical wounds, nasal packing
Si/Sx: Low blood pressure, fever, confusion, muscle aches, vomiting, rash resembling sunburn
Treatment:
- Remove foreign objects
- Aggressive hydration + vasopressor (dopamine)
- IV Nafcillin, oxacillin or cefazolin
- Vancomycin or linezolid, if MRSA is suspected

LYME DISEASE

Lyme disease is a bacterial infection caused by *Borrelia burgdorferi*, which is transmitted by a tick infected with *Borrelia burgdorferi*
Si/S: Classic sign of Lyme infection is **erythema chronicum migrans** (circular rash with central clearing, that is often described as " bull's eye); other symptoms may include fatigue, myalgia, headache, arthritis, neurologic abnormalities, myocarditis
Diagnosis:
- Best Initial diagnostic test is **ELISA**
- Confirmatory test is **Western blot**

Treatment:
- Oral doxycycline
- Pregnant women are usually treated with amoxicillin

- If a patients has neurologic abnormalities or 3rd degree heart block, then use **IV ceftriaxone**

ROCKY MOUNTAIN SPOTTED FEVER
Rocky Mountain spotted fever is bacterial infection caused by bacterium *Rickettsia rickettsii*, which is transmitted by a tick infected with bacterium *Rickettsia rickettsii*
Si/Sx: fever, chills, headache or malaise, followed by **centripetal rash** appears, which starts at wrist and ankle, and then spreads to trunk and face
Diagnosis: Serology
Treatment: Doxycycline, pregnant women are treated with chloramphenicol

CAT SCRATCH DISEASE
Cat scratch disease is a bacterial infection caused by Bartonella bacteria, which is transmitted by cat scratch or bite
Si/Sx: lymphadenopathy next to the site of scratch or bite, fever, fatigue, headache, sore throat
Treatment: usually no treatment is required, but in severe cases azithromycin may be helpful

OPHTHALMOLOGY

OPEN-ANGLE GLAUCOMA

Open-angle glaucoma accounts for more than 90% of glaucoma. It is caused by slow clogging of drainage canals. It is called open-angle glaucoma because the angle because angle where between the iris and cornea is wide and open.

Si/Sx: painless gradual peripheral vision loss (also known as tunnel vision), increased cup-to disc ratio on fundoscopy exam, increased intraocular pressure (20-30 mmHg),

Treatment:

- **Topical beta-blockers** (timolol, betaxolol), **prostaglandins** (latanoprost) **carbonic anhydrase inhibitors** (dorzolamide, brinzolamide) or pilocarpine.
- If medicines is ineffective or patients can't tolerate them, then surgery (laser trabeculoplasty) may be performed

ANGLE-CLOSURE GLAUCOMA

Angle-closure glaucoma is a less common form of glaucoma. It is caused by slow clogging of drainage canals. It is called angle-closure glaucoma because the angle because angle where between the iris and cornea is closed. It develops fast and requires immediate medical attention

Si/Sx: painful, sudden vision change, seeing halos around light, fixed dilated pupils, increased intraocular pressure >30 mmHg leads to

Treatment:

- **Immediate** treatment with **pilocarpine** to constrict the pupils, plus **topical timolol** and IV **acetazolamide**
- Definitive therapy is **laser iridotomy**

RETINAL DETACHMENT

Retinal detachment is condition in which retina gets separated from its underlying supporting layers

Si/Sx: sudden **painless unilateral vision** loss, **floater and flashes** of light, and blinding in a part of visual filed, which is often described by patient as **curtain falling down** in front of the eyes

Treatment: Immediate retinal reattachment or surgery

RETINAL ARTERY OCCLUSION

Retinal artery occlusion is a blockage of one of the small arteries that supply blood to the retina. It is common in temporal arteritis, emboli, and atherosclerosis

Si/Sx: sudden, acute and painless unilateral vision loss

Diagnosis: Funduscopy shows "**cherry red spot**" with surrounding pale retina

Treatment: Acetazolamide or paracentesis of anterior chamber

RETINAL VEIN OCCLUSION

Retinal vein occlusion is a blockage of small veins that take blood away from the retina. It is common in diabetes, glaucoma, HTN, atherosclerosis

Si/Sx: sudden, acute and painless unilateral vision loss

Diagnosis: Funduscopy shows tortuous retinal veins, **retinal hemorrhage**

Treatment: No specific treatment, treat the underlying cause

CATARACT

A cataract is a clouding of normal clear lens inside the eye that leads to painless vision loss.

Diagnose: opacification of the lens on slit-lamp exam. In advance stages red eye reflex become black

Treatment: Surgical removal of lens

MACULAR DEGENERATION

Macular degeneration is also known as age related macular degeneration is a painless vision loss in the center of the visual field due to damage of the retina

Type: two main types of macular degeneration are:

- **Dry (nonexudative) type** is caused by build up of drusen (cellular debris) between the retina and the choroid
- **Wet (exudative) type** is caused by neovascularization in choroid

Diagnosis:

- Dry type: Funduscopy exam shows **yellow white deposit** (drusen) in and around **macula**
- Wet type is diagnosed with fluorescein angiography

Treatment:
- **Dry type** is treated with laser photocoagulation
- **Wet type** is treated with injection of vascular endothelial growth factor inhibitors or thermal laser photocoagulation

DIABETIC RETINOPATHY

Diabetic retinopathy is a complication of diabetes, it usually occurs approximately 10 years after diabetes

Types: two main types of diabetic retinopathy are:
- **Nonproliferative** or background type is asymptomatic. It can only be detected by **fundoscopy exam**, which usually shows **microaneurysms, cotton wool spots, flame hemorrhages** on the retina.
- **Proliferative** type caused by **neovascularization** at the back of the eyes that can cause vitreous hemorrhages, which cause sudden vision loss, blurred vision floaters in the visual field. It is diagnosed with **fluorescein angiography**

Treatment
- **Dry type: strict glucose and HTN** control
- Wet type is treated with injection of **vascular endothelial growth factor inhibitors** in the eyes to control neovascularization

UVEITIS

Uveitis is an inflammation of uvea. It is associated with **autoimmune disease** (rheumatoid arthritis, reactive arthritis), **infections** (CMV, toxoplasmosis, syphilis), **ulcerative colitis**

Si/Sx: photophobia, blurry vision

Diagnosis: Slit lamp examination shows flare and cells in aqueous humor

Treatment: topical steroids and treat the underlying cause

CORNEAL ABRASION

Corneal abrasion is the most common eye injury from scratching or cutting

Si/Sx: pain, photophobia, foreign-body sensation, watery discharge

Diagnosis: Fluorescein satin with **wood lamp**

Treatment: No specific treatment

KERATITIS

Keratitis is an inflammation of the cornea. It is associated with multiple causes, but herpes simplex virus is most commonly asked on the boards

Si/Sx: pain, photophobia, tearing, decreased vision

Diagnosis: fluorescein stain shows dendritic branching

Treatment: oral acyclovir, famciclovir or valacyclovir

Note: Steroids are contraindicated in herpes keratitis because they can worsen the condition

CONJUNCTIVITIS

Condition	Bacterial conjunctivitis	Viral conjunctivitis	Allergic conjunctivitis
Si/Sx	• Unilateral • Purulent discharge • Rarely preauricular adenopathy (only in Neisseria gonorrhea) • Minimal pain • No vision change or pupillary change	• Bilateral • Watery discharge • Often preauricular adenopathy • Minimal pain • No vision change or pupillary change	• Bilateral • Watery discharge • Marked pruritus • No pain, vision change or pupillary change
Treatment	Topical antibiotics	Supportive	Antihistamine or steroid drops

PALPERBRAL INFLAMMATION

1. CHALAZION

Chalazion is a cyst in the eyelid that is caused by blockage and inflammation of internal meibomian gland

Si/Sx: Painless tender lump **away from the eyelid margin**

Treatment: Warm compression

2. HORDEOLUM

Hordeolum is a common disorder of eyelids, involving sebaceous glands of Ziess or sweat gland of Moll

Si/Sx: painful red tender lump **near the eyelid margin**

Treatment: Warm compression

3. BLEPHARITIS

Blepharitis is inflammation of the eyelids and eyelashes from infection
(S. aureus) or secondary to seborrhea
Si/Sx: red and swollen eyelids dry flaking on lids
Treatment: daily washing eyelids margin

4. ORBITAL CELLULITIS

Orbital cellulitis is an infection of the tissue-surrounding eye including
eyelids
Cause: Staphylococcus aureus, streptococcus pneumonia and H. influenza
type b
Si/Sx: red or purple eyelid, painful swelling of upper and lower eyelids,
eye pain, painful eye movement, limited eye movement
Treatment: Orbital cellulitis is medical emergency patient should be
immediately started on IV Vancomycin plus cefotaxime

5. PERIORBITAL CELLULITIS

Periorbital cellulitis is an inflammation of eyelid and skin around the eyes.
This condition can easily be **confused with orbital cellulitis**. The key
difference is in the symptoms; patient with periorbital cellulitis **do not
have pain with eye movement, vision change, and limited eye
movement.**
Treatment: warm to hot compress to reduce pain and inflammation, and
oral antibiotics

VISUAL FILED DEFECTS

Visual field defect	Location of lesion
Bitemporal hemianopsia	Optic chiasm
Right anopsia	Right optic nerve
Right homonymous hemianopsia	Left optic tract
Right upper quadrant anopsia	Optic radiation in **left temporal** lobe
Right lower quadrant anopsia	Optic radiation in **left parietal lobe**
Right homonymous hemianopsia with macular sparing	Left occipital lobe

BITES

HUMAN HAND BITE
Human bite is considered a high-grade bite. Patient should be given prophylaxis augmentation (amoxicillin + clavulanate), and then referred to a hand surgeon.

CAT BITE
Cat bite is considered a high-grade bite because their sharp teeth penetrate deeper. Patient should be given prophylaxis augment (amoxicillin + clavulanate)

DOG BITE
Dog bite is considered a low-grade bite, unless the dog is known to have rabies
Treatment: irrigation and proper wound care, observe the dog and treatment is given as follow:
- If the dog **doesn't develop** any symptoms of rabies, then **no vaccination** is needed
- If the dog **develops rabies symptoms** or **known to have rabies,** then give **vaccination** as follow:
    - If the patient **received** human diploid cell vaccine **(HDCV)** in the past, then give **rabies immunoglobulin**
    - If the patient **did not receive HDCV** in the past, then give **HDCV plus rabies immunoglobulin**

BAT BITE
- If the patient **received human diploid cell vaccine (HDCV)** in the past, then give **rabies immunoglobulin**
- If the patient **did not receive HDCV** in the past, then give **HDCV plus rabies immunoglobulin**

Note: there is a high incidence of rabies in the bats and they can spread it by saliva, as well. So if a person is exposed of bat's saliva or bit by a bat, then he should be treated as above. There is no need to locate and watch the bird for rabies symptoms

BLACK WIDOW SPIDER BITE

Symptoms: sharp pain at the site of the bite, deep burning aching pain, vomiting, headache, chest tightness, hypertension and abdominal muscle rigidity.

Treatment: maintain ABCs, tetanus prophylaxis, pain relievers, wound care and nitrate for HTN

BROWN RECLUSE SPIDER BITE

Symptoms: pain and necrosis at the site of bite, fever, chills, arthralgia, myalgia

Treatment: ice compress, oral erythromycin, wound care and plastic surgeons consult

SNAKE BITE

Symptoms: vomiting, diarrhea, restless, dysphagia, muscle weakness, fasciculation

Treatment: Advance cardiac life support (ACLS), tetanus prophylaxis, and type-specific antivenin.

HUMAN IMMUNODEFICIENCY VIRUS

HUMAN IMMUNODEFICIENCY VIRUS (HIV)

HIV is a slow replicating retrovirus that targets and destroys CD4 T cell. As CD 4 T cell declines below a critical level, cell-mediated immunity is lost and body becomes susceptible to opportunistic infection.

Si/Sx: some patients may develop symptoms shortly after the infection. However, it usually **takes years for a person to show symptoms** because a normal person has CD4 cells count of 600-1000 per µl, and CD 4 cells decreases at the rate of 50-100 cells per year. Therefore, on the average it takes 5-10 years for CD 4 T cells to decline below the critical level and show symptoms

Transmission: blood, semen, pre-seminal fluid, vaginal fluid, anal mucosa, needle stick injury, mother to child during breast milk

Diagnosis:

- Best **initial test is ELISA;** it detects HIV-1 antibodies in the blood, oral fluid or urine. It takes up to 2 weeks for the test results to be available. But sometimes, it may take up to six months for the antibodies to appear after acquiring infection
- If ELISA is positive, then it can be **confirmed** with **western blot**
- **PCR-RNA** test detects the viral genetic material in person. It is **useful in babies born to HIV positive mothers** because babies' blood can contain their mother's HIV antibodies for several months, but PCR-RNA can determine whether newborns have HIV genetic material in baby's genes.
  - o PCR also helps **determine the response and effectiveness of the treatment.**

Treatment: highly active antiretroviral therapy (HAART) is a combination of medicines that slow the rate of HIV virus to make its copies. HAART is started, when:

- Patient has an AIDS defining illness
- CD4< 500, or viral load > 100,000 µl

Any of the following HAART combination can be used:

- **Two nucleosides** combined with **a protease inhibitor** or Efavirenz
- **Two nucleosides** combined with **two protease inhibitors**
- **Once–daily a combined tablet** of emtricitabine, tenofovir and efavirenz

HAART THERAPY AND ITS SIDE EFFECTS

Type	Medicines	Side effects
Nucleoside reverse transcriptase inhibitors	• Zidovudine • Didanosine • Stavudine • Lamivudine • Abacavir • Emtricitabine • Tenofovir	• All of the nucleoside reverse transcriptase cause lactic acidosis • Zidovudine - **anemia** • Didanosine & stavudine - **pancreatitis and peripheral neuropathy** • Tenofovir – renal insufficiency
Protease inhibitors	• Indinavir • Ritonavir • Tipranavir • Lopinavir	• All protease inhibitor cause hyperglycemia hyperlipidemia, lipodystrophy • Indinavir – **needle shaped kidney stone**
Non-nucleoside reverse transcriptase inhibitors	• Efavirenz • Nevirapine • Efavirenz	

HIV PROPHYLAXIS

HIV prophylaxis medications are given in the following conditions:

1. Anyone exposed to **blood** or have **intercourse** with a **HIV-positive** patient, should receive 3-drug combination for **28 days**

2. Prophylaxis for pneumocystis carinii pneumonia **(PCP) is started** when **CD 4 T cell** counts **fall below 200/mm**. Treatment: Trimethoprim-sulfamethoxazole (TMP-SMX) or dapsone and/or pentamidine.

3. Prophylaxis for mycobacterium avium complex **(MAC)** is started, when CD **4 T cell** counts **fall below 100/mm**. Treatment: daily clarithromycin or weekly azithromycin. It is discontinued when CD 4 T cell goes above 100/mm

HIV-POSITIVE PREGNANT WOMEN MANAGEMENT

Start HAART in pregnant women:

- If CD4 count is <500, then start HAART regardless of gestational age
- If CD4 count is > 500, then start HAART in 2nd trimester

Note: HAART treatment regimen in pregnant women must include ZDV

HAART medicines **contraindicated** in pregnancy are:

- Nevirapine – side effects: fetal hepatotoxicity
- Efavirenz- side effects: neural tube defect
- Didanosine and stavudine – side effects: fetal lactic acidosis

Delivery options for a HIV-positive mothers are following:

- Women should be offered to have a C-section before 38 weeks of gestation, before the rupture of membrane
- Near-term women can have **elective C-section,** if she has high CD 4 T cell count and viral load <1,000 copies/ml
- Near–term pregnant women with **viral loads > 1,000 copies/ml** should have a C-section at 38 weeks gestation, before the rupture of membrane

OPPORTUNITISTIC INFECTIONS

1. PNEUMOCYSTIS CARINII PNEUMONIA (PCP)

PCP is **fungal pneumonia** that is caused fungus *pneumocystis jiroveci*. It is usually seen in HIV-positive patient with **CD 4 cells count < 200 cells/µL**

Si/Sx: **dry cough, shortness of breath** (SOB), fatigue

Diagnosis:
- Increased LDH
- Chest x-ray- shows **bilateral ground glass infiltrate**
- Most accurate test is **bronchoalveolar lavage**
- Pulmonary artery oxygen (p02)
- Alveolar–arterial gradient (A–a gradient) of oxygen

Treatment:
- 1st line of treatment is IV Trimethoprim/sulfamethoxazole (TMP/SMX)
  - If patient is **allergic to sulfa medicines** - Tx. Pentamidine or atovaquone

- 2nd line of treatment is pentamidine
  - Pentamidine causes low blood sugar, which can cause seizures

- If p02 < 70 or A–a gradient >35 mmHg, then **add prednisone** to the treatment

Prophylaxis treatment:
- Prophylaxis treatment for PCP is given to asymptomatic HIV-positive patient when CD4 cell count is < 200 **cells/µL**
  - 1st line of treatment is IV Trimethoprim/sulfamethoxazole (TMP/SMX)
  - If the patient is **allergic to sulfa medicine, then give** dapsone or aerosolized pentamidine

2. TOXOPLASMOSIS ENCEPHALITIS

Toxoplasmosis encephalitis is caused by toxoplasma gondii. It is the most common cause of encephalitis in **HIV-positive patient with CD 4 count < 200 cells/µL**

Si/Sx: **confusion, altered consciousness, seizures,** fever, headaches, and focal neurological deficits

Diagnosis:
- CT head shows **multiple ring enhancing lesions**
- Toxoplasmosis antibody test is **sensitive test**

Management:
- Standard care of toxoplasmosis encephalitis is **pyrimethamine plus sulfadiazine for 2 weeks, and then repeat CT of the head.**
  - If CT head shows that ring-enhancing lesions are resolving, then **continue treating the patient** with pyrimethamine plus sulfadiazine.
  - If CT head shows no improvement in ring-enhancing lesions, then **order brain biopsy**

Prophylaxis treatment:
- Prophylaxis treatment for toxoplasmosis is given to asymptomatic HIV-positive patient when CD4 cell count is < 100 **cells/μL**
  - 1st line of treatment is IV Trimethoprim/sulfamethoxazole (TMP/SMX)
  - If the patient is **allergic to sulfa medicine, then give** dapsone or pyrimethamine

3. CYTOMEGALOVIRUS ENCEPHALITIS

Cytomegalovirus is viral opportunistic infection that usually occurs when **CD4 cell count is < 50 cells/μL. It mostly affects the eyes**

Si/SX: confusion, **blurry vision**, oculomotor and cranial nerve palsies

Treatment: **Ganciclovir** or **Foscarnet**

4. CRYPTOCOCCUS MENINGITIS

Cryptococcal meningitis caused by **encapsulated yeast Cryptococcus neoformans.** It usually occurs in HIV- positive patient when **CD4 < 50** cell/mm3

Si/Sx: fever, headaches, nausea and vomiting, photophobia, stiff neck

Diagnosis:
- Best Initial test is **LP:** CSF stain with **India ink shows encapsulated yeast**
- Accurate test: **Cryptococcal antigen test**

Treatment:
- **Amphotericin B, and flucytosine** for 14 days
- Then **fluconazole** monotherapy and keep the patient on fluconazole until CD4 count rises
- If a patient present with **sudden vision loss** - Tx. Perform **serial LP** to keep CSF pressure < 200 mmH2O

5. PROGRESSIVE MULTIFOCAL LEUKOENCEPHALOPATHY

Progressive multifocal leukoencephalopathy is a fatal demyelinating disease that usually occurs in HIV-positive patient when **CD 4 cell count < 50**

Si/Sx: **focal neurological deficits, headaches, memory loss**
Diagnosis:
- MRI head shows **multiple demyelinating lesions**

Treatment: none, patients usually do not survive > 6 months after diagnosis

6. MYCOBACTERIUM AVIUM INTRACELLULAR

Mycobacterium avium intracellular also known as MAC (mycobacterium avium complex), is an atypical mycobacterial infection that usually occur in HIV-positive patient when **CD 4 cell count is < 50**
Mycobacterium avium affects the bone marrow and may cause **pancytopenia**

Si/Sx: persistent cough, anemia, recurrent infection
Diagnosis:
- Initial test: **Bone marrow biopsy**
- Accurate test: **Liver biopsy**

Treatment: **Clarithromycin** and **ethambutol**

Prophylaxis treatment:
- Prophylaxis treatment for MAC is given to an asymptomatic HIV-positive patient when CD4 cell count is < 50 **cells/μL**
  - 1st choice is **azithromycin**
  - 2nd choice is clarithromycin or rifabutin

TOXICOLOGY

1.   ANTICHOLINERGIC TOXICITY
Si/Sx
- Mydriasis
- Flushed skin
- Dry mouth
- Constipation

Diagnosis: Clinical
Treatment: Physostigmine

2. ORGANOPHOSPHATE POISONING
Si/Sx:
- Miosis
- Salivation
- Diarrhea
- Lacrimation
- Wheezing

Physiology: Organophosphate inhibits the metabolism of acetylcholine by inhibiting the acetylcholinesterase
Diagnosis:
- Clinical diagnosis
- Specific test is RBC cholinesterase level

Management:
- Respiratory support
- Atropine is the best initial treatment, and pralidoxime is the second choice

Note: Patient may have toxin on his or her clothes, so it is better to remove and wash all the patient's clothes to prevent further exposure of the toxin

3. ASPIRIN/ SALICYLATE OVERDOSE

Si/Sx: Tinnitus, nausea, vomiting, confusion that can progress to seizure and coma

Diagnosis:

- Labs show: Respiratory alkalosis with elevated anion gap channel acidosis, increased PTT and low glucose level
- **Most specific** test is **aspirin level**

Management:

- **Charcoal** to block absorption and alkalinization of urine with **D5W + 3amps bicarbonate**
- **Dialysis** is for severe cases

4. CARBON MONOXIDE POISONING

Si/Sx: **fatigue, headaches**, shortness of breath, disorientation, **cherry-red color skin or lips,**

Diagnosis: Co-oximetry

Treatment: 100% oxygen, severe cases are treated with **hyperbaric oxygen**

5. METHEMOGLOBINEMIA

Si/Sx: **cyanosis, shortness** of breath, **confusion** or **seizure,** after recent exposure of nitrate, dapsone, or anesthetics

Diagnosis: Metahemoglobin level

Treatment: 100% oxygen and methylene blue to restore hemoglobin

6. ACETAMINOPHEN TOXICITY

Si/Sx: nausea and vomiting starts within 2 hours of exposure, which usually resolves after first 24 hours and then hepatic failure develops

Diagnosis: Acetaminophen level

Treatment: Charcoal and N-acetyl cysteine within 8-10 hours

7. DIGOXIN TOXICITY

Si/Sx: GI disturbance, yellow " halos" around objects, paroxysmal atrial tachycardia

Diagnosis: blood level

Treatment: Digoxin-binding antibodies

8. ETHYLENE GLYCOL
Si/Sx: **Calcium oxalate urine crystals**, high anion gap metabolic acidosis
Dx: Urinalysis shows **envelope crystals**
Treatment: Fomepizole followed by dialysis

9. METHANOL
Si/Sx: **vision disturbance**, high anion gap metabolic acidosis
Diagnosis: blood level
Treatment: Fomepizole followed by dialysis

10. ALKALI BURN
Alkali burn are caused by ingestion dishwasher, detergent, drain cleaners, that can cause musical burn and respiratory compromise
Diagnosis: clinical
Treatment: Milk or water and NPO

Notes:

VITAMINS

Vitamin	Deficiency	Toxicity
Vitamin A	• Night blindness • Dry skin • Metaplasia of respiratory epithelium	• Pseudotumor cerebri • Hyperparathyroidism
Vitamin D	• Rickets in children • Osteomalacia in adults	• Kidney stones • Dementia • Abdominal pain • Depression
Vitamin K	• Clotting factor deficiency that leads to increased PT/INR	• Toxicity is rare
Vitamin B 1 (Thiamine)	• Wet beriberi (high cardiac output, cardiomyopathy) • Dry beriberi (neuropathy)	None
Vitamin B 2 (Riboflavin)	• Angular cheilosis • Stomatitis • Glossitis	None
Vitamin B 3 (Niacin)	• Pellagra (diarrhea, dementia and dermatitis)	None
Vitamin B 5 (Pantothenate)	• Dermatitis, enteritis	None
Vitamin B 6 (Pyridoxine)	• Peripheral neuropathy	None
Vitamin B 12 (Cyanocobalamin)	• Megalobalstic anemia • Peripheral neuropathy	None
Folic acid	• Megalobalstic anemia	None
Vitamin C	• Scurvy: bruising, anemia, poor wound healing, bone pain (seen in people on "tea and toast" or "hot dogs and soda" diet)	None

ADULT IMMUNIZATION

Influenza vaccine is given **yearly** to all patients > 65 years of age and those < 65 years of age with the risk factors such as health care workers, pregnant women, immunocompromised, chronic heart disease, diabetes mellitus, and COPD. It should be **avoided** in people with the history of **egg allergy**

Pneumococcal vaccine is given **once** to all patients > 65 years of age and those < 65 years of age with the risk factors (same as influenza). **Revaccination or second dose of pneumococcal vaccine** is only needed, if adults >65 years of age or immunocompromised patient received pneumococcal vaccine more than 5 years ago.

Hepatitis A vaccination is recommended to patients with chronic liver failure, IV drug abuse, chronic liver disease and men who have sex men.

Hepatitis B vaccination is recommended to all young adults and high-risk people such as health care workers, people with recent STD, IV drug abusers

MMR vaccination is recommended to everyone who is born after 1956. Rubella should not be given to pregnant woman. If a childbearing woman receives it, she should avoid for 3 months after the vaccination.

Varicella vaccination is recommended to people with high-risk such as health care workers, teachers, or childcare providers. It should be only given to HIV positive patient if CD 4 T cells are > 500.

Meningococcal vaccination is recommended to college dormitory residents, asplenic, and people with terminal complement deficiency

Tetanus vaccination is recommended to everyone, and then booster dose is given every 10 years. But, there are some other tetanus shot guidelines, which are as follow:

Type wound	Tetanus vaccination
Clean or dirty wound	If the patient received tetanus vaccination **within last 5 years**, then **no vaccination is needed**
Dirty wounds	If the patient received tetanus vaccination within last 5-**10 years**, then give **Td booster.** No vaccination is required for clean wounds
Clean and dirty wounds	If the patient received last tetanus vaccination **>10 years** ago, then give **Td booster plus Td immunoglobulin**

TRAVELER PROPHYLAXIS

Malaria
- **Mefloquine or atovaquone-proguanil** is recommended to people traveling to Asia, Africa. Chloroquine is not given to people traveling to these area because of high resistance rate
- **Chloroquine** is to recommended to people traveling to Caribbean, Mexico, and Central America

Typhoid prophylaxis is recommended to people traveling to India, Pakistan, Peru, Chile, and Mexico

Yellow fever prophylaxis is recommended to people traveling to South America and Africa

Meningococcus prophylaxis is recommended to people traveling to sub-Saharan Africa

Hepatitis A vaccination prophylaxis is recommended to all travelers planning to travel after 4 or more weeks, but if patient is planning on traveling within 4 weeks, then give **IVIG**

POSTOPERATIVE FEVER

MALIGNANT HYPERTHERMIA

Malignant hyperthermia is a life-threatening condition that is triggered by certain anesthesia or drugs. Patient usually develops a high fever (>104°F) **soon after exposure of anesthesia or drugs.**
Treatment: IV dantrolene, discontinue the known trigger, and supportive therapy such as 100% oxygen, correcting acidosis, hyperthermia and cooling measures
Complications: rhabdomyolysis, DIC, kidney failure, arrhythmia

BACTEREMIA

Bacteriemia is the presence of bacteria in the bloodstream. Bacteria can enter the blood during surgery, IV drug abuse. Patient usually develops high fever (>104°F) **30-45 minutes after procedure**
Diagnosis: blood culture
Treatment: empiric antibiotics until culture and sensitivity results are available

POSTOPERATIVE FEVER (101° - 103°F)

Most common causes of postoperative fever are known as mnemonic 5W's. Which stands for wind, water, walking, wound, and wonder (drug or abscess). These tend to occur at particular days after surgery

1. Wind

Fever presents **1-2 days** postoperatively. It is possibly caused by **lungs** condition such as atelectasis, pneumonia, or aspiration.
Diagnosis: chest x-ray followed by sputum culture
Treatment: antibiotic
Prevention: deep breathing, coughing, incentive spirometry or postural drainage after the surgery

2. Water

Fever presents **3-5 days** postoperatively. It is possibly caused by **urinary tract infection**
Diagnosis: urinalysis, urine culture and sensitivity
Treatment: antibiotics based on culture and sensitivity

3. Walking

Fever presents **4-6 days** postoperatively. It is possibly caused by **deep vein thrombosis**
Diagnosis: ultrasound of leg and pelvic veins
Treatment: Heparin and warfarin

4. Wound
Fever presents **5-7 days** postoperatively. It is possibly caused by **wound infection or cellulitis**
Diagnosis: physical exam shows erythema and tenderness at surgical site
Treatment: Incision and drainage followed by antibiotics

5.   **Wonder** (drug or abscess)
Fever presents **8-15 days** postoperatively. It is possibly caused by **drug fever or infection from intravenous line**
Diagnosis: CT
Treatment: CT-guided percutaneous drainage

PREOPERATIVE RISK FACTORS

CARDIAC

- Ejection fraction < 35% prohibits **non-cardiac surgery(s)**
- If patient has **a recent myocardial infarction, then:**
  - All surgeries should be **deferred for six months after MI**
  - **If surgery is necessary,** then the patient should be placed in **ICU the day before the surgery**
- Presence of JVD indicates congestive heart failure, **patient should be given ACE inhibitors, beta-blockers, digitalis and diuretics before the surgery**

PULMONARY RISK FACTORS

- Smoking is the most common cause of pulmonary complications
- If patient has a **history of smoking or** COPD, then evaluate the pulmonary function:
  - **Check FEV1,** if it is **abnormal, then** gets **ABGs**
- Patient are usually advised:
  - **Stop smoking at least 8 weeks before the surgery**
  - **Have pulmonary therapy after the surgery**

HEPATIC RISK FACTORS

- If **one of the below is** present, then **morality rate is~ 40%**
- If **≥ 3 of the below are present, then** mortality rate is **~80 to 85%**
  - Bilirubin >2.0
  - Prothrombin >16
  - Serum bilirubin <3.0
  - Encephalopathy

DIABETIC COMA

- Diabetic coma is absolute contraindication to surgery
- Tx. **Stabilize and hydrate** the patient **before the surgery**

NUTRITIONAL RISK FACTORS

- **If patient lost > 20% of the body weight** over several months before the surgery
- Anergy to skin testing
- Serum albumin < 3.0
- Serum transferrin <200 mg/dl.

Treatment: Provide 5 to 10 days of nutritional support before surgery

List of frequently tested CCS cases

- Abdominal Aneurysm
- Acetaminophen overdose
- Acute Asthma Attack
- Acute Bacterial Prostatitis
- Acute Cholecystitis
- Acute diarrhea
- Acute Hepatitis A
- Acute manic disorder
- Acute MI
- Acute pancreatitis
- Acute pericarditis
- Community-Acquired pneumonia
- Acute PID
- ADAPKD
- Adrenal Mass
- Acute lymphocyte leukemia (ALL)
- Alzheimer's Disease
- Anaphylaxis shock
- Atrial fibrillation
- Bacterial Meningitis
- Bipolar disorder
- Cardiac tamponade
- Cervical cancer
- Child abuse
- Chlamydia trachomatis urethritis
- Colon cancer
- Complete heart block
- Congestive heart
- Constitutional growth delay
- Cystitis
- Dehydration/ Hypernatremia

- Diverticulitis
- DKA
- Duodenal Atresia
- Dysfunctional uterine bleeding
- Eclampsia
- Endometrial carcinoma
- Erosive esophagitis/ GERD
- Folic acid deficiency
- Fracture of femoral neck
- G6PD deficiency
- Gastric carcinoma
- Gastritis secondary to NSAIDs
- Heat Stroke
- Hepatic encephalopathy
- Hypercalcemia secondary to primary hyperparathyroidism
- Hypertension
- Hypothyroidism
- Incomplete abortion
- Infective Endocarditis
- Inflammatory Bowel disease
- Intussusception
- Juvenile Rheumatoid Arthritis
- Minimal change disease
- Multiple sclerosis
- New Onset DM type II
- Obesity
- Osteoarthritis Arthritis
- Osteoarthritis of the Knee
- Osteoporosis
- Osteoporotic compression Fracture

- Ovarian Teratoma
- Pancreatic cancer

- Panic Attack
- Pericarditis
- Pneumocystis pneumonia (PCP)
- Polymyalgia rheumatica
- Postmenopausal bleeding
- Pregnancy
- Pregnancy with asymptomatic bacteriuria
- Pulmonary embolism
- Renal cell carcinoma
- Secondary Hypertension
- Septic arthritis
- Septic pulmonary emboli secondary to IV abuse.
- SLE
- Splenic rupture
- Stable Angina
- TIA
- Toxic Shock syndrome secondary to tampon use
- Tricyclic Overdose
- Turner's syndrome
- Urinary tract infection during pregnancy
- UTI/Sepsis
- Vaginal Bleeding secondary to Fibroids
- VSD

INDEX

Amoebic liver abscess, 339
Amphetamine intoxication, 374
Amphetamine withdrawal, 374
Amputated digits, 252
Amyotrophic lateral sclerosis, 204
Anaerobes, 289
Analgesic rebound headaches, 201
Anaphylaxis, 143
Anaplastic carcinoma, 114
Androgen insensitivity syndrome, 513
Anemia of chronic disease, 61
Anemia, 59, 421
Angelman syndrome, 438
Angle-closure glaucoma, 561
Ankylosing spondylitis, 232
Anorexia, 373
Anterior cruciate ligament, 253
Anterior shoulder dislocation, 248
Anterior spinal artery syndrome, 211
Anticholinergic toxicity, 575
Antiphospholipid syndrome, 237
Antisocial PD, 372
Anxiety disorders, 224
Aortic dissection, 6
Aortic regurgitation, 27
Aortic stenosis, 25
APGAR score, 389
Aplastic anemia, 75
Appendicitis, 340
Arrest disorder, 488, 489
Arterial ulcers, 41
Asbestos, 280
Ascending cholangitis, 338
Ascites, 327, 328
Asherman syndrome, 515, 516

Asperger syndrome, 386
Aspergillus, 293
Aspiration pneumonitis, 292
Aspirin/ salicylate overdose, 576
Asthma exacerbation, 275, 302
Asthma, 273
Astrocytoma, 209
Asymptomatic bacteriuria, 170, 482
Atonic seizures, 207
Atopic dermatitis, 554
Atrial fibrillation, 20
Atrial flutter, 22
Atrial septal defect, 394
Attention deficit hyperactivity disorder (ADHD), 386
Atypical depression, 364
Atypical pneumonia, 289
Autism, 386
Autoimmune hepatitis, 331
Autonomy, 543
Avoidant PD, 372

B

Back pain, 254
Back sprain, 210
Bacteremia, 582
Bacterial conjunctivitis, 564
Bacterial pneumonia, 410
Bacterial prostatitis, 129
Bacterial tracheitis, 408
Bacterial vaginosis, 498
Barrett's esophagus, 310
Basal cell carcinoma, 553
Bat bite, 567
Beat-thalassemia, 63
Behcet's disease, 242
Benign essential tremor, 191
Benign positional vertigo (BPV), 202

Ischemic stroke, 186

Membranoproliferative glomerulonephritis, 157
Membranous glomerulonephritis, 157
MEN Type 1 (Wermer's syndrome), 114, 115
MEN Type IIa (Sipple syndrome), 114, 115
MEN Type IIb, 90
Meniere's disease, 202
Meningioma, 209
Meningitis, 213
Meningocele, 418
Meningococcal vaccination, 580
Meningococcus, 581
Meniscal tear, 253
Menopause, 529
Mental retardation, 387
Metastatic malignancy of spine, 255
Methanol, 577
Methemoglobinemia, 276
Methemoglobinemia, 576
Microangiopathic hemolytic anemia, 72
Microcytic anemia, 60
Migraine headache, 198
Mild pre-eclampsia, 480
Milia, 391
Minimal change disease, 156
Missed abortion, 473
Mitral regurgitation, 27
Mitral stenosis, 28
Mitral valve prolapse, 29
MMR vaccination, 580
Molar pregnancy, 521
Mongolian spots, 391
Monteggia fracture, 250
Moribilliform rash, 557
Morton neuroma, 245

Müllerian agenesis, 513
Multifocal atrial tachycardia, 22
Multiple endocrine neoplasia syndromes (MEN), 114, 115
Multiple myeloma, 83
Multiple sclerosis, 203
Mumps, 441
Muscular torticollis, 413
Myasthenia gravis, 193
Mycobacterium avium complex, 574
Mycoplasma pneumonia, 410
Mycoplasma, 290
Myelodysplastic syndrome, 78
Myelofibrosis, 74
Myelomeningocele, 418
Myoclonic seizures, 207
Myxedema coma, 112

N

Nagele rule, 458
Narcissistic PD, 372
Narcolepsy, 377
Necrotizing enterocolitis, 398
Necrotizing fasciitis, 550
Neisseria meningitis, 214
Neonate acne, 391
Nephrogenic diabetes, 124
Nephrolithiasis, 161
Nephrotic syndrome, 156
Neuroblastoma, 428
Neurocysticercosis, 217
Neurofibromatosis, 418
Neurogenic shock, 142
Neuroleptic malignant syndrome, 359
Newborn jaundice, 433
Newborn screening, 389
Night terrors, 377

Vitamin D toxicity, 579
Vitamin K deficiency, 87, 579
Vitamin K toxicity, 579
Von Willebrand disease, 84, 422
Vulvar cancer, 505

W
Waldenstrom's
macroglobulinemia, 84
Wandering pacemaker, 22
Warm autoimmune hemolysis,
70
Wegner's granulomatosis, 153
Wernicke's aphasia, 186
West syndrome, 419
Whipple disease, 324
Wilms' tumor, 427
Wilson disease, 331
Wiskott-Aldrich syndrome, 440
Withholding and withdrawing
the treatment, 544
Withholding information from
patient, 544
Wolff–Parkinson–white
syndrome, 22

Y
Yellow fever, 581
Yersinia, 319

Z
Zenker diverticulum, 304
Zollinger-Ellison syndrome, 313

www.ingramcontent.com/pod-product-compliance
Lightning Source LLC
Chambersburg PA
CBHW031719210326
41599CB00018B/2436